The Book *of* Style
for Medical Transcription

THIRD EDITION

Author & Managing Editor
Lea M. Sims, CMT, FAAMT

Foreword By
John H. Dirckx, MD

ahdi

Published by the Association for Healthcare Documentation Integrity
(formerly AAMT)

The Book of Style for Medical Transcription, 3rd Edition

Author and Managing Editor
Lea M. Sims, CMT, FAAMT

Contributing Authors
Laura Bryan, MT (ASCP), CMT, FAAMT
Brenda Hurley, CMT, FAAMT

Copyediting
Kristin Wall, FAAMT

Proofreading
RuthAnne Darr, CMT, FAAMT

Foreword
John H. Dirckx, MD

ISBN 978-0-935229-58-5

©2008 Association for Healthcare Documentation Integrity (formerly AAMT)

Author credit for previous editions
The AAMT Book of Style for Medical Transcription ©2005
Claudia Tessier, CAE, CMT, RRA

The AAMT Book of Style for Medical Transcription, 2nd edition. ©2002
Peg Hughes, CMT; Linda A Byrne, CMT; Diane S. Heath, CMT; Brenda J. Hurley, CMT, FAAMT;
Kathy Rockel, CMT, FAAMT; Claudia Tessier, CAE, CMT, RRA

Custom publishing services provided by Network Design Group, *www.networkpub.com/ndg*

Indexing services provided by Indexing Research, *www.indexxres.com*

Association for Healthcare Documentation Integrity
A Nonprofit Professional Corporation
4230 Kiernan Avenue, Ste. # 130
Modesto, CA 95356
(209) 341-2449
ahdi@ahdionline.org
www.ahdionline.org

To all healthcare documentation specialists,
especially to those who place quality before quantity
and who apply their skills as both an art and a science.

Contents

Acknowledgments

It has been said that it *takes a village to raise a child*, and it certainly took an amazing team of experts and reviewers to "birth" this text. An overwhelming number of hours were spent compiling, drafting, reviewing, and redrafting the newly revamped style guide you now hold in your hands. The dedicated people who engaged in this labor of love represent every sector of our industry – language experts, educators, QA specialists/coordinators, private practice and acute care MTs, and association leaders with many years of collective experience and wisdom among them. Without their critical eyes and critical thinking, my task of creating a fresh, dynamic manual for our industry could not have been accomplished.

Thank you to the following individuals who contributed to this text by authoring key industry trends chapters found in Section 5:

Laura Bryan, MT (ASCP), CMT, FAAMT
Brenda Hurley, CMT, FAAMT

Thank you to the following individuals who served on the review team for this project:

Susan L. Aldous, CMT
Susan Bartolucci, CMT, FAAMT
Tamara Dicks, CMT
Sue Dickinson, CMT
Susan Dooley, CMT, FAAMT
Debora Eckelbarger, CMT

Melanie D. Gibbons, MA
Diane S. Heath, CMT
Evaleen Holden
Gregory J. Hillman, CMT
Kim Watts, CMT, FAAMT
Miriam Wilmoth, CMT, FAAMT

Any great style manual requires a keen editorial eye and great proofreading. Thank you to these two great editors who spent hours combing through proofs to ensure a quality outcome:

Kristin Wall, FAAMT (copyeditor)
RuthAnne Darr, CMT, FAAMT (proofreader)

Finally, for all his expertise, wisdom, and knowledge, I extend my heartfelt thanks to:

John Dirckx, MD

– Lea M. Sims, CMT, FAAMT
  Author and Managing Editor

Foreword

John H. Dirckx, MD

Since the publication of the second edition of this book in 2002, the name of the sponsoring organization has been changed from the American Association for Medical Transcription (AAMT) to the Association for Healthcare Documentation Integrity (AHDI) and major technical and administrative developments have arisen that challenge and threaten the very nature and structure of the medical transcription profession.

But the ideals and mission of the organization and of the profession it serves, as well as the rationale for this book of style, remain the same: to promote the well-being and preserve the safety of each and every patient whose story is documented initially in the form of dictation by ensuring that every transcribed healthcare record, whether in hard copy or electronic format, is exactly correct in accordance with known facts and circumstances and that it is clearly intelligible to all who need to review or consult it.

The word *style* has more meanings than you can count on your fingers. It can refer to distinctive features of a work of art, music, or literature, or of a car or a house. It can also mean the way you spend your time from day to day, the way you have your hair done, and all the other things that make you unique. With reference to writing styles we can distinguish between those of Dickens and Thackeray, between formal and colloquial, and between graceful and clumsy.

The style (or styling) of a body of text, as it relates to the editorial process, means its conformity to a set of standards established by a publisher, professional organization, or other authority. This book of style, sponsored by AHDI, is intended to support and facilitate the editorial role (often unsuspected or overlooked by outsiders) of medical transcriptionists (MTs).

People who compile books of style aren't motivated by pedantry, resistance to change, a compulsive mindset, or a need to control others. In every kind of communication you can imagine, from a prescription for a controlled substance to instructions for assembling a bicycle, from the dialogue in a comic strip to the phraseology of a federal law, the transmission of meaning demands consistency and precision in the use of language. In healthcare documentation, adherence to standard nomenclature, forms, formats, and practices becomes literally a matter of life and death.

Although this book supplies information on many points of spelling, meaning, and format that can be found in a general or medical dictionary, it goes far beyond the rigid, sterile realm of the dictionary, which after all merely codifies what "everybody" already knows. *The Book of Style* guides the user through the otherwise uncharted territory of recurring uncertainties and ambiguities, of common errors and misunderstandings peculiar to medical language, of words hovering between slang and technical terminology, of neologisms coined only yesterday that are suddenly everywhere today. It also alerts the user to standards of correctness that are not only linguistic but also technical, ethical, "political," or official.

When the umpire can't arrive at a decision, the ball game stops. Sometimes it's necessary to adopt an arbitrary stance on a constantly recurring topic of concern in order to establish and maintain the internal consistency without which a system of communication falters and fails. The user of this book can be assured that each entry dealing with a controversial topic presents a position or conclusion endorsed by AHDI after careful consultation and deliberation.

Once you become familiar with the many ways in which the *Book of Style* can help you on the job, there's little danger of its gathering dust on your shelf. But, valuable as it is, the book doesn't have everything. By the time any reference work makes its way through the press and the bindery, it's already drifting out of date. Every MT knows that maintaining proficiency means continual learning, upgrading, and updating in the dynamic field of medicine and its language. So fill in those wide margins with supplemental notes based on your own research and experience, and don't forget to share your findings with AHDI for possible inclusion in the next edition.

Just as change in language is unpredictable and inescapable, the field of medical transcription is in a constant state of flux both as a profession and as an industry, with this difference: that changes in the profession are driven by the pursuit of excellence, while changes in the industry are driven by the pursuit of financial gain. Naturally the two motivations seldom generate exactly the same kind of progress.

Quality assurance standards and safe practices are ubiquitous in today's world, and they exert an increasing influence on every aspect of medical transcription. Many of those standards (particularly the ones established to eliminate ambiguities and miscommunications arising from carelessly handwritten records and orders) ostensibly govern the actions of physicians, and yet it is the transcriptionist who assumes the burden of enforcing all of them at the keyboard.

The emergence of speech recognition technology, far from eliminating the role of the medical transcriptionist, has merely redefined it. If some transcriptionists now have less keystroking to perform, their editorial function has expanded as they are challenged to correct not only dictators' errors of commission and omission but also those perpetrated by the machinery.

Many aspects of the widespread change to electronic health records affect not merely the format of healthcare documents but even their content and their authenticity. Templates and point-and-click technology limit the user's choices and invite stereotyped, homogeneous, and ultimately sketchy record-keeping. What impact this evolving technology will eventually have on the MT remains to be seen, but certainly it portends no lessening of professional responsibility, nor does it herald any reduction in the demand for technical competence.

Even where verbatim transcription policies prevail—wildly irrational and seemingly unworkable though they are—the transcriptionist must still possess and employ a full complement of interpretive skills and linguistic acumen.

These and other changes looming on the horizon may seem to cast a shadow on your personal job security and indeed on the future of your profession. The thought of hardware and software sharing office space with human professionals and perhaps taking over their jobs like a gang of robots can be positively intimidating. It's true that these impersonal, mechanical, rigid, and often abstract entities with their *architecture* and *platforms* and *capture* are at times dizzyingly fast and efficient. But it's also true that they often act dumber than a keg of nails. They're going to need highly trained keepers and nursemaids for generations to come.

More significantly, you have assets and qualities that no electronic device or software program has ever had, or ever will have: commitment to a set of ideals, the determination to be the best you can be in your chosen profession, and the capacity to adapt, learn, and grow.

And you've got *style*!

Preface

As you can imagine, a project of this magnitude takes a great deal of research and planning. From the inception of a 3rd edition text, it was deemed critical that this text be entirely reorganized. The review team (listed on the *Acknowledgments* page) met to discuss the concept of layout and reorganization, and the most consistent feedback about the layout of the 2nd edition related to its alphabetical organization and the challenge of locating information. Standards related to a specific concept or clinical specialty were scattered throughout the text, making both research for the MT and training for the MT educator a significant challenge. MTs are trained to intellectually compartmentalize, certainly a natural inclination of the human brain when it comes to learning, and industry resources and textbooks that take a compartmental, topic-driven approach have proven to be the most valuable to the student MT and the working documentation specialist. To that end, this edition has been entirely reorganized to accomplish that same learning outcome for documentation standards.

What's New in This Edition?

- Reorganization of all content into topical sections and chapters
- A detailed content index at the beginning of each chapter
- A professionally drafted content index at the end of text
- Completely redrafted content sections throughout the text, particularly in *Section 2: General Standards of Style*
- More detailed, comprehensive content explanations and rationale for standards and style recommendations
- More and better style application examples taken from a clinical medicine context
- A complete chapter dedicated to medical record types and formats, including a new section addressing turn-around times (TATs)
- A complete chapter dedicated to medical record privacy, security, and integrity, including all standards and recommendations previously housed in AHDI's *HIPAA for MTs* paper
- A complete chapter dedicated to amending and modifying the patient record
- *Trend Notes* included throughout the text that alert the reader to the current and/or potential impact of emerging technologies (EHR/EMR, speech recognition, etc.) on a particular standard of style
- An entire section of chapters addressing trends and drivers in the industry, including:
    - *Chapter 25 – ASTM Standards for Healthcare Document Formats*
    - *Chapter 26 – CDA for Common Document Types (CDA4CDT)*
    - *Chapter 27 – Standardized Nomenclature for Medicine (SNOMED)*
    - *Chapter 28 – Speech Recognition and SR Editing*

- Medical specialty chapters with organized standards, including many new classification systems not included in the 2nd edition
- Cross-referencing throughout the text to redirect users to related information and standards
- Duplication of specific standards, where appropriate, in more than one chapter in anticipation of where users will most likely look for information

In addition to the changes and revisions to content, layout, and presentation as outlined above, many users will be anxious to know what changes have occurred in the arena of standards. There are a few notable standards updates and changes, as well as additional *Trend Notes* throughout the text that will alert users to the potential for a standard to evolve in a certain anticipated direction in the near future. Virtually all of the changes in standards outlined below have been adopted in compliance with the *AMA Manual of Style*, 10th edition, *The Gregg Reference Manual*, 10th edition, and the standards of style published under SI convention by the authorities governing the use of the International System of Units.

What Standards Have Changed in this Edition?

Per the sources indicated above, notable changes in standards in this edition include:

- Dropping the use of hyphens with numeric values and metric units when forming compound modifiers (*2 cm incision* rather than *2-cm incision*). *See 12.1.7 –Punctuation.*
- Dropping the use of periods in most lowercased Latin abbreviations, like legal abbreviations (*et al, eg, ie, viz, etc*), and literary reference abbreviations (*p, pp*). *See 6.1.1 – Periods.*
- Continued trend toward dropping the use of periods with abbreviated personal and courtesy titles unless it is known that the person in question prefers the inclusion of a period or periods (*Dr, Mrs, Jr, Sr*). *See 6.1.1 – Periods.*
- Dropping the use of a comma to separate a person's last name from titles such as *Jr, Sr*, or the roman numerals following a person's name (*John H. Smith III, George Baker Jr*). *See 6.2.7 – Titles.*
- The inclusion of a space between the numeric value and the degree symbol when expressing temperature values and their scales (*98 °F and 37 °C*) per SI convention. *See 12.2.6 – Temperature.*
- Dropping the space between parameters when expressing TNM staging for malignant tumors (*T2N1M0* rather than *T2 N1 M0* or *T2, N1, M1*). *See 16.2.1 – Cancer Staging and Grading.*
- Dropping the use of subscripts with EEG electrode references. *See 18.2.3 – Diagnostic Testing and Procedures.*

The vast majority of change to this text, as mentioned above, has been directed toward providing a more robust resource for the working medical transcriptionist. Each chapter is packed with organized, detailed information that goes far beyond information provided in any previous edition of this text. Certainly not all information related to terminology and applicable classification systems and diagnostic testing could possibly be included within the scope of this text, but every attempt has been made to address any area of clinical language about which there may be a question as to expression or style.

Given the ever-evolving nature of medical language and documentation standards, the need to stay on top of trends and changes in the industry never ends. AHDI continues to stay engaged in vigilant research and watchful oversight of emerging and evolving changes in both healthcare and documentation. To that end, we welcome ongoing feedback and insight into areas of research and discovery encountered every day by working MTs. "Trend watchers" can report their findings directly to the editor.

Lea M. Sims, CMT, FAAMT
AHDI Director of Publications & Communications
Author and Managing Editor – *The Book of Style for Medical Transcription*,
3rd edition
pubs@ahdionline.org

Section 1
The Legal Medical Record

CHAPTER

1

Types, Formats, and TATs

1.1 Report Types

While all documentation recorded of a patient's care is considered a legal part of the medical record, medical transcriptionists are responsible primarily for the narrative portions of the patient record that detail the diagnostic decision-making process surrounding a patient's care. In a private practice or clinical setting, this includes the history and physical report or letter generated on the patient's first visit to the office, followup visit notes, letters to referring physicians and third parties, and documentation of phone correspondence with the patient. In the acute care setting, however, this involves what is typically referred to as the "Basic Four"—i.e., admitting history and physical reports, consultations, operative reports, and discharge summaries. On a specialty basis, of course, transcription can cover radiology, special procedure, pathology (to include autopsies and gross and microscopic descriptions), and diagnostic testing reports.

Trend Note: For each of the report types outlined below, common content topics and headings are indicated. However, it is important to note that a great deal of effort in health information management is currently being directed toward standardization of report formats to facilitate interoperability and meaningful data exchange in the electronic health record. The headings indicated in this text are congruent with those recommended by the American Society for Testing and Materials (ASTM), and AHDI is working with other industry organizations on the *Clinical Documentation Architecture for Common Document Types (CDA4CDT)* project, in coordination with Health Level 7 (HL7), to establish standardized layout and data tagging formats for clinical documentation. *(Read more about ASTM, HL7, and CDA4CDT in Chapter 27—Standardized Templates and Nomenclatures).*

The following list of report types are provided in alphabetical order, but be aware that there is a chronology to how care encounters are documented. In virtually all settings, the initial History and Physical Examination is the first encounter documented. In the acute care setting, this will be followed by any preoperative and/or specialty consultations requested by the admitting physician, then by the operative report itself. Further consultations can be requested postoperatively for a variety of care management issues, of course. At the termination of care for the patient by that facility, either due to death or discharge, the death summary or discharge summary will be the final document entered into the record for that hospital stay. In the outpatient setting, the H&P is typically followed by progress, or followup, notes in either narrative or SOAP format.

1.1.1 Autopsy Report

An autopsy report is prepared by a pathologist, coroner, or medical examiner to document findings on examination of a cadaver. Not all deceased individuals undergo an autopsy, and often these are performed off-site by the county medical examiner. Typical content topics include:

- MEDICAL HISTORY
- COURSE OF TREATMENT
- EXTERNAL EXAMINATION
- INTERNAL EXAMINATION
- EVIDENCE OF INJURY
- MACROSCOPIC EXAMINATION
- MICROSCOPIC EXAMINATION
- GROSS FINDINGS (SYSTEMS AND ORGANS)
- SPECIAL DISSECTIONS
- PATHOLOGIC DIAGNOSIS
- CAUSE OF DEATH

1.1.2 Consultation Report

A consultation includes examination, review, and assessment of a patient by a healthcare provider other than the attending physician. The report generated is called a consultation report. The consulting specialist directs the report to the physician requesting the consultation, usually the attending physician. Often these are dictated in the form of a letter (*See 1.1.3 below*).

The history and physical sections of the report are highly repetitive of information provided in the original/admitting H&P, and in some cases, the transcriptionist is asked simply to duplicate those sections (*See content topics included under 1.1.6—History and Physical Examination*). Sometimes the dictating consultant will merely direct the transcriptionist to enter the statement "Please refer to the history and physical examination" or similar verbiage. In instances where the transcriptionist has access to the facility's chart management system and can pull up the previous report, the expectation may be that the transcriptionist will copy and paste those sections from the H&P into the consultation.

4

The transcriptionist should defer to facility policy in those instances.

A more detailed and focused review of systems and physical examination are often conducted by the consulting physician, particularly in the area(s) of concern or interest. Unique content topics found in a consultation report or consultative letter include:

- DIAGNOSTIC STUDIES
- ASSESSMENT, DIAGNOSIS, or DIFFERENTIAL DIAGNOSIS
- RECOMMENDATION or PLAN

1.1.3 Correspondence

In private practice and clinic settings, correspondence is commonly encountered, as providers will often dictate letters to referring and/or consulting physicians, insurance companies, employers, attorneys, etc. The content, style, and format of correspondence will vary from one facility to the next, and transcriptionists should focus primarily on internal consistency in these areas. Commonly, a consultation report by a specialist will be dictated in the form of a letter, and the transcriptionist should follow the same guidelines for content and format of a consultation report as outlined above in *section 1.1.2*, unless the provider/facility prefers that the consultation letter be transcribed entirely in narrative paragraph style.

1.1.4 Death Summary

Similar in format and outline as the discharge summary, a death summary deviates from that format, of course, in its ultimate disposition of the patient. In some instances, facilities use the term "clinical resume" to refer to the final summary, whether a discharge, transfer, or death summary.

1.1.5 Discharge Summary

The discharge report summarizes the entire course of a patient's stay in the hospital, including the reason for hospitalization, the significant findings, the procedures performed and treatment rendered, the condition of the patient on discharge, and the plan or recommended treatment upon discharge. Typical content headings include:

- ADMITTING DIAGNOSIS
- DISCHARGE DIAGNOSIS
- CHIEF COMPLAINT
- HISTORY or HISTORY OF PRESENT ILLNESS
- HOSPITAL COURSE

- PROGNOSIS
- PLAN, DISCHARGE PLAN, or DISPOSITION
- DISCHARGE INSTRUCTIONS
- CONDITION

Trend Note: While the use of the discharge summary as a comprehensive narrative document is still widely encountered in the acute care setting, most experts agree that this highly repetitive and redundant report will become obsolete in the electronic future, where all the information currently summarized in a discharge summary will be housed and accessible elsewhere in the electronic health record (EHR).

1.1.6 History and Physical Examination

The history and physical report is the foundational document of the clinical record, upon which all other documentation for a patient is built. Its presence in the patient record, either in paper or electronic format, is required upon admission before anything other than emergent treatment can be provided to the patient. It is the detailed and itemized summary of a patient's precipitating factors and history prior to arrival in a new physician's office or to the hospital via the emergency room or on direct admission. While this is typically abbreviated "H&P" (no periods or spaces), be aware that the ampersand (&) is an incompatible character in HL7, one that cannot be formatted. In those instances, the transcriptionist should spell out references to this document in the body of the report. Content headings can vary greatly from one facility to the next, but the standardized major content headings in a history and physical as outlined by ASTM (*E2184, Standard Specification for Healthcare Document Formats*) include the following:

- CHIEF COMPLAINT
- HISTORY OF PRESENT ILLNESS
- PAST HISTORY
- ALLERGIES
- CURRENT MEDICATIONS
- REVIEW OF SYSTEMS
- PHYSICAL EXAMINATION
- MENTAL STATUS EXAMINATION
- DIAGNOSTIC STUDIES
- DIAGNOSIS
- ORDERS

1.1.7 Operative Report

The operative report is a detailed, chronologic narrative summary of a surgical procedure or of multiple procedures performed during the same surgical session. Common section headings include:

- PREOPERATIVE DIAGNOSIS
- POSTOPERATIVE DIAGNOSIS
- REASON FOR OPERATION or INDICATIONS
- OPERATION PERFORMED or NAME OF OPERATION
- SURGEON
- ASSISTANTS
- ANESTHESIOLOGIST
- ANESTHESIA
- INDICATIONS FOR PROCEDURE
- FINDINGS
- PROCEDURE, OPERATIVE COURSE, or TECHNIQUE
- COMPLICATIONS
- TOURNIQUET TIME
- HARDWARE
- DRAINS
- SPECIMENS
- ESTIMATED BLOOD LOSS
- INSTRUMENT, SPONGE, AND NEEDLE COUNTS
- DISPOSITION OF PATIENT
- FOLLOWUP

Trend Note: Because of their highly repetitive nature, operative reports lend themselves quite readily to templates and normals. They have long been the sustaining bread and butter for MTs. However, industry experts agree that because of their repetitive nature, operative reports will likely be accessed via customized templates in the EHR, and only those complex and variable narrative exceptions will likely be traditionally transcribed.

1.1.8 Pathology Report

Any specimen that is sent for pathologic evaluation will undergo two distinct evaluations by the pathologist—a gross description and a microscopic description. These can either be dictated separately or together, as sometimes the gross descriptions will be dictated by a training pathologist, with the microscopic descriptions later dictated by a resident or chief pathologist. Both evaluations are included on the final report.
Common content sections include:

- SPECIMEN

- CLINICAL DATA or CLINICAL HISTORY
- GROSS or GROSS DESCRIPTION
- MICROSCOPIC or MICROSCOPIC DESCRIPTION
- DIAGNOSIS or MICROSCOPIC DIAGNOSIS

1.1.9 Progress Note

In the outpatient setting, progress notes (also called followup notes) are dictated by the physician on subsequent visits after the initial office evaluation/consultation. They can also be documented in the in-house acute care setting throughout the patient's stay. They can take the format of a SOAP note (*See section 1.1.10 below*) or they can take a simple narrative paragraph format, depending on facility preference. Other than the SOAP note format, progress notes have no standardized or common headings or subheadings.

1.1.10 SOAP Note

SOAP notes refer to progress notes that have a specific format with defined headings in keeping with the SOAP acronym. The headings are outlined below, with content descriptions in parentheses as clarification for those not familiar with this format:

- SUBJECTIVE (history)
- OBJECTIVE (physical exam)
- ASSESSMENT (diagnosis)
- PLAN

1.2 Formats

While various institutional formats are acceptable, standardized formats for many report types have been developed by the Healthcare Informatics committee of ASTM in a standard called *E2184, Standard Specification for Healthcare Document Formats*, which specifies the requirements for the sections and subsections, and their arrangement, in an individual's healthcare documents. Many formats are predetermined by the technology platform, and thus cannot be manipulated or changed by the transcriptionist. Refer to facility process and preference in these areas. Some of the formatting suggestions in this book—in particular H&Ps and similar reports—are consistent with those published in the ASTM standard. The standards and recommendations outlined below are organized in chronologic order from the start of the document to the end.

1.2.1 Margins

Leave half-inch to one-inch margins, top and bottom, left and right unless organizational letterhead or other exchange protocols dictate unique margins (defer to facility preference). Ragged-right margins are preferred over right-justified margins, with all lines flush left (block format).

The fonts, styles, and margins chosen for use in letters may differ from those used in other medical reports; each department (or client) will develop its own policies. Transcriptionists should refer to the guidelines outlined below in instances where facility preference has not been established. Margins for letters are often determined by the letterhead used. It is not uncommon in long letters that additional pages conform to different margins, depending on the paper used. Be sure to review the letterhead and continuation sheets (the paper used for additional pages after the first letterhead page) to adjust the left, right, top, and bottom margins as needed.

- In the full block format, all text begins flush with the left margin. This includes the date, address, reference line, salutation, the body of the letter with double spacing for each new paragraph, the complimentary close, and the signature line. Tabs are not used as all paragraphs are flush left.

EXAMPLE

January 5, 2007

John A. Smith, MD
1000 Doctor Blvd.
Ourtown, CA 55555

Dear Dr. Smith,

I saw your patient Mary Jones in the office today for followup after her surgery. Her wounds have healed nicely and I will be seeing her back on a p.r.n. basis.

Thank you for allowing me to participate in the care of this patient.

Sincerely,

Robert B. Williams, MD

- In the modified block format, the date, complimentary close, and signature line are placed just to the right of the middle of the page. An acceptable variation of the modified block allows each new paragraph within the text of the body of the letter to be double-spaced and indented five spaces or about 1/2 inch.

EXAMPLE

January 5, 2007

John A. Smith, MD
1000 Doctor Blvd.
Ourtown, CA 55555

Dear Dr. Smith,

I saw your patient Mary Jones in the office today for followup after her surgery. Her wounds have healed nicely and I will be seeing her back on a p.r.n. basis.

Thank you for allowing me to participate in the care of this patient.

Sincerely,

Robert B. Williams, MD

1.2.2 Salutation

The salutation is the greeting line utilized in correspondence, typically beginning with the word *Dear* and followed by the name of an individual or representative. Use courtesy titles (*Dr, Ms,* etc.), followed by a colon or a comma, according to facility preference. While salutation lines continue to be the preferred and common practice, it is acceptable to drop them in form letters or in those instances when the appropriate courtesy title is not known—for example, when you cannot determine whether the person is male or female. *To Whom It May Concern* is an alternative in that instance, but it is better to address correspondence to a specific individual unless that information is not available.

1.2.3 Paragraphs

Use paragraphs to separate narrative blocks within sections. In general, start new paragraphs as dictated except when such paragraphing is excessive (some originators start a new paragraph with every sentence or two) or inadequate (some originators dictate an entire lengthy report in one paragraph).

1.2.4 Type Style

Regular type: Type styles in clinical documentation are relatively straightforward and, with the exception of correspondence, do not tend to vary from one facility to the next. Also known as plain type, regular type is preferred throughout medical transcription, with just a few exceptions when bold type or italics may be preferred or required for emphasis or to conform to a facility's model or a client's personal style.

Font: Generally speaking, fonts are determined by the facility and often automatically formatted by the transcription software. In environments where the transcriptionist has to select font styles and sizes manually, facility preference should determine that selection.

Bold or Underlined type: In general, avoid bold type in medical transcription. Underlined type should also be avoided unless specifically dictated by the provider as a point of emphasis in the record. Avoid the use of either in electronic environments that do not support these type styles.

Note: ASTM's *E2184, Standard Specification for Healthcare Document Formats*, calls for all major headings in the report as well as allergies (the heading and the substance to which the individual is allergic) to be expressed in all capital letters but with regular type (not bold). While it is common practice in some facilities to put allergy references in bold type to ensure their emphasis, standards-setting organizations like ASTM and HL7 are encouraging facilities to discontinue this practice to promote interoperability and facilitate accurate file formatting and transfer.

Italics: Use regular type, not italics, for English and medical terms as well as for foreign words and phrases that are commonly used in the English language and in medical reports. This includes bacteria/virus genus and species names, which are typically expressed in italics in formal publication but should not be expressed in italics in clinical documentation. *(see examples next page)*

bruit
cul-de-sac
en masse
in toto
peau d'orange
poudrage

Use regular type as well in the following instances even though italics may be called for in manuscript preparation:

- abbreviations: AFO
- arbitrary designations: patient B
- chemical elements: boron
- Latin names of genera and species: Clostridium difficile
- letters indicating shape: T-bar
- names of foreign institutions and organizations

Superscripting and Subscripting: It is acceptable to use superscripting and subscripting in those areas of the report where doing so more clearly communicates meaning, as with exponential expressions and chemical nomenclatures; however, in electronic environments that do not support this formatting or where there is potential for conversion errors (105 instead of 10^5, for example), equivalent expressions should be used.

1.2.5 Character Spacing

When using a proportional-spaced font it is customary to mark the end of a sentence with a single space. Double-spacing is still used with nonproportional fonts, such as Courier, but with the migration toward environments built around Microsoft Word compatibility, few facilities have retained older, nonproportional fonts. While facility preference should be the guide, it is important to note that migration toward the electronic health record and interoperability protocols for standard data exchange will continue to dictate that single spacing be used with all proportionally spaced fonts. In environments where there is no preference, either spacing standard is acceptable. In any environment, character spacing is *not* considered a quality issue and should not be included in quality assurance measurements.

Use a single character space after:
- the end of a sentence, whether it ends in a period, question mark, exclamation point, quotation mark, parenthesis, bracket, or brace
- a colon used as a punctuation mark within a sentence

- each word or symbol (unless the next character is a punctuation mark)
- a comma
- a semicolon
- a period at the end of an abbreviation

Use a single character space before:
- an opening quotation mark
- an opening parenthesis
- an opening bracket or brace

Do not use a character space before or after:
- an apostrophe (except when the apostrophe ends the term, as in the plural possessive patients', in which case a space or another punctuation mark follows the apostrophe)
- a colon in expressions of time or clock or equator positions, e.g., 1:30
- a colon in expressions of ratios and dilutions, e.g., 1:100,000
- a comma in numeric expressions, e.g., 12,034
- a decimal point in numeric expressions (except in those rare instances when a unit less than 1 does not call for a zero to be placed before the decimal, e.g., .22-caliber rifle, in which instances a space precedes the decimal point but does not follow it)
- a decimal point in monetary expressions, e.g., $1.50
- a hyphen, e.g., 3-0 suture material
- a dash, e.g.: Episodes of dyspnea—usually without pain—occur on slight exertion.
- a virgule, e.g., 2/6 heart murmur
- a period within an abbreviation, e.g., q.i.d.
- an ampersand in abbreviations such as T&A, D&C

Do not use a character space after:
- an opening quotation mark
- an opening parenthesis, bracket, or brace
- a word followed by a punctuation mark

Do not use a character space before a punctuation mark (except an opening parenthesis, bracket, brace, or quotation mark).

1.2.6 Headings/Subheadings

Use headings and subheadings as dictated, unless you are following a standardized format. Institutional and client preferences should prevail, keeping in mind that adoption of standardized templates and formats across healthcare delivery will ultimately facilitate interoperability. Therefore, use standardized formats, including headings and subheadings, where able to do so.

- Use all capitals for major section headings.
- Use initial capitals for subheadings.
- List chief complaint, diagnoses, preoperative diagnoses, postoperative diagnoses, names of operations, and similar entries vertically.
- If the originator numbers some but not all items, be consistent and number all or none.
- When a single diagnosis is referred to as "number one," it is better to delete the number so that the reader is not led to believe that additional entries are missing.
- Change "diagnosis" to "diagnoses" when more than one diagnosis is provided.
- Obvious headings that are not dictated may be inserted, but this is not required. If the originator moves in and out of sections, insert the information into the appropriate sections. (Headings may be omitted where appropriate.)
- Double-space between major sections of reports.
- List subheadings vertically to assist the reader in identifying particular subsections.
- Do not use abbreviations or brief forms in headings except for such widely used and readily recognizable abbreviations as HEENT, if dictated.

Place the content on the next line following the section or subsection heading, if possible. The ASTM "Formats" standard calls for an extra line space between subheadings, as in the following examples.

EXAMPLE

HEENT
Within normal limits.

Thorax and Lungs
No rales or rhonchi.

Cardiovascular
No murmurs.

When the information following the section or subsection heading continues on the same line, use a colon (not a hyphen or a dash) after each heading.

> HEENT: Within normal limits.
> THORAX AND LUNGS: No rales or rhonchi.
> CARDIOVASCULAR: No murmurs.

Capitalize the word following the heading, whether or not a colon follows the heading. Exception: When quantity and unit of measure immediately follow a heading, such as estimated blood loss, use numerals.

> LUNGS: Within normal limits.
> ESTIMATED BLOOD LOSS: 10 mL.

End each entry with a period unless it is a date or the name of a person.

> ANESTHESIOLOGIST: Sharon Smith, MD
> ANESTHESIA: General.

1.2.7 Signature Block

Enter the signature block four hard returns below the final line of text, flush left. Use the originator's full name. If a title is given, place it directly below the originator's name; use initial capitals, unless institutional style calls for all caps. Signature lines are often preformatted; in that case, leave as formatted.

> Ruth T. Gross, MD
> Chief of Pediatrics

1.2.8 Dictator/Transcriptionist Initials

It is common practice to include originator and transcriptionist initials at the end of each report. When used, enter the initials flush left two lines below last line of text. Use either all capitals or all lowercase letters for both sets of initials, with a colon or virgule between them. Do not use periods. Do not include academic degrees, professional credentials, or titles.

> RH:ST or rh:st
> RH/ST or rh/st

There is no standard that requires or prohibits the inclusion of a transcriptionist's name or initials in the report. Some proprietary transcription systems include or exclude these automatically. Employed transcriptionists should defer to facility preference. Contracted transcriptionists or services should address this contractually. For audit trail and liability purposes, a contracted MT or service might wish to require the inclusion of this information on all reports that fall under the provision of services outlined in the contract, particularly if the facility contracts with more than one transcriptionist or service.

Some facilities may choose to identify the originators and MTs by other identifiers, such as a number or a number-letter combination, and system-generated reports may enter these identifiers automatically along with date, time, and place stamps.

> Dictated: D283, 02/02/2007, 2:35 p.m., Indianapolis, IN
> Transcribed: T149, 02/02/2007, 11:40 p.m., LaFayette, IN

1.2.9 Time/Date Stamping

For the sake of an audit trail, it is common practice to include the date and time of dictation and transcription at the end of each report. Use of either "Dictated" and "Transcribed" or "D" and "T" followed by a colon is acceptable. Enter the date and time flush left below the initials of the originator and transcriptionist. Use colons for the time unless military time is the preferred format.

> D: 05/10/2007, 11:40 p.m.
> Dictated: 05/10/2007, 11:40 p.m.
> D: 05/10/2007, 2340
> Dictated: 05/10/2007, 2340

Identification of the place of dictation and transcription may be required as well.

> D: 02/02/2007, 11:40 p.m., LaFayette, IN
> T: 02/03/2007, 8:45 a.m., Springfield, MO

1.2.10 Continuation Pages

When a transcript is longer than one page, enter *Continued* at the bottom of each printed page prior to the last, and repeat the patient's name and medical record number (where applicable), the page number, and the date of service on each continuation page. Additional identifying data may be noted, according to facility preference.

> Smith, Mary
> 99999
> 05/10/2007
>
> Page 2

Do not carry a single line of a report onto a continuation page. Do not allow a continuation page to include only the signature block and the data following it. When the printing is done by someone other than the medical transcriptionist, or when it is programmed into the system, these guidelines should still be followed. Follow facility guidelines for including other headings or designated material on subsequent pages after the first.

Trend Note: The guidelines above cannot be applied in electronic environments where formatting is automatically generated by the technology. In those instances, the MT should follow facility guidelines for allowing text to wrap and flow from start to finish without formatting for page breaks.

1.2.11 Copy Designation

The copy designation, often referred to as the carbon copy area, is a notation of those to whom copies of a report or letter are to be distributed.
A carbon copy is increasingly known as a courtesy copy. Abbreviated *cc*.
A blind copy designation is noted only on the file copy and on the copy to whom it is sent; other recipients' copies do not indicate the blind copy (thus its name). Abbreviated *bc* or *bcc*. Place copy designations flush left and two

line spaces below the end of the report. These designations should be followed by a colon.

bc	blind copy
bcc	blind courtesy copy
c	copy
cc	courtesy copy, carbon copy
pc	photocopy

Trend Note: The above guidelines are only relevant to environments where transcriptionists are still manually entering this kind of information into the record. In electronic environments and on most transcription platforms, the document is electronically tagged for fax and email copies via data entry fields outside the record itself, and in those instances, the transcriptionist would not transcribe copy designations directly into the record. Defer to facility technology and preference.

APPENDICES: See sample reports for each of the report formats discussed in this chapter in *Appendix A.*

1.2.12 Diagnosis

When only one diagnosis is given, it is preferable not to number it, even if a number is dictated, because the number gives the appearance that there are additional diagnoses.

DIAGNOSIS
Appendicitis.

preferred to:

DIAGNOSIS
1. Appendicitis.

In section headings, when *diagnosis* is dictated, it may be changed to the plural form *diagnoses* if more than one is listed. If there are several diagnoses, it is preferable to number them even if numbers are not dictated. Enumerating diagnoses promotes clarity and more readily facilitates the coding and reimbursement process.

Dictated:
DIAGNOSIS: Appendicitis, history of myocardial infarction, and chronic sinusitis.

Transcribed:
DIAGNOSES
1. Appendicitis.
2. History of myocardial infarction.
3. Chronic sinusitis.

1.3 Turn-Around Times

Turn-around time, or TAT, in transcription refers to the window of time between the dictation of a report and when it is transcribed and returned to the author for authentication. This includes the period of time the report is pending transcription on the dictation system, the time it is checked out or routed to the transcriptionist, the time it is checked out or routed to a QA coordinator or editor, and any other time or delay between dictation and delivery to the author or facility.

1.3.1 Acute Care TATs

Most facilities have established their own TAT policies, but for acute-care facilities some of those TAT requirements are shaped by Joint Commission standards.

History and Physical Examinations: Joint Commission standard PC.2.120 defines in writing the time frame(s) for conducting initial assessments for hospital admission.

Elements of Performance for PC.2.120
The hospital specifies the following time frames for these assessments:

- A medical history and physical examination is completed within no more than 24 hours of inpatient admission.
- A registered nurse completes a nursing assessment within 24 hours of inpatient admission
- A nutritional screening, when warranted by the patients' needs or condition, is completed within no more than 24 hours of inpatient admission.
- A functional status screening, when warranted by the patient's needs or condition, is completed within no more than 24 hours of inpatient admission.

Some of these elements may have been completed ahead of time, but must meet the following criteria:

- The history and physical must have been completed within 30 days before the patient was admitted or readmitted.
- Updates to the patient's condition *since* the assessment(s) are recorded at the time of admission.

Operative Reports: Joint Commission standard IM.6.30 outlines the elements of performance for documenting operative or other high-risk procedures.

Elements of Performance for IM.6.30

- The licensed independent practitioner (responsible for the patient) records the provisional diagnosis before the operative or other high-risk procedures.
- Operative or other high-risk procedure reports dictated or written immediately after an operative or other high-risk procedure record the name of the licensed independent practitioner and assistants; procedure(s) performed and description of the procedure; findings; estimated blood loss; specimens removed; and postoperative diagnosis. *The exception to the requirement is when an operative or other high-risk procedure progress note is written immediately after the procedure, in which case the full operative or other high-risk procedure report can be written or dictated within a time frame defined by the organization.*
- An operative or other high-risk procedure progress note is entered in the medical record immediately after the procedure, if the full operative or other high-risk procedure report cannot be entered into the record immediately after the operation or procedure.
- The completed operative or other high-risk procedure report is authenticated by the licensed independent practitioner and made available in the medical record as soon as possible after the procedure.
- Postoperative documentation records the patient's vital signs and level of consciousness; medications (including intravenous fluids) and blood and blood components administered; unusual events or complications, including blood transfusion reactions; and the management of those events.
- Postoperative documentation records the patient's discharge from the postsedation or postanesthesia care area by the responsible licensed independent practitioner or according to discharge criteria.
- The use of approved discharge criteria to determine the patient's readiness for discharge is documented in the medical record.
- Postoperative documentation records the name of the licensed independent practitioner responsible for discharge.

- The history and physical examination and the results of indicated diagnostic tests are recorded before the operative or other high-risk procedures.

Based on the requirements above, most facilities mandate that a surgeon must enter some form of documentation about the procedure into the record *immediately after the procedure*. In many facilities, this means the surgeon will write a brief summary note into the record after the procedure, which will suffice until the fully transcribed report is returned within 24 hours. While the Joint Commission does not have a TAT requirement for the transcription of that record, most facilities operate under a 24- to 48-hour TAT policy for operative reports.

Consultation Reports: There presently is no standard or requirement for consultation turn-around times, though given their direct correlation to continuity of care and ongoing treatment decisions for inpatients, most facilities establish a 24-hour-or-less TAT policy for these reports.

Discharge Summaries: Per Joint Commission standard IM.6.30 above, there are specifications about what type of information needs to be record in a discharge summary, but there are no turn-around time requirements specifically indicated as part of the standard. However, Joint Commission regulations about delinquent records require that less than 50% of previous-month discharged patient records be incomplete during the current month. Therefore, most internal hospital policies and procedures require that the recorded discharge summary needs to be transcribed and signed, the chart coded, all nurses' notes signed, all labs filed on the chart, and all physical therapy, occupational therapy, consultations, and operative reports be assembled and in order *within 30 days of discharge*.

1.3.2 Outpatient TATs

Since outpatient and private practice facilities fall outside the auspices of the Joint Commission, there are no regulations or standards related to turn-around times for documentation in those facilities. There is, in fact, a great deal of variance in expectation where TAT is concerned in the outpatient setting. In general, a 24- to 48-hour turn-around time expectation prevails in most of the private sector for transcription. There is often a 24-hour-or-less TAT expectation for unique reports – such as new patient H&Ps, consultation letters, notifications to insurance companies, or other documents considered of high priority to the provider or facility. Turn-around times for priority documents in those settings are established between the facility and the transcriptionist or service owner.

Resources

Joint Commission. *Comprehensive Accreditation Manual for Hospitals: The Official Handbook.* Oakbrook Terrace, IL: Joint Commission on Accreditation of Healthcare Organizations, 2007.

CHAPTER

2

Chapter 2: Editing the Record

Introduction

If transcriptionists were only required to "type what they hear" and apply the standards as outlined throughout this book, the role would be a relatively straightforward and unencumbered one. There are some in health care who advocate this kind of restricted role for documentation specialists, embracing a "verbatim" transcription policy that limits the MT to transcribing only what is dictated, whether right or wrong, and flagging discrepancies for review by the dictator. In most environments, however, there is the expectation that the MT will be actively engaged in the diagnostic story-telling of the patient encounter, noting discrepancies in grammar, style, and clinical information, and correcting those discrepancies that fall within the scope of the MT's knowledge and informed judgment. Certainly, routing discrepancies back to the dictator that could have been reasonably corrected by the transcriptionist has a direct impact on turn-around time and reimbursement. Such a restrictive policy for editing and correction can be costly to the facility and burdensome to the medical records department who has to facilitate those corrections. A skilled, engaged MT partners with the physician to ensure an accurate, timely, and secure record.

AHDI recognizes that MTs are *not* engaged in provision of patient care and cannot be expected to have insight into the patient encounter beyond what is provided by the dictator. However, many discrepancies encountered in dictation represent areas of obvious error where correction falls within the scope of the interpretive skill set and clinical knowledge of the MT. (*See Appendix B—Statement on Verbatim Transcription.*)

Transcriptionists who find themselves in a verbatim environment will have no choice but to comply with facility policy, and the ability of those MTs to engage in informed editing and impact risk management will be extremely limited. In those settings, an MT must stay within the guidelines of the verbatim standard, but AHDI urges even those MTs to be proactive in advocating for the role of the skilled MT in ensuring accurate capture and formatting of healthcare data.

2.1 When to Edit

A patient's record is an important story, one that needs to accurately reflect the exchange of information that occurred between the provider and the patient during that encounter. Preserving the tone and scope of that encounter, while ensuring the accuracy of the data being captured, is critical to creating a long-term care record that is historically and clinically meaningful. The *art* of managing information that ensures this outcome falls within the skill set of the transcriptionist. Honoring a physician's dictation style, recognizing error or inconsistency in the record, correcting errors appropriately, refraining from correcting or altering what cannot be confirmed, and notifying the provider of errors that cannot be corrected are all part of protecting the *integrity* of the patient care encounter.

Trend Note: The computerized translation by a speech recognition engine of dictated material results in text that usually needs considerable editing. This is sometimes done on the front end by the originator but more often by a back-end speech recognition editor (an experienced medical transcriptionist) who will review the text while listening to the original audio file to ensure that the data has been captured and formatted appropriately. The same editing guidelines outlined below that apply to transcription editing equally apply to editing a speech-recognized draft.

2.1.1 Grammar/Punctuation

Edit errors in grammar and punctuation, including dictator-provided instructions related to paragraph breaks and punctuation. Dictators, especially those who speak English as a second language, may struggle with effective grammar and appropriate punctuation. Common errors include poor subject-verb agreement and transposition of personal pronouns. Be careful also to listen for errors in pluralization, especially where Latin and Greek plurals are concerned, and edit appropriately.

EXAMPLE

> D: The anterior and posterior views of the chest was normal.
> T: The anterior and posterior views of the chest were normal.
>
> D: The patient had multiple diverticuli in the transverse colon.
> T: The patient had multiple diverticula in the transverse colon.

2.1.2 Syntax

Syntax refers to the appropriate arrangement of words in a sentence. Word order is important to ensuring clarity of communication. Often, in the haste of dictation, providers will unwittingly dictate sentences with gross errors in syntax. While the result can be humorous, it is critical for the transcriptionist to edit these errors so that they do not lead to misinterpretation of meaning. ESL physicians are particularly prone to errors in syntax, as their native grammar structures often vary greatly from English syntax. While the vocabulary and concepts may be accurate, they will often need assistance from the MT in ensuring appropriate word order and avoiding misplaced modifiers. Edit errors in syntax to ensure clarity of communication.

EXAMPLE

D: The patient developed a puffy right eye that was felt to be secondary to an insect bite by the ophthalmologist.
T: The patient developed a puffy right eye; this was felt by the ophthalmologist to be secondary to an insect bite.

D: CT scan showed there was nothing in the brain but sinusitis.
T: CT scan of the brain showed only sinusitis.

2.1.3 Spelling

While electronic spell checkers can be tremendously helpful in identifying and correcting misspelled words in the record, transcriptionists should not rely on those resources alone, nor should the transcriptionist rely on dictator spelling of new terms, medications, equipment, or instruments *unless* that term cannot be located or verified in any reputable resource. In that instance, it is best to spell the term as provided by the dictator and flag the report for verification (*See 2.4.3—Flagging the Report*). For all misspelled words for which a correct spelling can be verified, the transcriptionist should edit that term appropriately.

2.1.4 Slang, Jargon, and Brief Forms

Modern medicine is constantly evolving and so is its language. In addition, with the fast pace of American health care, clinicians sometimes find themselves dictating their notes on the fly, before they have had a chance to put their thoughts together. The result may be an awkward use of language and frequent neologisms. Edit inappropriate slang words and phrases, keeping in mind that many words start out as coined or slang terms but later evolve through usage to eventually become acceptable words in the American medical lexicon.

To include a list of acceptable and unacceptable slang word, brief form, or jargon would be virtually impossible. Transcriptionists should consult a reputable industry reference book or resource to verify what terms are acceptable in their shortened or altered forms and which terms should be edited.

Sometimes a noun or adjective is used as a verb. If possible, edit awkwardly created verbs.

EXAMPLE

D: Stool was guaiac'd.
T: Stool guaiac test was done.

Likewise, if possible, edit proper nouns dictated as verbs.

EXAMPLE

D: The baby was de-lee'd on the abdomen.
T: The baby was suctioned on the abdomen using a DeLee.

Jargon refers to special language that is used and fully understood only by members of a particular craft, trade, or profession. Like other jargons, that of healthcare professions parallels, but only slightly overlaps, formal technical terminology. It consists partly of lay and technical terms to which special meanings are assigned. It is largely unrecorded in reference books and is highly informal, including some expressions that are slangy and humorous. Medical jargon tends to be particularly imprecise and may be offensive and derogatory.

EXAMPLE

D: urines
T: urine samples

D: premie
T: premature infant

D: orthopod
T: orthopedic surgeon

Leave blank and flag obscenities, derogatory or inflammatory remarks, and double entendres (words or word combinations, symbols, and abbreviations that have varying, and usually inappropriate, meanings) except when these are purposefully dictated by the author as part of a direct quote. In instances where the inclusion is easily edited, do so to avoid misinterpretation or the retention of an inappropriate abbreviation or term.

EXAMPLE

> D: He is complaining of some SOB.
> T: He is complaining of some shortness of breath.

Brief forms are shortened forms of common words that are acceptable to transcribe in abbreviated format. These are discussed more fully in Chapter 9. Consult a reputable industry reference or resource when attempting to determine whether a dictated abbreviated form is an acceptable brief form or is potentially an unacceptable slang, jargon term, or back formation.

Examples of acceptable brief forms:

EXAMPLE

> exam
> lab
> monos, basos, lymphs, eos
> prep

Examples of unacceptable brief forms:

EXAMPLE

> appy (appendectomy)
> crit (hematocrit)
> epi (epinephrine)

2.1.5 Back Formations

Back formations are new words formed by altering an existing word (usually a noun). Back formations are often verbs but may appear as adjectives or adverbs. They are frequently encountered in medical dictation. Use dictated back formations if they have become acceptable through widespread use. Avoid absurd back formations or ones that will be confusing to the reader. It is difficult to say which back formations will become accepted; this is ultimately determined by usage. False verbs and other back formations are increasingly prevalent in the communications industry and technical world, but they should be used judiciously in transcribed health records.

Examples of back formations that have evolved to acceptable and common usage:

> diagnosis—to diagnose
> Bovie—bovied

Examples of back formations that are not acceptable and should be edited appropriately:

> adhesion—to adhese
> cardioplegia—to cardioplege
> liaison—to liaise
> orchiopexy—to pex

2.1.6 Incorrect Terms

Edit incorrectly dictated English and medical terms when the intended meaning is unquestionably clear. This requires a transcriptionist to have skilled interpretive judgment and the ability to recognize any ambiguity related to a dictated term or phrase *(See 2.2.1—Critical Thinking versus Guessing)*. If there is any doubt, leave a blank and flag the report.

> D: At the time of discharge, the patient was feeling much better and no longer had a temperature.
> T: At the time of discharge, the patient was feeling much better and no longer had a fever.

Note: In the above example, temperature was changed to fever because it would be clinically erroneous to describe a patient, particularly one being discharged, as having no temperature. While it is common for people, even dictators, to use these terms interchangeably, clarity of communication dictates that the appropriate word (in this case *fever*) be used instead.

> D: The baby was delivered over an intact peritoneum.
> T: The baby was delivered over an intact perineum.

2.1.7 Contextual Inconsistencies

Many contextual inconsistencies have to be flagged and referred to the dictator for verification, but some contextual inconsistencies can be resolved by a critically thinking transcriptionist. If, for example, the physician clearly identifies the patient as a female in the opening statements of the history, accidental references to the patient as "he" or "him" elsewhere in the report should be edited by the transcriptionist and do not require notification of the dictator. Some ESL dictators (for example, those who are native to the Philippines) struggle with personal pronouns because such pronouns do not exist in their native languages. Likewise, it is common for a dictator to dictate erroneous directional and positional terms (like *left* and *right*), and when a clear delineation is evident in the record, the transcriptionist should edit appropriately. Do not guess. If in doubt, leave a blank and flag the report.

2.1.8 Transposition of Terms and Values

It is not uncommon for a dictator to accidentally transpose words or values in the haste of dictating. When it is extremely clear that those terms have simply been flipped or transposed, edit them appropriately. If there is any ambiguity or doubt about the transposition of those terms or the correlation of values to the appropriate terms, leave a blank and flag the report. Many transposed terms can be left unedited, as they do not alter meaning, nor do they impact grammatical structure. However, some clinical and diagnostic phrases are typically expressed in a specific order and have common abbreviations associated with that word order. When those types of phrases contain transposed terms, edit them appropriately to reflect the common phrase.

EXAMPLE

> D: Hemoglobin 42, hematocrit 17.
> T: Hemoglobin 17, hematocrit 42.
>
> D: Vaginal laparoscopic-assisted hysterectomy
> T: Laparoscopic-assisted vaginal hysterectomy (LAVH)

2.1.9 Demographics

Accurate patient demographics are critical to managing health information, and every attempt should be made to ensure that accurate patient demographics (as defined by the facility) have been captured in the documentation process. Some demographics, like medical record number and date of service, are manually entered by the dictator via the technology interface. Others are dictated by the physician. Both capture methods are fraught with error, and in settings where the transcriptionist has access to the patient chart, chart management system, or Admission/Discharge/Transfer (ADT) data, the transcriptionist should refer to that data when selecting or transcribing demographics. Do not rely solely on dictator spelling of patient names nor the dictated or manually entered medical record numbers, chart numbers, dates of birth, or dates of service.

Trend Note: With most modern dictation platforms and many ASP models, the demographic or ADT information is captured automatically by the system at the point of dictation and electronically associated with the transcribed record. Transcriptionists working under those models are often required to verify what has been captured by the ADT feed against the information being dictated by the physician to ensure accurate demographic mapping. In settings where this is not automatic, the MT may have to manually access this information to verify demographics.

2.2 How to Edit

Error recognition is only the first step in ensuring accurate data capture. Managing those errors requires the transcriptionist to be engaged in critical thinking that has been shaped by knowledge of clinical terminology and the diagnostic process. The skilled, engaged transcriptionist should engage all of the strategies below for appropriate and informed editing.

2.2.1 Critical Thinking versus Guessing

Transcriptionists should approach the editing process from the position of informed judgment. An MT should never guess when interpreting what has been dictated or the accuracy of a term, phrase, or reference in the record. Only in instances where the transcriptionist's interpretive skill and experience have shaped a high degree of accuracy and confidence in the appropriate areas of editing (as outlined above in section 2.1) should the MT be permitted to proceed with editing those areas. Postgraduate transcriptionists and new hires should be watched closely to evaluate consistency in error recognition and interpretive judgment. In instances where even a skilled transcriptionist cannot confidently edit an error or inconsistency, the MT should leave a blank and flag the report.

2.2.2 Clarifying Content

Be proactively engaged in capturing a patient encounter by paying close attention to the entire narrative and the information that has been relayed about the patient. Encountered errors or questionable inclusions can often be clarified by content elsewhere in the report. When attempting to interpret a dictated term or phrase, search for context clues that will facilitate an informed editing decision.

2.2.3 Dictator Style

Editing what has been dictated to reflect grammatical or clinical accuracy should be done in a subtle and nonintrusive manner. In general, MTs should not edit syntax or diction unless it represents an error or potential for misinterpretation. Just because a sentence can be better worded does not mean that it is wrong. When editing phrases, terms, and syntax, do so with respect for dictator style and employ the least intrusive strategy for correction.

2.2.4 Access to Ancillary Records

Refer to the patient's record to clarify or correct content in dictation. In settings where the transcriptionist has access to the patient chart or previous records, refer to those records for verification of information when needed. In settings where access to those records is restricted, the transcriptionist should leave a blank and flag the report.

2.3 When Not to Edit

As important as the ability to accurately edit errors and inconsistencies in the record is the ability to recognize and acknowledge those instances when it is inappropriate for a transcriptionist to engage in editing or altering the dictated record. The objective of quality assessment programs is to ensure that transcriptionists not only know when and how to edit, but when *not* to edit, and confidence in the skills of an MT is often based on whether that MT knows what to do when he/she cannot edit or are unsure of how to handle a questionable area of the record.

2.3.1 Missing/Inaudible Dictation

In any area of the record where the dictation is missing, has been cut off, is complicated by extraneous noise, is inaudible, or is hindered by the speed or poor articulation skills of the dictator, the transcriptionist should not attempt to guess unless the missing term or phrase is extremely obvious (see below). In most instances, the only option is to leave a blank and flag the report.

D: Temperature 98.6, pulse 60, and <garbled dictation> 122/77.
T: Temperature 98.6, pulse 60, and blood pressure 122/77.

D: The patient was sent home on <garbled dictation> and will follow up
   in the office.
T: The patient was sent home on _____ and will follow up in the office.

2.3.2 Irreconcilable Words and Phrases

When every attempt has been made by the transcriptionist to research a questionable term or phrase and reputable resources have been consulted with no verification, the transcriptionist should leave a blank and flag the report, even in instances where the term or phrase was specifically dictated and/or spelled by the physician.

2.3.3 Contradictory Information

In instances where there is clearly contradictory information in the record that cannot be clarified contextually or in ancillary records, the transcriptionist should leave a blank and flag the report.

2.3.4 Direct Quotes

When the dictator provides information in the form of a direct quote, the transcriptionist should be careful not to edit that information, as the dictator may be intentionally including incorrect terms or references that were stated by the patient.

D: The patient believes her husband may have early quote old timer's
   disease unquote.
T: The patient believes her husband may have early "old timer's disease."

not:
T: The patient believes her husband may have early "Alzheimer disease."

2.3.5 Negative Findings

Never delete negative or normal findings if dictated. To do so could potentially imply that those areas were not evaluated. Remember that a negative or normal finding *is* a finding, often as diagnostically significant as a positive finding.

2.4 Notification and Flagging

The standard process for notifying either the quality assurance department or the provider of an error or inconsistency in the record is to leave a blank and flag the report to the attention of an accountable party who will need to review that blank and correct it.

2.4.1 Blanks

Leave a blank space in a report rather than guessing what was meant or transcribing unclear or obviously incorrect dictation. In many instances, leaving a blank means including an underlined section equivalent to the perceived length of questionable content. In other instances, it may mean leaving a blank space or a text marker or tag that can be searched for by the QA person who will review the flag (see examples below). Transcriptionists should defer to facility/client preference for managing flagged areas of the record.

EXAMPLE

The patient came in today complaining of _____ for the last 3 days.
The patient came in today complaining of   for the last 3 days.
The patient came in today complaining of ### for the last 3 days.

2.4.2 Audio Indexing

With many dictation systems, it is now possible to index the dictation or audio file at points where there is a question or potential error in the record. This enables QA personnel to jump quickly to that portion of the dictation to resolve flagged issues. On proprietary transcription systems, it is also possible for the indexed audio file to be automatically linked to the blank or tag in the record. This greatly facilitates the QA and review process, and transcriptionists should defer to company or facility procedures for audio indexing.

2.4.3 Flagging the Report

At one time, flagging simply referred to the process of leaving a note at the end of the record that would draw the attention of medical records personnel and/or the physician to a blank or inconsistency in the record. The term has taken on the additional meaning of electronically marking a report for review. When flagging a report to draw attention to unclear or incorrect dictation, cite the page, section, and line number, tagging the error on paper or electronically.

If the word or phrase is unfamiliar, note what it sounds like. If the term is inconsistent, briefly state why, as below.

EXAMPLE

A left below-knee amputation is later referred to as a right BK amputation. Please review and verify.

CHAPTER

3

Chapter 3: Record Privacy, Security, and Integrity

Introduction

To provide effective treatment, healthcare providers must have comprehensive, accurate, and timely medical information. The automation of medical information permits the collection, analysis, storage, and retrieval of vast amounts of medical information that is not only used but also shared with other providers at remote locations. The increasing demand for access to medical information by providers and others, such as insurance companies, has led to increasing concern about patient privacy and confidentiality, resulting in the enactment of the privacy and security provisions of the Health Insurance Portability and Accountability Act of 1996 (HIPAA). HIPAA, and its implementing regulations, requires providers and certain others who maintain health information to put in place measures to guard the privacy and confidentiality of patient information. Before HIPAA, patient privacy was only sporadically protected by various state laws but never so dramatically as it is by the HIPAA statute and its accompanying regulations.

3.1 Record Privacy

Medical transcriptionists who are employees of healthcare providers or other HIPAA "covered entities" (as defined in this chapter) are affected by HIPAA, but they should go to their employers for guidance regarding HIPAA compliance. However, even these MTs should also be aware of the issues, in case they consider going into business for themselves, even on a part-time basis, at some point in the future. Consider the fact that "doing a little work on the side" makes one an independent contractor and thus a business owner if that work does not fall under an employment relationship. MTs who are subcontractors to MT businesses will be required to agree contractually to essentially the same restrictions and conditions that apply to MT businesses with respect to handling patient information.

3.1.1 Confidentiality

Patients have a legal and ethical right to the reasonable expectation that their private information will not be disclosed except for the purposes for which it was provided (such as receiving healthcare services). Medical transcriptionists share with other healthcare personnel the responsibility to respect the confidentiality of medical records. Federal and state laws govern the extent of confidentiality required and the exceptions under which appropriate disclosures can be made.

3.1.2 Protected Health Information

The privacy rule regulates the use and disclosure of *protected health information*, or PHI, by certain entities. Protected health information is information transmitted or maintained in any form—by electronic means, on paper, or through oral communications—that:

- Relates to the past, present, or future physical or mental health or condition of an individual, the provision of healthcare to an individual, or the past, present, or future payment for the provision of healthcare to an individual.
- Identifies the individual or with respect to which there is a reasonable basis to believe the information can be used to identify the individual.

Information that has been de-identified in accordance with the rule's stringent de-identification criteria is not considered protected health information and is not subject to the rule.

3.1.3 Accountable Parties under HIPAA

The HIPAA privacy rule is almost 100 pages long, yet never once is the term "medical transcriptionist" used. Organizations *directly* subject to the HIPAA privacy rule are those that typically generate individually identifiable patient health information and therefore have primary responsibility for maintaining the privacy and confidentiality of such information. These *covered entities*, as defined by HIPAA, are:

- Most health plans.
- Healthcare clearinghouses.
- Healthcare providers that transmit any health information in electronic form in connection with certain administrative transactions related to payment for health care (i.e., most healthcare providers, such as hospitals, nursing homes, clinics, and physician offices).

Employees of covered entities generally are not themselves covered entities but effectively must comply with the rule because improper uses and disclosures of information by employees may be imputed to employers. Thus, medical transcriptionists who work as employees of hospitals, clinics, private physician offices, and other covered entities should follow the policies and procedures established by those organizations with respect to the handling of protected health information.

3.1.4 Permitted Disclosure

Disclosure, historically referred to as *release of information*, involves both legal requirements and professional responsibility. MTs should not release information except as authorized by institutional policies and procedures, and consistent with the law. The patient's rights to personal and health information privacy and confidentiality must be respected. Courts and others may have legitimate rights to health information. HIPAA privacy regulations indicate that a covered entity may use or disclose protected health information only:

- After first obtaining an individual's "authorization" for "treatment, payment, and healthcare operations" with an individual's written "authorization" for certain purposes unrelated to treatment, payment, or healthcare operations.
- Without an individual's authorization for certain other purposes enumerated by the rule, such as for certain research and public health purposes, but only if specified conditions are met.

Prior to 2002, the privacy rule required covered entities to obtain "consents" from individuals in order to use their health information for treatment, payment, or health operations purposes. Although such "consents" were easier to obtain than written "authorizations" under the rule, this requirement was nevertheless onerous, and it was eliminated by HHS in an August 2002 amendment to the privacy rule, though it is important to note that many state laws still require authorization/consent. As a result, covered entities now can use or disclose protected patient information for treatment, payment, or healthcare operations without any prior consent or authorization from the patient; however, a covered entity still must furnish patients with a notice of its privacy practices and must use its best efforts to obtain from patients written acknowledgment of the receipt of that notice. Except for disclosures made to healthcare providers for treatment purposes and certain other disclosures identified by the rule, a covered entity may use or disclose only the "minimum necessary" protected health information needed to accomplish the intended purpose. The rule also generally requires covered entities to grant individuals access to records containing protected health information about them, as well as the opportunity to request amendments to such records. In addition, covered entities also must comply with a host of administrative requirements intended to protect patient privacy. For instance, each covered entity must appoint a privacy officer who is responsible for ensuring that the entity develops and implements written policies and procedures designed to safeguard the privacy of individual health information.

3.1.5 Reporting of Disclosures

An important requirement of contractors and service owners under HIPAA is the reporting of disclosures. This requirement is included within the written BAA and is usually stated like this: *Report to the covered entity any use or disclosure of PHI not permitted by this agreement.* Covered entities and their business associates who are responsible for an inappropriate disclosure must be able to account for such disclosures for a period of at least six (6) years. Reports of disclosure are needed by covered entities as patients have a new right under HIPAA for an accounting of their disclosures. In order for the covered entity to fulfill its obligation, they must receive from their business associates any disclosures that occur so those can be included in their full disclosure record.

The contractor or service owner should have written policies and procedures (P&Ps) in place for this type of incident. Written P&Ps will help to ensure a standard process will be used each time and that steps will be executed in a well-planned and thoughtful manner, rather than reactionary for each individual occurrence. The first step is to ensure that the disclosure has been identified and contained, thereby mitigating any further or continued risk of disclosure as a result. After this has been accomplished, the MTSO will need to provide a report of the disclosure to the covered entity to which the record belongs. When reporting disclosures, include the following information and maintain this documentation for 6 years:

- Date of disclosure
- Name, address, or identifying information of the patient
- Brief description of information disclosed
- Where did the PHI go that was disclosed (i.e., wrong hospital, wrong referring physician, etc.) and its location
- Brief statement of cause for disclosure
- Actions taken
- Remedies implemented to avoid future disclosures

3.1.6 Penalties

The deadline for covered entities to be in compliance with HIPAA privacy regulations was April 14, 2003. Failure to comply with HIPAA requirements and standards can result in civil monetary penalties of up to $100 for each violation. It is not clear how "violations" may be counted, so a repeated mistake could result in significant liability. The total amount of civil penalties imposed on a covered entity in any calendar year could climb as high as $25,000 for all violations of a single HIPAA requirement or prohibition. Civil penalties may be applied whether the violation is accidental or intentional. While business associates are not directly subject to these penalties, they are subject to breach of contract actions by covered entities for violations of their business associate agreements. In addition to civil penalties, under certain circumstances violation of the rule may result in stiff criminal penalties, including fines of up to $250,000 and/or imprisonment for up to 10 years.

3.1.7 Precedence of State Laws

The HIPAA privacy rule does not preempt state law provisions related to the privacy of health information if such provisions are "more stringent" than the privacy rule. Some states are believed to have more stringent privacy requirements than those contained in the HIPAA privacy rule. It behooves every medical transcription business owner to understand the applicable state laws and make a determination as to which is more stringent—the state laws or HIPAA—and the business owner should seek the advice of an attorney in this regard. Because a medical transcription business may have customers in more than one state, and may have the work transcribed in yet other states, it is important to identify which state laws apply to each client. Generally, a covered entity is governed by the laws of the state in which it is located.

3.1.8 Audit Trails

The HIPAA security rule requires covered entities to use audit controls to protect health information pertaining to an individual that is electronically maintained or transmitted. In addition, under the privacy rule, covered entities are required to track and account for disclosures of protected health information (regardless of medium) made for purposes *unrelated* to treatment, payment, or healthcare operations. A business associate is required to provide information as necessary to assist the covered entity in fulfilling this requirement. Thus, if the business associate, acting on the covered entity's behalf, makes a disclosure for which an accounting is required, the business associate must keep track of such disclosures. Satisfying the accounting requirement will be made easier with the use of audit trails.

3.1.9 Retention of PHI

For the medical transcriptionist, this retention of protected health information generally refers to dictation (whether analog tapes or digital voice files), transcribed reports (whether print or electronic), and patient logs (again, print or electronic). AHDI recommends that MT businesses retain such information only as long as is absolutely necessary to conduct business; that is, no longer than necessary for verification, distribution, and billing purposes. This opinion is shared by the authors of ASTM's *Standard Guide for Management of the Confidentiality and Security of Dictation, Transcription, and Transcribed Health Records, E1902.*

As noted above, the privacy rule generally requires covered entities and their business associates to allow a patient access to records containing protected health information about that patient which are maintained by the covered entity or business associate, as well as the opportunity to request amendments to such records. Since the true patient record should reside with the originator, or the healthcare provider (the covered entity), AHDI views patient access to records retained by an MT business as an unfortunate opportunity for confusion. If the record has not yet been returned to the originator for authentication, then it is not yet truly the patient record. And if it *has* been authenticated, then the copy retained by the transcription business is also not the authenticated version; it is only a preliminary copy.

Destroying records as soon as is practical will serve the MT business well in situations where patients request access to records containing protected health information about them. If the MT business owner does not keep the records, patients will simply have to be referred to their healthcare providers, who are, after all, the appropriate caretakers of patient files. Moreover, once records are destroyed, they obviously are not subject to unintentional or otherwise impermissible disclosures.

3.1.10 Inclusion of PHI in the Record

Although HIPAA does not specifically mention the practice of using patient names within a report, it does require that healthcare providers strictly control the privacy of protected health information (PHI). Should a transcribed medical report be chosen for use as an example or for research or case-study purposes, all PHI must be deleted in order to "de-identify" the report. However, if identifying data is included within the body of the report, such facts are difficult to remove. Therefore, AHDI recommends omitting patient names; names of relatives, employers, or friends of the patient; names of places; and other identifying information within the report when it is transcribed.

Trend Note: It is important to note that the above recommendation to exclude PHI from the body of the report is not without controversy. While it is inarguably the safest way to guard PHI from being accidentally retained in a report that has been de-identified for nonsecure use and distribution, there are many who argue that retention of dictated PHI in the body of the report serves several important purposes. First, many providers purposefully include identifying data in the report as a means of conveying a familiar and a personal connection to the patient. More important is the argument that many risk managers and compliance officers are making on behalf of inclusion due to technology concerns. Stripping all identifying data from the body of the report, they argue, potentially puts the record at risk in the event of a data transfer problem or error. Often for security reasons, the file containing captured demographics is saved, encrypted, and uploaded separately from the file containing the body of the report. The files are reassociated with each other in the chart management system after delivery and decryption. In the event that there is an upload or transfer error where these files do not get matched back up in the system, the body of the report could only be tracked back to the demographic file by matching identifying PHI in the body of the report to the available demographics. Inclusion of PHI, therefore, is considered by some to make the record more secure. Transcriptionists should consider both arguments above and defer to facility policy about the retention of PHI in the body of the report.

3.2 Business Associates

The HIPAA privacy rule also applies indirectly to business associates of covered entities. Business associates are individuals and organizations who are not employees of covered entities but who provide certain services on behalf of covered entities that involve the receipt or disclosure of protected health information. An MT business that provides transcription services for a covered entity (including "sole practitioner" MTs who furnish transcription services on an "independent contractor" basis directly for a covered entity) is a business associate of that covered entity.

3.2.1 Subcontractors
Subcontractors of business associates are not themselves considered "business associates" and do not enter into "business associate agreements." As indicated below, however, subcontractors must contractually agree to essentially the same conditions and restrictions as business associates with respect to the use and disclosure of protected health information.

3.2.2 Business Associate Agreements
The privacy rule requires covered entities to enter into a written agreement with each business associate—known as a "business associate agreement"—that limits the ability of the latter to use and disclose the protected health information and that includes numerous other provisions. Significantly, the business associate may not use or disclose the protected health information

other than as permitted or required by the business associate agreement or as required by law. Thus, an MT business generally may not use or disclose protected health information for a purpose unrelated to the provision of transcription services—unless the covered entity authorizes the MT business through the agreement to make uses or disclosures for that purpose.

The privacy rule is clear regarding requirements for business associates. Covered entities are required to have written agreements with their business associates whereby the business associate agrees that it will (among other things):

- Not use or disclose protected health information other than as permitted by the agreement or as required by law.
- Use appropriate safeguards to protect against unauthorized uses or disclosures of the information.
- Report to the covered entity any use or disclosure not permitted by the agreement.
- Ensure that any agents or subcontractors will agree to the same restrictions and conditions as the business associate.
- Make available protected health information as necessary for the covered entity to comply with its obligations to patients and others under HIPAA, including the covered entity's obligations to allow individuals to access and to request amendments of protected health information about them.
- Make available to the Office for Civil Rights the business associate's internal practices, books, and records relating to the use and disclosure of the protected health information.
- Destroy or return to the covered entity the protected health information once the agreement is terminated, if feasible. If it is not possible to return or destroy the information because of other obligations or legal requirements, the protections of the agreement must continue to apply to the information for so long as it is retained by the business associate, and no uses or disclosures of the information may be made except for those purposes that make its return or destruction unfeasible.

3.2.3 Data Aggregation Services

While business associates are generally prohibited from making uses or disclosures of protected health information that would be prohibited if done by the covered entity, an exception exists for the provision of data aggregation services relating to the healthcare operations of the covered entity. "Data aggregation" means the combining by a business associate of protected health information created or received as a business associate of one covered entity with protected health information received from another covered entity to permit data analyses related to the healthcare operations of the respective covered entities. The business associate agreement must specifically authorize the business associate to conduct data aggregation services on behalf of the covered entity.

With the increased use of XML (extensible markup language) in medical transcription, there is a potential for offering data aggregation services to clients, perhaps to evaluate clinical practices with respect to the treatment of specific conditions. In the absence of a business associate agreement involving data aggregation, the ability of the participating hospitals, as covered entities, to share protected health information with one another for data analysis purposes would be restricted under HIPAA.

3.2.4 Offshore Transcription

An increasing amount of medical transcription is being performed in locations outside the United States, and it should be noted that the privacy laws of other nations also may apply (e.g., the EU Data Privacy Directive). An attorney experienced in the privacy laws of the nation where the business is located should be consulted.

The offshore MT business is also a business associate if it contracts directly with a covered entity. The requirements for business associates do not vary, regardless of where work is transcribed. Full disclosure to the covered entity about where the transcription is done is strongly recommended. If the offshore MT business is a subcontractor to an American business associate, it will still have to agree contractually to essentially the same restrictions as those imposed by the business associate agreement on the business associate.

3.2.5 Breach and Termination

Under the privacy rule, if a covered entity knows of a pattern of activity or practice of a business associate that is a material breach or violation of the business associate's obligations under the business associate agreement, the covered entity must take "reasonable steps" to cure the breach or end the violation. If these measures are unsuccessful, then the covered entity must terminate the agreement, if feasible, or if termination is not feasible, report the problem to the Office for Civil Rights. The termination provisions of the business associate agreement should reflect these requirements. MT businesses should prepare to answer the following questions asked by their potential and current covered entity clients:

- Do you have written agreements with every subcontractor who receives protected health information from you by which the subcontractors agree to protect the integrity and confidentiality of protected health information exchanged between you?

- Do you have a contingency plan in place that provides for a (1) data backup plan, (2) disaster recovery plan, and (3) emergency mode operation?
- Do you have written policies and procedures establishing rules for granting access (both inside and outside your organization) to protected health information?

3.2.6 Indemnification

Indemnification refers to a provision in a contract whereby one party agrees to be financially responsible for specified types of damages, claims, or losses. There is no legal requirement that a business associate agreement contain specific indemnification provisions, but given the prominence of privacy issues in the public, legislative, and judicial arenas, it is advisable for both the covered entity and the business associate to give this issue detailed review. Generally, it is advisable to include either no indemnification or a mutual, partial indemnification clause, whereby each party agrees to indemnify and hold harmless the other party only for its mistakes. Because indemnification provisions are at the heart of allocations of liability under an agreement, they tend to vary greatly from contract to contract and should be negotiated to suit the specific arrangement.

3.3 Record Security

Because a security breach can result in a privacy violation, an integral part of protecting the privacy of individually identifiable documents involves the secure handling of such documents. The privacy rule requires business associates to use commercially reasonable efforts to maintain the security of the protected health information and to prevent the unauthorized use and/or disclosure of such information. The following advice, while not specifically stated as such in the HIPAA privacy rule, nor even in the security rule, constitutes good business practice for MTs and is included here for that reason.

This relates to the security of all types of protected health information—whether paper or electronic—that contains patient-identifiable information. This includes, but is not limited to, print and electronic patient records, daily schedules, surgery lists, patient sign-in sheets; computer files of any type, whether document, database, or voice; floppy disks, compact disks, zip disks, removable zip drives; analog audio tapes and voice files created on digital dictation systems.

It is important to remember that MTs routinely receive this kind of documentation via fax, courier, the US Postal Service, and computer file transfer. The privacy rule prohibits the disclosure by the covered entity of the entire patient chart, except where the entire chart is specifically justified as the amount of protected health information reasonably necessary to accomplish the purpose of the disclosure. If this "minimum necessary" standard is met, consider using the security measures suggested below for patient charts as well.

3.3.1 Physical Transport of PHI

Use a bonded commercial courier for transport of patient records, and consider having the courier sign a HIPAA compliance and confidentiality contract to ensure understanding of these regulations as they pertain to handling of patient records. It's a good idea to notify clients of the individual courier or courier service being used and inform them of the contract between the MT and courier. When shipping out of town, use a service whose packages can be traced and that requires a signature by the recipient. Whether the MT is transporting patient information personally or having it delivered by an employee, a subcontractor, or a courier, the material should be transported in a sealed or locked and tamper-proof container that is accessible only by the business associate and the designated party to whom the material is being sent. No patient identifiable information should be visible by the courier or any other third party. If a courier or other properly permitted third party routinely picks up work from the MT's establishment at a specified location, particularly if that location is on the outside of a building, the container should be secured in a locked, tamper-proof area. Leaving envelopes, boxes, or containers on a porch, in an open basket, or in an unlocked mailbox is not sufficient for security. A pick-up container should be not accessible by anyone but the MT and the courier or other properly designated third party.

Trend Note: AHDI strongly recommends against physical transport of PHI unless absolutely necessary. Given the innumerable secure, electronic options for transfer of patient records, the practice of manually picking up and delivering patient-sensitive material is rapidly becoming an outdated and questionably secure method. Independent contractors who are providing this kind of door-to-door service should engage in a risk management dialogue with clients and services to relay the HIPAA concerns inherent in physical transport. Cost-effective, secure electronic solutions are available and should be instituted.

3.3.2 Sending and Receiving Faxes

Although HIPAA does not have official regulations for paper faxes, it is suggested that the following precautions be taken into consideration:

- A fax machine used for sending protected health information should

be located in a secured area of the business or office that is inaccessible by any individual not bound to a HIPAA compliance contract. The area should be locked when the fax machine is unattended.
- A faxed document containing protected health information should be accompanied by a cover sheet that includes language clearly outlining the confidential nature of the information being faxed and provides a warning to any recipient who is not authorized to have access to that information. The following language is suggested to serve this purpose:

The information contained in this facsimile message is privileged, confidential, and only for the use of the individual or entity named above. If the reader of this message is not the intended recipient, or the employee or agent responsible to deliver it to the intended recipient, you are hereby notified that any dissemination, distribution, or copying of this communication is strictly prohibited. If you have received this message in error, please immediately notify us by telephone and return the original message to us at the address listed above via the US Postal Service. Thank you for your cooperation.

- The MT should consider pre-programming frequently dialed client fax numbers in order to avoid potential dialing errors that could result in protected health information being erroneously sent to an unauthorized third party.
- If protected health information is erroneously sent via fax to an unauthorized third party, the covered entity (or the client if the client is a business associate of the covered entity) must be notified immediately of the infraction in accordance with the notification requirements of the business associate agreement, and the appropriate steps followed for the reporting of a disclosure followed to include the filing of a disclosure report with the covered entity who originated the patient health information.

3.3.3 Electronic System Security

Protected health information may be found on computers in document and database files as well as voice files created on digital dictation systems. Make sure all files and folders containing protected health information are secure from unauthorized access.

- For the home-based MT, the computer that is used for work should not be accessible to unauthorized individuals (e.g., family members). The computer should be password-protected and kept in a separate, locked room in order to adequately prohibit access to protected health information files by unauthorized individuals. Simply partitioning the hard disk—creating an "invisible" drive onto which health information files are stored—is not enough. This type of partition is very difficult to create and yet too easy to break into. Having two computers in the home—one for work and one for family—may seem like an unnecessary expense, but the importance of security cannot be overestimated. In addition, keeping computers separate in the home protects the transcriptionist from accidental data loss or deletion/disabling of programs and files that are critical for provision of services.

- When password-protecting a computer, dictation equipment, or software applications, the password should be changed approximately every 30 days to prevent access by individuals who may have once been authorized but are no longer contracted or employed by the MT.
- Passwords themselves should be protected from unauthorized access as well. A valid password should be a combination of uppercase and lowercase letters, numbers, and symbols and be at least 8 digits in length.
- When connected to the Internet, whether through dial-up, cable modem, DSL, network, or T-1 connection, the MT should utilize firewall protection software to protect all computers, and thus individuals' health information files, from being accessed by unauthorized individuals through their Internet connection. This risk is greatest with an uninterrupted connection (cable modem, DSL or T-1), and it is therefore important to use software that makes the computer's IP address "invisible" to anyone who might try to access it through the uninterrupted connection.

3.3.4 Electronic File Transfer

When transferring protected health information files through the Internet, whether uploading to or downloading from a Web server or attaching to an email, the MT should utilize encryption software to ensure the security of files over the connection. It is recommended that the business associate use software structured on a 128-bit, random-algorithm encryption standard. Consider also using a zipping utility program if a batch of files is being sent with a single email. In addition to encryption, the MT should make sure that files are password-protected prior to transfer and that only authorized individuals at the points of origin and termination have password access to those files. When transferring files via direct connection to another computer, the MT should use software that provides encryption and password protection. Software on the host computer should provide password protection for both remote control and file transfer, and the password should be changed approximately every 30 days. The MT may also want to consider using the activity-logging feature common with these programs for tracking who has accessed the host computer and when.

3.3.5 Storage of PHI

The following considerations need to be followed with regard to short- and long-term storage of PHI:

- The MT should survey computer system settings to ensure that the voice and text files are not retained longer than necessary and to ensure that user profiles are set up with limited access to parts of the system not deemed appropriate or necessary for the user. In other words, the MT should make sure that originators and transcriptionists do not have user profile settings that allow them access to the dictation or transcription of other originators or transcriptionists unless they are given authorization (such as providing access to a transcriptionist who also checks for quality assurance and requires access for review purposes).
- Paper media containing protected health information should not be left unattended on a desk or in a workspace if the person working with the material is interrupted or has to leave the work area. Likewise, all patient-sensitive documents should be covered when an unauthorized person enters the work area.
- For short-term storage, all paperwork, audio tapes, floppy disks, compact disks, zip disks, and removable drives containing patient files should be kept in a locked, secured container or cabinet, and no unauthorized person should have access to the key or combination. The password-protected computer hard disk should be utilized for short- and long-term data storage to avoid having to secure disks and removable drives.
- The MT should return all media containing protected health information to the covered entity or client (or destroy it) as soon as possible. That is, once the completed transcription has been returned to the originator and the MT has been paid, there should be no need to retain patient records. The healthcare provider—the covered entity—is the long-term caretaker of patient records. If the MT must retain logs or lists, they should be kept in a locked container or file cabinet to which no unauthorized person has access by either key or combination.
- If longer retention is permitted—or required—under the terms of the service contract, all protected health information in the possession of the MT should be destroyed or returned to the covered entity or client at the termination of the agreement.
- Before reusing or discarding tapes and disks, the information on them should be erased. All old disks containing patient files should be erased and reformatted when the information on them is no longer needed.
- When deleting or purging electronic files, the MT should make sure that such files are completely purged from computer hard drives and cannot be restored. The MT might even consider moving the files to a separate or removable drive that can be reformatted after the files are deleted.

3.4 Information Integrity

Data integrity refers to the validity of data. Data integrity can be compromised in a number of ways, to include human error when data is entered, errors that occur when data is transmitted from one computer to another, software bugs or viruses, hardware malfunctions such as disk crashes, or natural disasters such as fires and floods. All of those involve the vigilant physical protection of data that was covered in section 3.3. However, data integrity also involves ensuring that the *information* is not compromised or put at risk in any way, and a critically thinking transcriptionist needs to be mindful of potential data integrity risks at the point of dictation, during transcription, with author authentication, and where amending and revising the record are concerned.

3.4.1 Problem Dictation

In the AHDI *Dictation Best Practices Tool Kit*, the association addresses the impact of problem dictation as it relates to documentation errors and critical flaws affecting patient safety, the potential for sentinel events, the effects on turn-around time, and the resulting increased cost. These were separated into (a) critical errors impacting patient safety and (b) major errors that involve document integrity. Transcriptionists should be actively engaged in identifying and recognizing potential errors and risk management issues related to dictation, including:

- A provider dictating under the wrong author ID number.
- A provider dictating patient demographic information that does not match what has been manually entered into the dictation system and/or provided to the transcriptionist via the ADT feed.
- A provider dictating a patient encounter or procedure *prior* to its occurrence, especially in the instance of operative reports, special procedures, and discharge summaries, which legally can *only* be dictated at the time or shortly after those events occur.
- The obvious omission of critical information in the report *(Example: an operative report that is missing critical sequential steps, like the opening or closure of incisions, mention of anesthesia, or the required end-of-report counts)*.
- The inclusion of wrong words, phrases, or contradictory information as outlined in Chapter 2 of this text.
- The inclusion of statements in the record that could represent a risk management concern *(Example: indication by the dictator that the patient was not informed of surgical risks and benefits or that the patient left without signing a surgical consent)*.
- Rambling, disjointed dictation that lacks cohesion and raises an information integrity concern with the transcriptionist.

- A request on the part of the dictator to alter or falsify audit trail information, such as the date of service, date of dictation, or date of transcription.

In any of the instances above where the transcriptionist deems there to be an information-integrity or risk management concern, the report needs to be flagged and routed to the appropriate quality assurance and/or risk management personnel for review.

3.4.2 Authentication Issues

Authentication refers to the process by which the provider verifies what has been captured in the record and affixes his or her signature to the report as proof of that verification. According to the Joint Commission, authentication must be done by the author of the record and cannot be delegated to anyone else, regardless of the process for inclusion of signature. The Joint Commission further defines authentication as: *to prove authorship*. Therefore, the legal responsibility for ensuring that all information in the record represents an accurate reflection of the patient encounter falls to the author of that record, *not* to the transcriptionist or any other ancillary personnel. Given this clear directive, there are several authentication concerns with which the transcriptionist must be familiar:

Electronic signatures: It has become an increasingly common practice for providers to request that their signatures be electronically dropped into the record, a practice that, it has been argued, facilitates the unhindered forward progress of the record for both inclusion in the patient record and processing for reimbursement. It also inarguably relieves providers of the burden of having reports backlogged for physician authentication and signature. Both the Joint Commission and AHDI oppose the practice of autosignatures, whereby electronic signatures are dropped into the record automatically or by a third party. Only in the instance where the author assumes the responsibility of authenticating the report and dropping in his/her own electronic signature do the organizations support this practice. Automated or third-party inclusion of electronic signatures generates a critical risk management concern, where the assumption has been made that the transcribed report is without error or inconsistency, leaving the transcriptionist to unfairly shoulder the burden for the accuracy of the report—something the MT, who is clearly not the *author* of the record, is not legally qualified to do.

The US Department of Health and Human Services (HHS) has likewise established clear policies defining record authentication [42CFR 482.24(c)]:

- All entries must be legible and complete and must be authenticated and dated promptly by the person (identified by name and discipline) who is responsible for ordering, providing, or evaluating the service furnished.
- The author of each entry must be identified and must authenticate his or her entry.
- Authentication may include signatures, written initials or computer entry.

Dictated but Not Read: Similar to the scenario above is the unfortunate practice of many providers who direct that the statement "dictated but not read" or similar statements be entered at the end of the report in an attempt to waive the author's responsibility for reviewing the report and confirming its accuracy. It is not appropriate for an MT to enter this statement into the record because, like third-party electronic signatures, it creates a scenario where the unauthenticated report becomes a finalized entry into the patient record and creates the assumption of accuracy that unfairly holds the transcriptionist responsible. Where both of these scenarios are concerned, the underlying risk management issue involves a provider who is not reading and authenticating his or her records, and this is a practice that a transcriptionist should never facilitate or support.

Employed transcriptionists who are asked to drop in electronic signatures or include statements like "dictated but not read," or they discover that these are included in the record without provider authentication, should address this risk management concern with their supervisors. If the facility will not alter this practice, the MT may wish to (a) request that his/her name or initials be omitted from the report as an accountable party and (b) request a statement in writing that protects him/her from any liability or accountability with regard to the accuracy of the reports they are asked to transcribe. Independent contractors and transcription service owners should likewise require that such statements be included in their business contracts.

3.4.3 Corrections, Revisions, and Addenda

The primary consideration for regulatory authorities who have addressed and/or developed standards related to modifying the patient record involve stipulations outlined in the Uniform Rules of Evidence, which stipulate what kind of information can be placed into evidence in a court of law. Generally speaking, statements made outside of the court that are offered into evidence are considered hearsay and are typically not admissible. In order to admit outside statements, such as a medical record, into evidence, there has to be substantive proof that the record and the information contained within it are reliable. Medical records fall under the business record hearsay exception if the following conditions can be demonstrated:

- The record was made in the regular course of business.
- The entries in the record were made at or near the time the matter was recorded.
- The entries were made by the individual within the enterprise with firsthand knowledge of the acts, events, conditions, and opinions.
- Process controls and checks must exist to ensure the reliability and accuracy of the record.
- Policies and procedures must exist to protect the record from alteration and tampering.
- Policies and procedures must exist to prevent loss of stored data.

The Federal Rule of Evidence 803 and other state laws and regulations likewise govern the modification of a medical record and outline strict criteria for any modification of the record that might be deemed fraudulent. HIPAA, ASTM, and HL7 have all provided guidelines and standards to assist healthcare workers in managing the record correction and modification process.

HIPAA Privacy Final Rule—Amendment of Protected Health Information
This privacy rule outlines the process by which an individual can allow a covered entity to correct or amend PHI or medical records as long as the information falls within the designated record set, which is defined by HIPAA as a group of records maintained by or for a covered entity that includes medical and billing records and any other information required by the covered entity for provisions of services. This process requires:

- That the records affected by the amendment be identified and appended or otherwise linked to the location of the amendment.
- That the covered entity make a reasonable effort to inform individuals impacted by the amendment within a reasonable time and to provide the amendment within a reasonable time.
- That the covered entity which is informed by another covered entity of an amendment to the original record amend the protected information in their records.

ASTM E31 Standards
This standard [E1762-95, Section 8—*Electronic Authentication of Health Care Information*] provides three methods for correcting and amending the record:

- Addendum Signature: The signature on a new amended document of an individual who has corrected, edited, or amended an original health information document.
- Modification Signature: The signature on an original document of an individual who has generated an amended document.

- Administrative (Error/Edit) Signature: The signature of an individual who is certifying that the document is invalidated by error(s) or was placed in the wrong chart.

Health Level Seven (HL7)
HL7 is primarily concerned with the kind of audit trail communication that needs to exist in electronic environments where health data is exchanged between and within healthcare facility systems. To that end, HL7 standards address the types of errors and/or corrections that might occur in a record and provide associated electronic messaging for tagging and identifying these errors:

- Creating an addendum: HL7 recommends that in instances where the author comes back to dictate additional information into the record that this new information be transcribed in a new document with its own document ID number that can later be linked to the original document and "parent ID" number.
- Correcting errors in a document not yet made available for patient care: HL7 recommends that the errors or corrections be made and a notification sent (per the HIPAA privacy rule outlined above).
- Correcting errors in a document that has been made available for patient care: HL7 recommends that the errors or corrections be made, that the original document be replaced with the new document (which would have its own unique document ID number linked to the original). The original document would be marked as obsolete in the system to avoid confusion as to its availability and use but should be retained for record-keeping purposes.
- Notification of a canceled document: HL7 recommends that in instances where a patient report is erroneously tagged and routed to another patient's record, a cancellation notice should be sent to remove the report from general access in the wrong patient's record. Where the document is retained for historical reference in the wrong patient's record, the identifying information from the original patient should be removed to protect his/her privacy.

When it comes to revisions or corrections made to the record *before* the report is authenticated by the provider, there are no standards or guidelines for how those revisions are entered and tracked, since they will all be authenticated and signed off by the author. For audit trail purposes, it is recommended that each access to the record for corrections and revisions, including those made by quality assurance coordinators and reviewers, be identified separately in the date/time stamp area, with separate entry of reviewer initials. This puts it in the record that the report was modified after the original transcriptionist signed off on the report prior to it being forwarded for authentication.

What is relevant to the transcriptionist in these standards is the need to make sure that there is a clear indication in the record of any correction or amendment that is made, including the date, time, and identification of the person who accessed the record to make the modification. A paper or electronic trail of original and amended reports should be retained, and all recipients of the original health information should be notified of the correction or change.

References

Final Privacy Rule, as published in the Federal Register, August 14, 2002: <http://www.hhs.gov/ocr/hipaa/privrulepd.pdf>

Office of Civil Rights—Privacy Questions & Answers: <http://answers.hhs.gov/cgi-bin/hhs.cfg/php/enduser/std_alp.php>

Office of Civil Rights—HIPAA Assistance: <http://www.hhs.gov/ocr/hipaa/assist.html>

AHIMA Practice Brief: Facsimile Transmission of Health Information: <http://library.ahima.org/xpedio/groups/public/documents/ahima/pub_bok2_000116.html>

Tessier, Claudia. "What's Wrong with This Picture?" *Journal of the American Association for Medical Transcription*, Vol.12, No. 4, July-August 1993, pp. 3, 32-33,36-38.

Rhodes, Harry. "Modifying the Patient Record: Corrections, Revisions, Additions and Addenda" *The AAMT Book of Style, 2nd Edition*, Appendix G, pp. 481-488.

Section 2
General Standards of Style

CHAPTER

4

Grammar

Introduction

Strong language skills are critical to the skilled MT, and they will often make the difference between an average transcriptionist and an excellent one. An understanding of language structure and the rules related to sentence construction and agreement, for example, will be essential to identifying grammatical errors in dictation and correcting them in the transcribed record.

It is the reality of the profession that transcriptionists will encounter variable language skills among the dictators for whom they provide transcription services. Many dictators have poor fundamental grammar themselves; others speak English as a second language and possess only a rudimentary grasp of grammar. Still others will be careless or hurried and will make errors that an MT will be expected to recognize and correct. The transcriptionist will not always be able to rely on the skills of the dictator. If the provider dictates, "Lungs is clear," the MT will be expected to recognize the error in grammar and correct it.

4.1 Parts of Speech

Understanding the role and function of each word in a sentence will empower the MT to recognize faulty grammar, erroneous words, and misplaced modifiers. It is also important to have a strong knowledge of parts of speech to later apply rules, such as those outlined for compound modifiers, which are built around the function of words in the sentence.

4.1.1 Nouns

A noun is a word used to name a person, place, thing, or idea.

Proper nouns name a particular person, place, or thing and are typically capitalized.

White House
St. Mary's Hospital
Kleenex
Jell-O
Band-Aid

Common nouns are nouns that do not name a particular person, place, or thing.

woman
city
building
patient
doctor
president

Abstract nouns name qualities, characteristics, or ideas.

beauty
strength
love
courage

Concrete nouns name objects that can be perceived by the senses.

pen
desk
chart
medication

Collective nouns name a group of persons/things regarded as a unit.

EXAMPLE

> board (of directors)
> committee
> pair
> couple
> family
> staff

Compound nouns are nouns composed of more than one word.

EXAMPLE

> St. Joseph's Medical Center
> Oakdale Cancer Treatment Clinic
> First National Bank

4.1.2 Pronouns

A pronoun is a word used in place of a noun or of more than one noun.
The word to which a pronoun refers is called the *antecedent* of the pronoun.
Pronouns are classified as personal, reflexive, intensive, relative, interrogative,
demonstrative, and indefinite.

Personal pronouns reflect person and number and can function as the subject of
a verb (nominative form), as the object of a verb or preposition (objective), or
to show possession (possessive).

EXAMPLE

> Nominative forms: I, you, he, she, it, we, they
> Objective forms: me, him, her, us, them
> Possessive forms: my, mine, your, yours, his, her, hers, its, our, ours, their, theirs

Reflexive pronouns are personal pronouns combined with –*self* or –*selves* that
reflect action expressed by the verb back to the subject.

EXAMPLE

> The patient injured <u>himself</u> while mowing the lawn.
> She insisted on feeding <u>herself</u>.

Intensive pronouns are used to emphasize a noun or pronoun already expressed.

> Robert <u>himself</u> was not hurt.

Do not use reflexive or intensive pronouns unless the noun or pronoun to which it refers is expressed in the same sentence.

> D: The discharge instructions were given to the patient's daughter and <u>herself</u>.
> T: The discharge instructions were given to the patient's daughter and <u>her</u>.
>
> *better:*
> T: The discharge instructions were given to the patient and her daughter.

Do not use reflexive or intensive pronouns in the objective case *(See 5.2.2— Pronoun Usage—Objective Case)* where a personal pronoun should be used.

> D: The patient was last seen by <u>myself</u> in February of 2006.
> T: The patient was last seen by <u>me</u> in February of 2006.

Relative pronouns are used to introduce independent/subordinate clauses and reflect back to previous nouns or pronouns. The most common relative pronouns are *that, who, whom, what, which,* and *whose.* Other variations include *whoever, whomever, whosoever, whatsoever,* and *whichever.*

> Dr. Smith is a physician <u>whom</u> we can trust.
> The medication was one <u>that</u> she had not heard of before.

Interrogative pronouns are relative pronouns used to introduce a question.

> <u>Who</u> brought the patient to the emergency room?
> <u>What</u> is the name of your primary care physician?

Section 2: General Standards of Style

Demonstrative pronouns are used to point out persons or things. The common demonstrative pronouns are *this, that, these,* and *those.*

EXAMPLE

> <u>That</u> is an excellent question.
> <u>This</u> seems to be my lucky day.

Indefinite pronouns are pronouns that do not fall into any of the classifications above. Most of them express the idea of quantity. The most commonly used indefinite pronouns are *all, another, any, anybody, anyone, both, each, either, everybody, everyone, few, many, most, neither, nobody, none, no one, one, other, several, some, somebody, someone,* and *such.*

EXAMPLE

> <u>All</u> of us are here.
> <u>Few</u> of the cars were new.

Do not confuse those compound indefinite pronouns that function differently when separated.

EXAMPLE

> <u>Anyone</u> can succeed with passion and determination.
> <u>Any one mistake</u> can lead to disaster.
> <u>No one</u> knows how hard her recovery has been.
> <u>No one person</u> can possibly do that much work.

4.1.3 Adjectives

An adjective is a word used to modify a noun or a pronoun. *To modify* means "to limit" or to make more definite the meaning of a word. Adjectives may modify nouns or pronouns in any one of three different ways:

- By telling *what kind*
- By pointing out *which one*
- By telling *how many*

EXAMPLE

> <u>loose</u> stools, <u>shotty</u> nodes, <u>noncompliant</u> patient (what kind)
> <u>this</u> patient, <u>that</u> treatment (which one)
> <u>numerous</u> complaints, <u>several</u> days, <u>two</u> dogs (how many)

Typically, adjectives are positioned directly before the word or words they modify. Occasionally, however, adjectives can be positioned after the words they modify.

EXAMPLE

> The patient, <u>disoriented</u> and <u>confused,</u> was unable to provide a meaningful history.

Predicate adjectives are separated from the words they modify by the verb.

EXAMPLE

> The patient was <u>alert</u> and <u>oriented</u>. (modify the subject "patient")
> Her palms and soles were <u>red</u> and <u>warm</u>. (modify the compound subject "palms" and "soles")

Pronouns used as adjectives—a word may be used as more than one part of speech. This is especially true of the words in the following list, which may be used as both pronouns and adjectives: *all, another, any, both, each, either, few, many, more, neither, one, other, several, some, that, these, this, those, what,* and *which.*

EXAMPLE

> <u>Which</u> medication did you give the patient? (adjective modifying the noun "medication")
> <u>Which</u> do you want? (pronoun taking the place of a noun previously mentioned)
> I need <u>this</u> information. (adjective modifying the noun "information")
> I need <u>this</u>. (pronoun taking the place of a noun previously mentioned)

Nouns used as adjectives—occasionally, nouns will function in the role of an adjective in a modifying relationship with another noun.

EXAMPLE

> <u>sofa</u> cushion
> <u>hospital</u> pharmacy
> <u>glass</u> beads

4.1.4 Verbs

A verb is a word that expresses action or otherwise helps to make a statement. Some verbs express action that is physical (*hit, play, move*) and others express action that is mental (*think, know, imagine*). Action verbs may or may not take an object—a noun or pronoun that completes the action by showing who or what is affected by the action.

Transitive verbs are verbs that have an object.

EXAMPLE

> The patient <u>gave</u> consent for treatment. ("consent" is the object of "gave")
> Demerol <u>relieved</u> her symptoms. ("symptoms" is the object of "relieved")

Intransitive verbs are verbs that express action without an object.

EXAMPLE

> The girl <u>smiled</u>.
> His employee <u>quit</u>.

While some verbs are always transitive (*ignore, complete, give*) and others are always intransitive (*arrive, sleep*), most verbs in the English language can be either.

EXAMPLE

> I <u>explained</u> the procedure to the patient. (transitive)
> She questioned the course of treatment, and I <u>explained</u>. (intransitive)

Linking verbs are intransitive verbs that make a statement without expressing action. They express, rather, a state or condition. These verbs link back to the subject a noun, pronoun, or adjective that describes or identifies it. The word that is linked back to the subject is called the subject complement. The most common linking verbs are those that are derived from the verb *to be* (*am, is, are, was, were, be, being, been*) as well as verb phrases ending in these forms (*can be, have been, is being, could have been*). They are only considered linking verbs when they (a) modify or describe the subject and (b) when they are followed by a noun or adjective. When these verbs are followed by an adverb or adverb phrase, they are not considered linking verbs because they do not reflect back to the subject.

EXAMPLE

> The patient <u>looked</u> unhappy and depressed. ("unhappy" and "depressed" modify "patient")
> She <u>was being</u> evasive in her answers. ("evasive" modifies "she")

Keep in mind that many linking verbs can also be used as action verbs without a subject complement. It is only when they have a complement that they are said to "link" the complement to the subject.

The patient <u>looked</u> depressed. (linking)
The patient <u>looked</u> for her daughter. (action)

Helping verbs are verbs that help the main verb express action or make a statement. Together with the action verb, they form a verb phrase. Common helping verbs are *am, are, is, was, were, do, did, have, has, had, can, may, will be, will have, has been, can be, can have, could be, could have, will have been, might have, must, must have.*

has arrived
should have called
will be going
must have been injured

Often, the parts of a verb phrase are separated from each other by other words.

She <u>had</u> finally <u>completed</u> her course of treatment when I saw her in November.
He <u>will</u> definitely <u>be seen</u> in the office on Friday.

Split verbs are verb phrases in which a word (usually an adverb) has been inserted between parts of the verb phrase. Splitting infinitives or other forms of verbs used to be considered grammatically incorrect. Traditionalists still hold to this view, but pragmatists recognize that such splits are appropriate if they enhance meaning (or at least do not obstruct it). Transcribe split verbs as dictated provided they do not obstruct the meaning.

The test was intended <u>to</u> definitively <u>determine</u> whether he has an infectious process.
He <u>will</u> routinely <u>return</u> for followup.

4.1.5 Adverbs

An adverb is a word used to modify a verb, adjective, or another adverb. The adverb is the most commonly used modifier of a verb. It may tell *how, when, where,* or *to what extent* (how often or how much) the action of the verb is performed. Some, but not all, adverbs end in *–ly.*

EXAMPLE

> The patient takes her medication <u>faithfully</u>. (how)
> The patient takes her medication <u>early</u> and <u>late</u>. (when)
> The patient brings her medication <u>everywhere</u> with her. (where)
> The patient <u>barely</u> remembers to take her medication. (to what extent—how much)
> The patient takes her medication <u>daily</u>. (to what extent—how often)

Some adverbs, such as *really, actually, truly, indeed,* are used mostly for emphasis and are classified as verbs of extent *(to what extent).*

EXAMPLE

> Her brother has <u>really</u> been a great help to her.
> She has <u>truly</u> been a great patient to care for.
> The patient believes the medication has <u>actually</u> made her feel worse.

An adverb may modify an adjective.

EXAMPLE

> She complained that the cream made her face <u>really</u> red.

An adverb may modify another adverb.

EXAMPLE

> Despite the injury, she spoke <u>very</u> well.
> He says he wakes up at night <u>quite</u> frequently to urinate.

Keep in mind that the word *not* is classified as an adverb of extent or degree.

EXAMPLE

> He is <u>not</u> eating as often as he should be. (modifies the verb "eating")
> The patient is <u>not</u> compliant with her medications. (modifies the predicate adjective "compliant")

Squinting modifiers are adverbs that are placed in such a way that they can be interpreted as modifying more than one word. If the intended meaning can be determined, recast the sentence so that the modifier clearly relates to the appropriate word.

> He only walked 2 blocks. (He only walked, not ran.)
> Only he walked 2 blocks. (Only he, not anyone else, walked 2 blocks.)
> He walked only 2 blocks. (He didn't walk more than 2 blocks.)

The transcriptionist should listen carefully when squinting modifiers are erroneously dictated to ensure that the intended meaning is captured. When in doubt, transcribe as dictated. Otherwise, edit appropriately.

> D: The patient says he had only walked 2 blocks when he felt a sharp pain in his chest.
> T: The patient says he had walked only 2 blocks when he felt a sharp pain in his chest.

In the example above, it should be assumed that the patient was referring to the distance he walked, not the manner in which he did so.

Nouns used as adverbs—Sometimes nouns can be used adverbially.

> I called her yesterday. (when)
> She will be discharged tomorrow. (when)
> The patient will follow up in my office Monday. (when)

4.1.6 Prepositions
A preposition is a word used to show the relation of a noun or pronoun to some other word in the sentence.

> The rash on her left hand has improved significantly. ("on" shows the relationship between "rash" and "hand")

A preposition always appears in a phrase, usually at the beginning. The noun or pronoun at the end of the prepositional phrase is the *object* of the preposition that begins the phrase. Commonly used prepositions are *about, above, across, after, against, along, amid, among, around, at, before, behind, below, beneath, beside, besides, between, beyond, but (meaning "except"), by, concerning, down, during, except, for, from, in, into, like, of, off, on, over, past, since, through, throughout, to, toward, under, underneath, until, unto, up, upon, with, within,* and *without.*

4.1.7 Conjunctions

A conjunction is a word that joins words (nouns, verbs, adjectives, or adverbs), phrases, or clauses (independent and dependent). There are three kinds of conjunctions: coordinating, correlative, and subordinating.

Coordinating conjunctions are the most common conjunctions that form a linking or joining relationship. They are *and, but, or, nor,* and *for.*

EXAMPLE

> Mrs. Smith was told to bring her medication list <u>and</u> previous films.
> She can either wait here <u>or</u> come back in an hour.
> His chest pain was mild <u>and</u> intermittent.
> The patient <u>nor</u> her mother were able to accurately describe the incident.

Correlative conjunctions are always used in pairs. The most common are *either...or, neither...nor, both...and, not only...but (also),* and *whether...or.*

EXAMPLE

> The medication is <u>not only</u> fast-acting <u>but also</u> inexpensive.
> Do you know <u>whether</u> the patient is coming alone <u>or</u> with family?

Subordinating conjunctions begin adverb clauses and join the clause to the rest of the sentence. Common subordinating conjunctions are *after, although, as, as if, as long as, as though, because, before, if, in order that, provided that, since, so that, than, though, unless, until, when, whenever, where, wherever, whether,* and *while.*

EXAMPLE

> <u>After</u> arriving in the emergency room, the patient's symptoms seemed to diminish.
> The patient left the waiting room <u>before</u> we could see her.

4.2 Parts of a Sentence

For a fundamental understanding of English sentences, it is important not just to know the parts of speech but how they function in coordination with each other to form a complete thought or sentence. With only two terms, *subject* and *predicate*, one could begin to describe most sentences, but the composition of sentences is complex and variable, so it is important to understand the role of other simple sentence parts, including the *predicate nominative, predicate adjective, direct object,* and *indirect object*.

4.2.1 Subject and Predicate

A sentence consists of two parts: the *subject* and the *predicate*. The *subject* of the sentence is that part about which something is being said. The *predicate* is that part which says something about the subject. These two parts may consist of single or many words. The whole subject is called the *complete subject*; the whole predicate, the *complete predicate*.

EXAMPLE

SUBJECT	PREDICATE
The patient and her daughter	met with me in my office.

The *simple subject* is the principal word or group of words in the subject.

EXAMPLE

The efficacy of her course of treatment has yet to be determined.
("The efficacy of her course of treatment" is the subject and "treatment" is the simple subject)

The *simple predicate*, or *verb*, is the principal word or group of words in the predicate.

EXAMPLE

She and her husband plan to seek genetic counseling. ("plan to seek genetic counseling" is the predicate and "plan" is the simple predicate)

A *compound subject* consists of two or more subjects that are joined by a conjunction and have the same verb, with the usual connecting words being *and* and *or*.

> Her <u>gentamicin</u> and <u>ampicillin</u> were started this morning.

A *compound verb* consists of two or more verbs that are joined by a conjunction and have the same subject.

> She <u>was given</u> discharge instructions and <u>was told</u> to call her physician's office.

4.2.2 Direct and Indirect Objects

Some sentences express a complete thought by means of a subject and verb only. Most sentences, however, have in the predicate one or more words that complete the meaning of the subject and verb. These completing words are called *complements*. Only nouns, pronouns, and adjectives can act as complements. Adverbs modify the verb and do not function as complements. Complements that receive or are affected by the action of the verb are called *objects*, of which there are two kinds: *direct* and *indirect*.

The *direct object* of the verb receives the action of the verb or shows the result of the action. It answers the question *what?* or *whom?* after an action verb.

> I called <u>Dr. Smith</u> about the surgery. (called *whom?*)
> The radiologist wrote a <u>note</u> for the surgeon. (wrote *what?*)

The *indirect object* of the verb precedes the direct object and tells *to whom* or *for whom* the action of the verb is performed.

> I wrote the <u>patient</u> a prescription for Diflucan. ("patient" is the indirect object; "prescription" is the direct object)

4.2.3 Subject Complements

Complements that refer to (describe, explain, or identify) the subject are *subject complements*. There are two kinds: the *predicate nominative* and the *predicate adjective*. Subject complements follow linking verbs only.

A *predicate nominative* is a noun or pronoun complement that refers to the same person or thing as the subject of the verb.

EXAMPLE

> The patient is a pleasant, cooperative <u>woman</u>. ("woman" refers to the subject "patient")
> The medications she takes are <u>Prevacid</u> and <u>allopurinol</u>. ("Prevacid" and "allopurinol" refer to the subject "medications")

A *predicate adjective* is an adjective complement that refers to, and in this case modifies or describes, the same person or thing as the subject of the verb.

EXAMPLE

> The patient was <u>alert</u> and <u>oriented</u>. (modify the subject "patient")
> Her palms and soles were <u>red</u> and <u>warm</u>. (modify the compound subject "palms" and "soles")

4.3 The Phrase

Words in a sentence not only act individually but also in groups. The grouped words act together as a unit which may function as a modifier, a subject, a predicate, an object, or a predicate nominative. A phrase is a group of words not containing verb and its subject. A phrase is used as a single part of speech. There are two kinds of phrases: prepositional phrases and verb phrases.

4.3.1 Prepositional Phrases

A prepositional phrase is a group of words beginning with a preposition and usually ending with a noun or pronoun. The noun or pronoun that concludes the prepositional phrase is the object of the preposition that begins the phrase.

in the examining room
under the microscope
on further examination
without explanation

Prepositional phrases are usually used as modifiers—as adjectives and adverbs. Occasionally, they are used as nouns.

After dinner will be too late. (prepositional phrase as subject)

Adjective phrases are prepositional phrases that modify a noun or pronoun.

The right upper abdomen is the location of her pain. (modifies "location")
The sensation in her fingers has completely returned. (modifies "sensation")

Adverb phrases are prepositional phrases that modify a verb, adjective, or another adverb.

The incision was made over the symphysis pubis (where).
On admission (when) the patient complained of blood (what) in her stool (where).

4.3.2 Verbal Phrases

Verbal phrases are named as such because the most important word in the phrase is a verbal, or verb form, and they are formed from verbs. They may express action and have modifiers, and they may be followed by complements, but they do not function as verbs, or predicates, in the sentence. They are phrases containing verb forms that function as other parts of speech—noun, adjective, or adverb. These include participial phrases, gerund phrases, and infinitive phrases.

A *participle* is a verb form that is used as an adjective. There are two kinds of participles: present participle (ends in *–ing*) and past participle (ends in *–ed*, *–d, –t, –en,* or *–n*).

> The developing infection was cause for concern.
> Developing rapidly, the infection was cause for concern.
> The infection, developing rapidly, was cause for concern.

In the examples above, "developing," which is formed from the verb "develop," is used as an adjective modifying the noun "infection."

> When I entered the room, I found the patient crying. (modifies "patient")
> The patient, awakened, began to complain about her IV. (modifies "patient")

Although participles are formed from verbs, they are not used alone as verbs. Be careful. When the word combines with a helping verb, it is then part of the predicate and *not* a participle.

> The restrained patient was transferred to another floor. (participle modifying "patient")
> The patient was restrained and transferred to another floor. (verb phrase)

A *participial phrase* is a phrase containing a participle and any complements or modifiers.

> Complaining of abdominal pain x2 days, the patient presented to the ER.
> Her husband, appearing uncomfortable with the interview, chose to leave the room.

A *gerund* is a verb form ending in *–ing* that is used as a noun.

> Walking was very painful for the patient. (gerund as subject)
> She felt the pain while swimming. (gerund as object of preposition)

A *gerund phrase* is a phrase consisting of a gerund and any complements or modifiers.

EXAMPLE

> The clinic advises making an appointment in the next 3 days. (gerund phrase as direct object)
> Her primary goal in therapy is walking without a limp. (gerund phrase as predicate nominative)

An *infinitive* is a verb form, usually preceded by the word *to*, which is used as a noun or modifier. It is generally used as a noun but may also be used as an adjective or adverb.

EXAMPLE

> To wait for surgery can be stressful. (noun subject)
> He lacked the strength to stand. (adjective modifying "strength")
> Healthy patients eat to live. (adverb modifying "eat")

An *infinitive phrase* is a phrase consisting of an infinitive and any complements or modifiers.

EXAMPLE

> The nurse intended to give the patient another dose of Demerol. (infinitive phrase as direct object of "intended")
> There must be a way to solve her problem. (infinitive phrase modifying the noun "way")

4.4 The Clause

In addition to words and phrases, clauses are essential word group elements that add dynamic detail to a sentence. A clause is a group of words containing a subject and a predicate and used as part of a sentence. Clauses are classified according to grammatical completeness. Those that can stand alone if removed from their sentences are called independent clauses. Those that do not express a complete thought and cannot stand alone are called dependent, or subordinate, clauses.

4.4.1 Independent Clauses
The *independent clause*, when removed from its sentence, makes complete sense and can stand alone. When written with a capital at the beginning and

a period at the end, it becomes a simple sentence. It is an independent clause only when combined with one or more additional clauses, either independent or subordinate.

> Despite being told she needed to be admitted, the patient signed out of the emergency room against medical advice.

When two or more independent clauses are joined by a conjunction, the result is a compound sentence.

> The patient was taken to the operating room, and she was prepped and draped in the usual sterile fashion.

4.4.2 Dependent/Subordinate Clauses

Subordinate clauses, which cannot stand alone as sentences, are used as nouns or modifiers in the same way as single words and phrases. A subordinate clause is always combined in some way with an independent clause.

> who was the patient's previous doctor
> which could have been the cause of his symptoms
> as I had suspected

When combined with an independent clause, the subordinate clause plays its part in the sentence.

> Dr. Green, who was the patient's previous doctor, had believed her symptoms to be psychosomatic.
> I cautioned him about eating spicy foods, which could have been the cause of his symptoms.
> As I had suspected, the patient had been miscalculating her insulin doses.

4.4.3 Adjective Clauses

The *adjective clause* is a subordinate clause that, like an adjective, modifies a noun or pronoun.

EXAMPLE

> The clinic where she was treated is in Phoenix. (modifies "clinic")
> The patient's sister, who accompanies her today, also has a history of breast cancer. (modifies "sister")
> The surgery, which is scheduled for Friday afternoon, will be done on an outpatient basis.

Adjective clauses often begin with the pronouns *who, whom, which,* or *that.* These pronouns refer to, or are related to, a noun or pronoun that has come before, they connect their clauses to the rest of the sentence, and serve as the subject or object of the subordinate clause.

EXAMPLE

> I referred the patient to Dr. Smith, who specializes in upper extremity surgery. (refers back to "Dr. Smith")

4.4.4 Noun Clauses

A *noun clause* is a subordinate clause used as a noun. The noun clause can serve as the subject of the sentence, object of a preposition, predicate nominative, or direct object just like a noun.

EXAMPLE

> This is what she does. (noun clause as predicate nominative)
> Do you know what the patient's allergies are? (noun clause as direct object)
> I gave her an overview of what I would do during the procedure. (noun clause as object of the preposition "of")

4.4.5 Adverb Clauses

An *adverb clause* is a subordinate clause that, like an adverb, modifies a verb, an adjective, or an adverb. Adverb clauses often begin with a subordinating conjunction *(See list under 4.1.7)*

EXAMPLE

> The patient takes her medications whenever she can. (when)
> The patient takes her medications with her wherever she goes. (where)
> The patient takes her medications because she knows it is important. (why)
> The patient takes her medications if she remembers. (under what conditions)

Adverb clauses may also modify adjectives and other adverbs.

EXAMPLE

> The patient is confident that the surgery will benefit her. (modifies "confident")

4.4.6 Elliptical Clauses

Elliptical clauses, or *incomplete clauses*, are adverb clauses that contain missing words, often commonly omitted in writing and in speech. Because they are implied and readily understood, they do not need to be included, even if omitted when dictated.

EXAMPLE

> I am stronger than you [are].
> While [I was] waiting on the phone for her test results, I was told by the nurse that they had arrived by fax.

4.5 Sentence Classification

Sentences are classified by structure and purpose. Sentence structure relates to the complexity of the sentence in terms of the number of independent and/or dependent clauses that are contained within it. Sentence purpose relates to the intention of the sentence in communicating its information.

4.5.1 Simple Sentence

A *simple sentence* is a sentence with one independent clause and no subordinate clauses.

EXAMPLE

> The patient's past medical history is unremarkable.
> Immediate treatment is critical to her prognosis.

4.5.2 Compound Sentence

A *compound sentence* is a sentence composed of two or more independent clauses but no subordinate clauses.

EXAMPLE

> The patient presented to the ER with chest pain, and an EKG was significant for an acute MI.
> I explained the risks and benefits of the procedure, and the patient consented to the surgery.

4.5.3 Complex Sentence

A *complex sentence* is a sentence that contains one independent clause and at least one subordinate clause.

EXAMPLE

> The patient presented to the ER with chest pain, which had been intermittent over the previous 12 hours.
> Despite aggressive resuscitative efforts, we were unable to initiate a pulse.

4.5.4 Compound-Complex Sentence

A *compound-complex sentence* is a sentence that contains two or more independent clauses and at least one subordinate clause.

The patient presented to the ER with chest pain, which had been intermittent over the previous 12 hours, and EKG was significant for an acute MI. (two independent clauses and one subordinate clause)

Despite aggressive resuscitative efforts, we were unable to initiate a pulse, and the patient was pronounced at 2250. (two independent clauses, and one subordinate clause)

After explaining the risks and benefits of the procedure to the patient, she consented to the surgery, which will be scheduled for this week, and I told her to follow up with my scheduling coordinator. (two independent clauses and two subordinate clauses)

4.5.5 Declarative Sentence

A *declarative sentence* is a sentence that makes a statement. This is the predominant sentence type found in clinical documentation.

She is a well-developed, well-nourished white female.
Repeat blood cultures were ordered.

4.5.6 Imperative Sentence

An *imperative sentence* is a sentence that gives a command or makes a request. These would rarely be encountered in transcription unless in a direct quote.

Take these specimens to the laboratory.
Squeeze my hand.

4.5.7 Interrogative Sentence

An *interrogative sentence* is a sentence that asks a question. Again, unless in a direct quote, this sentence type would rarely be encountered in clinical documentation.

EXAMPLE

> Are you allergic to anything?
> When was the last time you ate?

4.5.8 Exclamatory Sentence

An *exclamatory sentence* is a sentence that expresses strong feeling. Like the imperative and interrogative sentence types, exclamatory sentences are encountered only in direct quotes in transcription.

EXAMPLE

> The other guy ran the red light and slammed right into me!

CHAPTER

5

Usage

Introduction

Usage, quite simply, refers to the way language is used by those who speak it and express it in written form. In conversation, we tend to concern ourselves with appropriate usage only when the manner in which a person chooses to use the language strikes us as clearly unsuitable, where we become distracted from *what* is being said by *how* it has been expressed. In formal writing, of which healthcare documentation is a part, it is essential that usage complies with the guidelines of Standard English—the language of most educational, legal, governmental, and professional documents, thereby being the model by which most professionals shape not only their understanding of language but their *usage* of that language. While a transcriptionist may encounter nonstandard forms of the English language, and retention of those nonstandard forms may be appropriate in the context of a direct quote, part of the analytical and editorial process of transcription includes ensuring appropriate usage in capturing the meaning of what has been dictated.

5.1 Verb Usage

Verbs express action or being. Verbs have tense, mood, and voice.

5.1.1 Tense

Verbs change in form to show the time of their action or of the idea they express. The time expressed by a verb (present, past, future, etc.) is its *tense*. The six tenses are outlined below.

The *present tense* is used to express action (or to help make a statement about something) occurring now, at the present time. The present tense can be expressed as a general action, a progressive action, or with a helping verb as an emphatic action, but all of them occur, or are occurring, in the present. *(see examples next page)*

I work here. (general)
I am working now. (progressive)
I do work. (emphatic)

The *historic present tense* uses the present tense to relate past events in a more immediate manner. In dictation, it is common to use the historic present tense to describe patient information or treatment in the present rather than in the past. In other words, unless a physician dictates the record while actually providing care for the patient, any dictation of the present tense to represent the patient encounter would be classified as the historic present tense.

On examination, the patient <u>is sitting</u> upright on the examining table and <u>appears</u> to be alert, oriented, and in no acute distress.

The *universal present tense* uses the present tense to state something that is universally true or that was believed to be true at the time. The universal present is not the same as the historic present.

Traditional treatment modalities were used because <u>they are</u> so effective.

The *past tense* is used to express action (or to help make a statement about something) that occurred in the past but did not continue into the present. The past tense is formed in regular verbs by adding *–d* or *–ed* to the verb.

The patient <u>worked</u> for the government for 10 years.
I <u>closed</u> the wound with interrupted sutures.
She <u>did take</u> her medication. (emphatic)

Section 2: General Standards of Style

The *future tense* is used to express action (or to help make a statement about something) occurring at some time in the future. The future is formed with *will* or the increasingly less common word *shall*.

EXAMPLE

> The patient <u>will return</u> to the clinic on Monday for wound check.
> She <u>will be taking</u> her baby to a genetic specialist.
> He <u>is about to leave</u> for college next week.

The *present perfect tense* is used to express action (or to help make a statement about something) occurring at no definite time in the past. It is formed with *have* or *has*. It is also used to express action occurring in the past and continuing into the present.

EXAMPLE

> He <u>has worked</u> for us many times.
> She <u>has been treated</u> with 5-FU for the last 6 weeks.

The *past perfect tense* is used to express action (or to help make a statement about something) completed in the past before some other past action or event. It is formed with *had*.

EXAMPLE

> When he <u>had taken</u> all of his medication, he <u>called</u> my office for a refill. (the "taking" preceded the "calling")
> After she <u>had decided</u> to go ahead with the surgery, she <u>changed</u> her mind. (the "deciding" preceded the "changing" of her mind)

The *future perfect tense* is used to express action (or to help make a statement about something) which will be completed in the future before some other future action or event. It is formed with *will have* or, less frequently, with *shall have*.

EXAMPLE

> By the time she <u>returns</u> to my office, her pain <u>will have diminished</u> significantly. (the "diminishing" precedes the "returning)
> When she <u>sees</u> me next year, she <u>will have been</u> cancer-free for greater than 5 years. (the "being" cancer-free precedes the "seeing")

In transcription, maintain uniformity of tense, but keep in mind that tense may vary within a single report or even within a single paragraph, depending on the time being referenced. A provider may dictate the history of present illness and past medical history in the past tense, then may dictate the review of systems and physical exam in the present tense, and later dictate the plan or recommendations in the future tense. This is usually a representative chronology of the diagnostic process, and the transcriptionist should capture that chronology just as it is dictated. Varying tenses may also be used within the same paragraph, even in the same sentence. As long as there is no ambiguity, the transcriptionist should record this as dictated. It is not uncommon to hear the provider say, "Her vitals signs *have returned* to baseline, and she *will be discharged* tomorrow." This is a consistent representation of chronology and should be captured as such.

It's also important to note that some providers are attempting to dictate material from a previously documented encounter (such as dictating certain information into the discharge summary that is extracted from the admitting H&P). What may have appropriately been dictated in the present tense on an admitting H&P may be inappropriate to retain in the present tense for a discharge summary, where the historical information on a discharge summary is clearly in the past tense. Defer to facility policy for modifying the tense in those instances.

5.1.2 Mood
Verbs may be in one of three moods: *indicative, imperative,* or *subjunctive.*

The *indicative* mood makes factual statements and is most common.

EXAMPLE

The patient <u>returned</u> on schedule for a followup visit.

The *imperative* mood makes requests or demands.

EXAMPLE

<u>Come</u> here now.

The *subjunctive* mood expresses doubt, wishes, regrets, or conditions contrary to fact. It is the most difficult and most formal mood and usually relates to the past or present, not the future. The use of the subjunctive mood usually applies to only one verb form—*were* or forms of *be*.

EXAMPLE

> I suggested that she <u>be</u> admitted to the emergency room.
> If I <u>were</u> her, I would have the lesion on her back evaluated by a dermatologist.
> She spoke as though she <u>were</u> a physician or someone who worked in health care.

5.1.3 Voice

A verb is in the *active voice* when it expresses action performed *by* its subject. A verb is in the *passive voice* when it expresses an action performed *upon* its subject or when the subject is the result of the action.

EXAMPLE

> The car <u>hit</u> a tree. (active voice)
> The tree <u>was hit</u> by a car. (passive voice)

Most communication guidelines urge use of the active voice except when it is more important to emphasize *what* was being acted upon and that it *was* acted upon. In transcription, the active voice is more common in reporting observations, e.g., in history and physical reports, while the passive voice is more common in describing the healthcare provider's actions, e.g., hospital treatment and surgery.

EXAMPLE

> The abdomen is soft and nontender.
> The patient was given intravenous aminophylline.
> The incision was made over the symphysis pubis.

It is important to note that the transcriptionist should never recast the sentence from passive to active voice except in awkward or unclear constructions. To recast a passive construction may erroneously assign action to an unintended subject.

EXAMPLE

> D: The wound was closed with interrupted Vicryl sutures.
> T: The wound was closed with interrupted Vicryl sutures.
> *not:*
> T: I closed the wound with interrupted Vicryl sutures.

In the example above, even in an instance where the physician has used a predominantly active voice throughout the dictation of the operative note, to recast this type of sentence to the active voice could erroneously assign action to the physician. The use of the passive voice is often used, particularly in operative reports, simply to indicate that action was performed upon the patient by a member of the surgical team. The wound in the example above could have been closed by an assisting surgeon or a physician's assistant, and to recast the sentence could create an error in assignment of action.

5.2 Pronoun Usage

The function of a pronoun in a sentence is demonstrated by the case form of the pronoun. Different functions demand different forms.

5.2.1 Nominative Case
A pronoun that acts as the subject is in the *nominative case*. The nominative pronouns are *I, you, he, she, it, we, you,* and *they.* Since the subject of the verb is always in the nominative case, use the nominative form of a pronoun when it is used as the subject. When the subject is compound, it is particularly important to be careful to use a nominative pronoun.

EXAMPLE

> She and I are good friends.
> Neither Dr. Jones nor he was on call this evening.

Remember that pronouns used as predicate nominatives, even though they follow the verb, are in the nominative case.

EXAMPLE

It might have been she.
This may be he coming to pick up the patient.

5.2.2 Objective Case

A pronoun that acts as the object is in the *objective* case. The objective pronouns are *me, you, him, her, it, us, you,* and *them.* Since the object of the verb or
preposition is always in the objective case, use the objective form of a pronoun
when it is used as the direct or indirect object of the verb or the object of a
preposition.

EXAMPLE

I saw <u>him</u> sitting next to the patient's bed. (direct object)
The patient gave <u>me</u> a friendly smile. (indirect object)
When I asked about her husband, the patient said she was afraid of <u>him</u>.
(object of the preposition)

Like the nominative forms of pronouns, the objective forms are troublesome
principally when they are used in compounds. Keep in mind that the use of
an objective pronoun does not change just because it exists in a compound
expression.

EXAMPLE

I saw <u>him</u> and his wife in the emergency room. (I saw <u>him</u> in the emergency
room)
not:
I saw <u>he</u> and his wife in the emergency room. (I saw <u>he</u> in the emergency
room)

When the compound occurs as the object of a preposition, be particularly
careful to select the objective pronoun.

EXAMPLE

D: The house belongs to <u>she</u> and her husband.
T: The house belongs to <u>her</u> and her husband.

5.2.3 Who vs. Whom

Like the personal pronouns, the pronouns *who* and *whoever* have three different case forms. *Who* and *whoever* are the nominative forms, *whom* and *whomever* are the objective forms, and *whose* and *whosoever* are the possessive forms.

Who and *whom* are in the *interrogative* case when they are used to ask a question. Like the pronouns discussed in sections 5.2.1 and 5.2.2 above, these pronouns follow the same rules for nominative and objective case.

EXAMPLE

> <u>Who</u> gave the patient her discharge instructions? (nominative case; "who" is the subject)
> <u>Whom</u> did Mary call? (objective case; "whom" is the object of "did call")
> She asked <u>who</u> the doctor on call was. (subjective case; though it follows the verb "asked" and appears to be the object of the verb, "who" functions as the predicate nominative of the linking verb "was")
> They asked <u>whom</u> she had met. (objective case; "whom" is the direct object of the verb "had met")

Who and *whom* (*whoever* and *whomever*) are relative pronouns when they are used to begin a subordinate clause. Their case is governed by the same rules that govern the use of personal pronouns for use in the nominative and objective case. The case of the pronoun beginning a subordinate clause is determined by its use in the clause, not by the words around it. *(See 4.4.2— Dependent/Subordinate Clauses)*. It is often helpful when analyzing a who-vs.-whom scenario to follow these steps:

- Pick out the subordinate clause.
- Determine how the pronoun is used in the clause—i.e., subject, predicate, nominative, object of the verb, object of the preposition—and decide its case according to the rules.
- Select the correct form of the pronoun.

EXAMPLE

> This pleasant, cooperative patient, <u>(who/whom) was referred to me by Dr. Green</u>, comes in today seeking surgical consultation.

- "who/whom was referred to me by Dr. Green" is the subordinate clause
- within this clause, the pronoun serves as the subject of the verb "was referred"
- the subjective form "who," not "whom," is the correct pronoun usage here

> This pleasant, cooperative patient, who was referred to me by Dr. Green, comes in today seeking surgical consultation.

In determining whether to use *who* or *whom*, do not be misled by a parenthetical expression like *I think, he said,* etc.

> He is the physician who, I believe, performed her cataract surgery. ("who" performed her cataract surgery)
> This is the patient who Dr. Green thinks should be included in my case study. ("who" should be included in my case study)

5.2.4 Incomplete Constructions

An *incomplete construction* occurs most commonly after the words *than* and *as*.

> I like Jim better than he. (than he likes Jim)
> I like Jim better than him. (than I like him)

After *than* and *as* introducing an incomplete construction, use the form of the pronoun you would use if the construction were completed. Listen carefully for faulty dictation when it comes to incomplete constructions, and accurately capture the intended meaning.

> D: I told the husband that at this point a nursing home could provide better care for the patient than him.
> T: I told the husband that at this point a nursing home could provide better care for the patient than he.

In the example above, what is dictated implies that the nursing home could provide better care for the patient than it could provide for him, the husband. Obviously, the physician was referring to the nursing home's ability to provide better care of the patient than the husband was capable of providing for her himself. Again, expanding both sentences to their complete construction makes the choice obvious *(see examples next page)*:

I told the husband that at this point a nursing home could provide better care for the patient than [it could provide for] him.
I told the husband that at this point a nursing home could provide better care for the patient than he [could provide].

5.3 Agreement—Subjects and Verbs

Some words in English have matching forms to show grammatical relationships. Forms that match in this way are said to "agree." For example, a subject and verb agree if both are singular or both plural.

5.3.1 Basic Rule of Agreement
A verb must agree with its subject in number and person. Use a singular verb with a singular subject and a plural verb with a plural subject.

I hope to see improvement in her symptoms over the next week.
Her pain seems rather vague and difficult to qualify.
She is coming in to the office next week.
The lungs are clear.

5.3.2 Compound Subjects
Subjects joined by "and"—If the subject consists of two or more words joined by *and*, the subject is plural. Use a plural verb.

Bedrest and elevation are recommended. (not "is")
The hospital staff and the patient's family were surprised by her rapid recovery. (not "was")

Use a singular verb when the compound subject refers to the same person or thing.

Her companion and healthcare surrogate is her husband. (not "are")
Red beans and rice was the cause of his heartburn. (not "were")

Use a singular verb when two or more subjects joined by *and* are preceded by *each, every, many a,* or *many an.*

Each medication, wound care instruction, and postoperative precaution was carefully explained to the patient. (not "were")
Every verbal response, facial expression, and body movement was recorded under her mental status examination. (not "were")

Subjects joined by "or"— If the subject consists of two or more singular words connected by *or, either…or, neither…nor,* or *not only…but also,* the subject is singular and requires a singular verb.

Either chemotherapy or chemotherapy with concomitant radiation therapy <u>is</u> the course I would recommend.
Not only pain but also suffering is considered when awarding compensatory damages in a malpractice case.

If the subject consists of two or more plural words that are connected by *or, either…or, neither…nor,* or *not only…but also,* the subject is plural and requires a plural verb.

Neither headaches nor vision problems were noted on her review of systems.
Muscle spasms or cramps are common in the later months of pregnancy.

If the subject consists of both singular and plural words connected by *or, either…or, neither…nor,* or *not only…but also,* the verb agrees with the nearest subject.

The patient's husband or her daughters are going to stay home with the patient next week.
I believe his ulcers or his recent anxiety is the cause of his worsening symptoms.

5.3.3 Intervening Phrases and Clauses

Disregard any phrases or clauses that interrupt the flow from subject to verb. These can often be distracting and misleading when trying to determine subject-verb agreement. Always be careful to question *what* is performing the action of the verb.

EXAMPLE

> The x-rays the patient brought with her from her referring physician showed severe chronic sinusitis.
> Only one of her sisters has a history of breast cancer.

When a compound subject has both a positive and a negative component, the verb should agree with the positive subject.

EXAMPLE

> The patient, but not her daughters, is convinced her chest pain is due to anxiety.
> His postoperative swelling, not his pain medications, is causing his temporary loss of sensation.

Phrases that interrupt the flow from subject to verb that begin with expressions such as *along with, together with, and not, as well as, in addition to, accompanied by, plus, besides, including, except, rather than,* and *not even* do not change the agreement of the subject to its verb. In other words, be careful not to assume that these intervening phrases represent a compound subject.

EXAMPLE

> The patient, along with his wife and sons, presents to the office today.
> Mrs. Smith, accompanied by her husband, presents for cardiac consultation.

5.3.4 Indefinite Pronouns

Pronouns like *everybody, someone, everything, all,* or *none* can present some special usage challenges. Some of them are always singular and require singular verbs. Some are always plural and require plural verbs. Yet others can be either singular or plural, depending on the meaning of the sentence. They are also commonly followed by intervening phrases.

Always singular—The following indefinite pronouns are always singular: *each, either, neither, one, no one, every one, anyone, someone, everyone, anybody, somebody,* and *everybody.*

> Each <u>does</u> his own work.
> Every patient <u>is treated</u> equally.
> Anyone that has been through the training course <u>is</u> a candidate for this project.

Always plural—The following indefinite pronouns are always plural: *both, few, many, others,* and *several.*

EXAMPLE

> Few <u>are chosen</u> for that position.
> Several of her friends <u>have told</u> her that she is too thin.

Singular or plural—The indefinite pronouns *all, none, any, some, more,* and *most* may be singular or plural depending on the nouns they refer to.

EXAMPLE

> Some of her symptoms <u>are</u> ambiguous.
> Some of her pain <u>is</u> difficult to describe.
>
> Most of the group <u>is going</u> to eat after the meeting.
> Most of the people <u>are going</u> to eat after the meeting.

5.3.5 Unusual Nouns

Some nouns are unique in their expression and can present a particular problem in determining subject-verb agreement. It is important to learn those nouns and whether they take a singular or plural verb.

Nouns ending in "s"—Some nouns appear to be plural because they end in "s" but are, in fact, singular. Therefore, they require singular verbs.

EXAMPLE

> news
> measles
> lens
> ascites
> lues
> pons
> facies

Some nouns are always considered plural, even though they refer to a single thing. Therefore, they require plural verbs.

adnexa
assets
credentials
dues
odds
premises
fauces

Some nouns have the same form in the plural and in the singular form. When they function as subjects, they take singular or plural verbs depending on their meaning.

series
species
means
gross
corps
biceps
forceps
scissors
sheep, deer, moose, etc.

This particular species of bacteria <u>causes</u> cellular destruction.
Many species of bacteria <u>cause</u> cellular destruction.

The left biceps <u>was</u> weaker than the right.
The left and right biceps <u>were</u> equally strong.

An Allis forceps <u>was used</u> to grasp the muscle.
Both forceps <u>were required</u> to elevate the muscle.

Nouns ending in "ics"—Many nouns ending in "ics" take singular or plural verbs depending on usage. When they refer to a body of knowledge or a course of study, they are singular. When they refer to qualities or activities, they are plural.

Genetics <u>is</u> his area of research.
Her genetics <u>indicate</u> the potential for breast cancer.

Statistics <u>has</u> been a difficult class for her to pass.
The statistics <u>show</u> this type of protocol to be reasonably effective.

Foreign nouns—Some nouns have foreign plural endings, which are discussed in greater detail in Chapter 8, and they require plural verbs.

On spinal films, the vertebrae <u>are</u> intact.
On spinal films, the vertebra <u>is</u> intact.

There <u>were</u> scattered diverticula in the ascending colon.
There <u>was</u> a single diverticulum in the ascending colon.

The word *data* has been a subject of controversy where subject-verb agreement is concerned. Since it is technically plural, it is requires a plural verb. However, usage now dictates a unique consideration of agreement with this word. When *data* is used to refer to "information" in the collective sense, a singular verb should be used. When used to refer to "distinct bits of information," it is followed by a plural verb.

Her laboratory data is within normal limits.
That data gathered by the task force are being analyzed and compared.

5.3.6 Collective Nouns

A *collective noun* represents a group of persons, animals, or things that is expressed in a singular form. Agreement between a collective noun and its verb is determined by meaning. If the group is deemed to be acting as a unit, use a singular verb. If the members of the group are deemed to be acting individually, use the plural verb.

EXAMPLE

The Board of Directors meets every month. (meet as a unit)
The Board of Directors are not in agreement on this issue. (disagree individually)
better:
The members of the Board of Directors are not in agreement on this issue.

A number vs. the number—The collective noun *number* can be either singular or plural depending on whether it is preceded by the articles *the* or *a*. *The number* is specific and therefore singular in meaning and requires a singular verb. *A number* is general and therefore plural in meaning and requires a plural verb.

EXAMPLE

The number of times she has called my office over the last 2 weeks is considerable.
A number of possible diagnoses associated with these symptoms come to mind.

5.3.7 Organizational Names

Like collective nouns, organizational names are treated as either singular or plural depending on whether the collective or individual nature of the organization is emphasized. Typically, organizational names are expressed as singular entities and require singular verbs. However, when wishing to emphasize the individuals who make up an organization, a plural verb should be used. Either way, consistent usage of the selected form should continue within the same context.

EXAMPLE

Smith, Myers & Goldman has collected extensive data under this protocol. (the practice has collected)
Smith, Myers & Goldman have collected extensive data under this protocol. (the individuals have collected)

5.3.8 Geographic Names

Treat geographic names as singular entities when they refer to only one thing. When it is obvious that the geographic name is being referred to collectively, use a plural verb.

EXAMPLE

The Virgin Islands is a popular honeymoon destination.
The Virgin Islands are positioned in close proximity to each other.

The United States has been a member of the United Nations since 1945.
These United States have been unified in the belief that freedom is a human right.

5.3.9 Units of Measure

Though they represent a plural quantity, units of measure are collective singular nouns and take singular verbs.

EXAMPLE

After the lab report came back, 20 mEq of KCl was added to her treatment.
Then 3 mL was injected.

When combined medications are given to the patient and dictated together, subject-verb agreement with those units of measure can be tricky. When the medications are joined by the conjunction *and*, the expression is compound and requires a plural verb.

EXAMPLE

Then 1% Xylocaine without epinephrine and 20 mg of Aristospan were injected into the carpal tunnel.

When the medications are joined by the prepositions *plus* or *with*, the expression is read as a single unit and requires a singular verb.

EXAMPLE

Then 1% Xylocaine without epinephrine plus 20 mg of Aristospan was injected into the carpal tunnel.

5.3.10 Time, Money, and Quantity

When subjects refer to periods of time, amounts of money, or quantities, they can be either singular or plural depending on whether the subject represents a total amount or a number of individual units. Subjects representing total amounts should be treated as singular subjects with singular verbs. Subjects representing individual units should be treated as plurals requiring plural verbs.

EXAMPLE

Three weeks <u>is</u> a long time.
Five days <u>have</u> passed.
In all, 4 doses <u>were given</u>.

5.3.11 Inverted Sentences

When the verb precedes the subject, make sure the subjects and verbs agree.

EXAMPLE

<u>Attached is</u> (verb) a <u>copy</u> (subject) of the patient's liver function tests.
Happy <u>are</u> (verb) <u>they</u> (subject) who can easily forgive.

Sentences that begin with *there is, there are, here is, here are,* etc., represent constructions that result in the subject following the verb. Use *is* when that subject is singular and *are* when that subject is plural.

EXAMPLE

There <u>is</u> usually significant <u>pain</u> (singular) after this kind of procedure.
There <u>are</u> often many <u>complications</u> (plural) after this kind of procedure.
Here <u>is</u> five dollars (singular) to buy lunch.
Here <u>are</u> ten candidates (plural) for that new position.

5.4 Agreement—Pronouns and Antecedents

An antecedent is a person or thing to whom the pronoun refers. In some instances, pronouns do not have antecedents, as in the use of the first-person personal pronoun I. But in most cases, pronouns have antecedents, either mentioned within the same sentence or in a previous one.

5.4.1 Basic Rules of Agreement

A pronoun must agree with its antecedent in number, gender, and person.

EXAMPLE

I (antecedent) can only render my professional opinion.
Dr. Adams (antecedent) indicated he would be willing to assist in this surgery.
The surgical team (antecedent) has completed its preoperative evaluation.

Use a plural pronoun when the antecedent is a compound expression.

EXAMPLE

Dr. Smith and I (antecedent) believe we can help this patient.
You and the baby (antecedent) should follow up with your pediatrician next week.

When the antecedent is a compound expression joined by *or* or *nor*, use a singular pronoun when both antecedents are singular and use a plural pronoun when both antecedents are plural. When the antecedent consists of both a singular and a plural noun, use the pronoun that agrees with the nearest subject.

EXAMPLE

The patient or her daughter (antecedent) will have to drive her car.
Neither the patients nor the doctors (antecedent) want their pictures in the paper.
Neither the doctor nor his patients (antecedent) are unhappy with their treatment outcomes.

5.4.2 Common-Gender Antecedents

A common-gender noun is one that applies to both males and females. When these occur as antecedents, it can be challenging to select the appropriate pronoun genders to accompany them. When the gender of the antecedent is known, or *definite*, select the appropriate gender pronoun.

EXAMPLE

> Her doctor needs to give <u>her</u> consent. (if known to be a female)
> The CEO of AHDI will give <u>his</u> annual report in the next issue of the association's journal. (if known to be a male)

When the gender of the antecedent is unknown, or *indefinite*, there are several options for ensuring that the meaning is clear without guessing or venturing into politically incorrect waters. In transcription, the choice will be obvious based on what is dictated unless the physician has dictated an awkward or unclear construction, in which case the transcriptionist should choose from the options below, being careful to pick the one that is less intrusive to the physician's style.

EXAMPLE

> The physician of a fearful patient should use <u>his or her</u> most comforting bedside manner. (use of "his or her")
>
> Physicians of fearful patients should use <u>their</u> most comforting bedside manner<u>s</u>. (recast from singular to plural to avoid "his or her")
>
> The physician of a fearful patient should use the most comforting bedside manner. (recast to avoid using a generic pronoun)

5.4.3 Indefinite Pronoun Antecedents

When the antecedent is an indefinite pronoun *(See 4.1.2—Indefinite Pronouns)*, use a singular pronoun.

EXAMPLE

> <u>Every</u> obstetrical patient has <u>her</u> own story to tell. (not their)
> <u>Another</u> antibiotic has run <u>its</u> course without much effect. (not their)

Some indefinite pronoun antecedents will require the application of strategies outlined in 5.4.2 above.

> Everyone should submit his or her insurance information on the first visit.
> All patients should submit their insurance information on the first visit.

5.5 Diction

Diction refers to *word choice*, whose determination is entirely dependent on *meaning*, in the sentence. It can refer to the application of the correct article preceding a noun or pronoun, the correct use of the appropriate part of speech or form of a word, and it can refer to the use of the correct word in the instance where two or more words sound and look alike.

> a, an
> affect, effect
> bizarre, bazaar
> callous, callus
> patients, patience
> a lot, allot
> ensure, insure, assure

The terms above are just a small sampling of the many instances in the English language when usage comes down to proper word choice, or diction. There are innumerable examples in clinical medicine of words and phrases that can be confused for each other and certainly many instances where even the dictator may be unsure of the correct word in a given setting. Transcriptionists should refer to reputable dictionaries and industry resources to be certain the word or phrase being captured is appropriate to the context.

For a detailed listing of common errors in word usage and words that sound or look alike, refer to *Appendix C—Usage Glossary* at the back of this book.

CHAPTER

6

Punctuation

Introduction

Punctuation marks function to make the expression of language more easily read and understood. Unlike all other elements of language, punctuation only asserts itself in the written word and thus plays a vital role in the *visual* expression and interpretation of language. In many instances, punctuation marks serve to separate or otherwise clearly delineate the appropriate flow of words, thoughts, and concepts, in many instances functioning to set apart certain information from the rest of the sentence or to indicate a connection between two or more concepts. Punctuation also functions to convey tone in written language, as in the use of question marks and exclamation points, to provide the emphasis normally intoned in the spoken language.

The role of punctuation in clinical documentation is no different than in any other form of written expression. Clarity of communication should always be the guide in the application of concepts in this chapter. The unique challenge faced by the transcriptionist is in exercising informed judgment when punctuating. Unlike other standards outlined in this text, appropriate punctuation is expected of the MT even in a verbatim environment, whether dictated by the provider or not. It is also important to note that while providers may attempt to provide appropriate punctuation as part of the dictation process, a transcriptionist should never rely on the provider in the decision to include or exclude punctuation marks—again, even in a verbatim environment.

A Note About Quality Assurance: While punctuation errors have their place in all quality measurement systems, including the guidelines outlined by AHDI in the *Metrics for Measuring Quality in Medical Transcription* standard, there are very few instances when the inclusion or omission of punctuating marks results in a compromise of clinical clarity or a potential risk to patient safety. Transcriptionists should *not* be unreasonably penalized for errors in punctuation that do not compromise the integrity of the document. Punctuation is not an absolute science, and there are many areas (particularly in the application of commas) where the process is somewhat subjective and there-

continued next page

fore open to interpretation and debate. Where punctuation is concerned, feedback given to transcriptionists in a quality-driven environment should focus primarily on clarity of communication and secondarily on mentoring MTs toward enhanced understanding of the principles and nuances of this complex arena of language.

Trend Note: The migration toward an electronic environment, where clinical data will be increasingly captured via disparate methodologies (i.e., speech recognition, point-and-click templates, etc.) will likely result in decreased focus/emphasis on extraneous symbols and punctuation marks in the record. In environments where the data being tagged and captured will be accessed, used, and displayed in user interfaces that are field-driven, the use/inclusion of punctuation will become irrelevant and unnecessary. AHDI maintains that regardless of the capture method, any resulting *documentation* created from captured data should continue to reflect not only clinical accuracy but also the application of quality standards outlined in this text, including the appropriate placement of punctuation. Transcriptionists working with emerging/enabling technologies in an electronic environment should defer to facility policy for the use/inclusion of symbols and certain punctuation marks, while still advocating for the preservation of quality standards in any resulting useable document.

6.1 Terminal Punctuation

Terminal punctuation refers to punctuation marks that terminate an independent clause or sentence. Each of the terminal punctuation marks—period, question mark, and exclamation point—serves to create a separation between one thought and the next. The period and question mark have other uses and applications outside of the terminal role, particularly in clinical language, and those uses are likewise outlined below.

6.1.1 Period
Use a period to mark the end of a sentence, either statement or command.

EXAMPLE

> The patient presents to my office today for followup.
> Pick up the pen, please.
> She was prepped and draped in the usual sterile fashion.

Use a period at the end of an *indirect* question.

> The patient asked whether she would have to be out of work for more than a week after the surgery.
> He was less concerned about the details of the procedure; his question was about how his insurance would be billed.

Use a period to separate a whole number from a decimal fraction.

> 3.344
> 0.12
> $5.30

Use periods after the numbers or letters used to enumerate items in a list *unless* the numbers/letters are enclosed in parentheses.

> DISCHARGE MEDICATIONS
> 1. Protonix daily.
> 2. Xanax p.r.n. nightly.
> 3. Allegra-D p.r.n. seasonal allergies.
> *but:*
> In contemplating tubal ligation, the patient should determine whether she (a) is confident she does not desire future pregnancy and (b) wants to have the procedure performed at the time of her C-section.

Use periods at the end of each item in a list when those items are essential to the grammatical completeness of the statement introducing the list.

> The patient is instructed to:
> 1. Go home and elevate the arm for the next 24-36 hours.
> 2. Take Darvocet q.4 h. p.r.n. pain.
> 3. Follow up in my office on Monday for bandage check.

In the list above, each item completes the opening sentence introduced by the word *to*. Often the physician will transition away from a list like that above and return to dictating in narrative sentences. When that occurs, the transcriptionist should begin a new paragraph or express the list above in paragraph form.

The patient is instructed to:
1. Go home and elevate the arm for the next 24-36 hours.
2. Take Darvocet q.4 h. p.r.n. pain.
3. Follow up in my office on Monday for bandage check.

I have told her that she should expect to return to work within a week unless there are unforeseen complications. She understands these instructions and will follow up as indicated.
or:
The patient is instructed to: (1) go home and elevate the arm for the next 24-36 hours, (2) take Darvocet q.4 h. p.r.n. pain, and (3) follow up in my office on Monday for bandage check. I have told her that she should expect to return to work within a week unless there are unforeseen complications. She understands these instructions and will follow up as indicated.

Periods are not needed at the end of each item in a list that does not represent a grammatical connection to the introductory statement.

The benefits of exercise are many:
1. Weight loss
2. Heart health
3. Stress relief
4. Improved sleep

In clinical documentation, lists like the one above are rarely encountered. The vast majority of enumerated lists seen in the health record represent information that follows a major report heading. In those instances, the heading functions as an implied form of an introductory statement for which each enumerated item is a grammatical completion. Thus, all enumerated lists in clinical documentation should include terminal periods at the end of each entry. In the list below, each item completes the opening sentence *implied* by the heading (*The discharge diagnoses are…*).

EXAMPLE

DISCHARGE DIAGNOSES
1. Status post myocardial infarction.
2. Status post balloon angioplasty with stent placement.
3. Chronic renal insufficiency, stable.
4. Chronic rheumatoid arthritis.

Likewise, when only one item follows the header, it serves the same role and should include a terminating period. In the example below, the item completes the opening sentence *implied* by the heading (*The discharge diagnosis is…*).

EXAMPLE

DISCHARGE DIAGNOSIS
Status post myocardial infarction with balloon angioplasty and stent placement.

The only exception to this rule is when the single-item or enumerated list represents a list of people's names, such as physicians, surgeons, specialists, etc. Do *not* include a period in those instances.

EXAMPLE

ATTENDING PHYSICIAN
George A. Smith, MD

SURGEONS
1. John D. Frazier, MD
2. William Douglas, DO

Use periods with lowercased abbreviations and acronyms, whether English or Latin.

EXAMPLE

etc.
p.r.n.
pp.
q.6 h.
et al.

Trend Note: Many language and style sources, including the *AMA Manual of Style*, have transitioned to dropping periods in most lowercased Latin abbreviations, like legal abbreviations (*et al, eg, ie, viz, etc*), and literary reference abbreviations (*p, pp*), but recommend the retention of periods in abbreviations used in treatment and drug dosing instructions (*p.r.n., q.i.d., q.4 h.,* etc.). Transcriptionists should defer to facility preference.

Do *not* use periods with uppercase abbreviations and acronyms, including titles and credentials that may have required periods at one time. It is no longer common practice to include periods with those abbreviations.

EXAMPLE

MD
CMT
CABG
CAD
aVL

Do *not* use periods with abbreviated personal and courtesy titles unless it is known that the person in question prefers the inclusion of a period or periods. While the use of periods in these instances is still acceptable, there continues to be a strong trend toward dropping them and their omission is now preferred. Defer to facility preference.

EXAMPLE

John A. Smith Jr
Ms Emily Williams
Dr Edward Jones
Walter W. Adams III

Do *not* use periods with abbreviated units of measure.

EXAMPLE

mg
g
mL
mmHg
mm/h

6.1.2 Question Mark

Use a question mark at the end of a direct question.

> Are you sure you need this procedure?
> Does he want to go with us?
> Who is responsible for this catastrophe?

Use a question mark to indicate a question within a direct quote.

> The patient asked me, "How long will I be out of work?"
> He merely said "huh?" when I asked him to describe his symptoms.

Do *not* use a question mark within a quotation if it is the overall sentence that poses the question and not the direct quote itself. Place the question mark at the end of the sentence, not the end of the quoted material.

> Did she really say "leave me alone"?
> How many times did he yell "help"?

In healthcare documentation, it is common for a provider to indicate the use of a question mark to imply uncertainty about a diagnosis. This should be transcribed as dictated, using an actual question mark in the area indicated.

> D: Diagnosis...question mark idiopathic thrombocytopenic purpura.
> *Transcribed:*
> DIAGNOSIS
> ?idiopathic thrombocytopenic purpura.

Do *not* use the question mark when the physician dictates "question of" or "questionable."

> There is a question of pigmented nevus versus melanoma.
> *not:*
> There is ?pigmented nevus versus melanoma.

6.1.3 Exclamation Point

The use of exclamation points in health records is extremely rare, except in the instance of a direct quote, and the use of them outside of a direct quote, even if dictated, is discouraged since they tend to inject an inflammatory tone to the record that is inappropriate and informal. In dictation, the only time this would require editorial insight is if the physician actually dictates the words "exclamation point" at the end of a sentence (as opposed to discerning that implication from his/her tone).

EXAMPLE

> D: The patient is 103 years old!
> T: The patient is 103 years old.
>
> D: I strongly advised that she be admitted for testing, but the patient signed out against medical advice!
> T: I strongly advised that she be admitted for testing, but the patient signed out against medical advice.

6.2 The Comma—Separating

Commas essentially serve two purposes in the English language: (a) to set off nonessential elements (*See 6.3 The Comma—Setting Off*) and (b) to *separate* elements of an expression in order to clarify their relationship with each other. A separating comma is a *single* comma that serves as a divider between two elements—digits, words, phrases, and clauses.

6.2.1 Adjectives

Use a comma to separate two or more adjectives modifying the same noun.

EXAMPLE

> This well-developed, well-nourished woman presented to my office for evaluation. (two adjectives modifying "woman")
> I explained that we would be using a safe, quick-acting anesthesia for her outpatient procedure. (two adjectives modifying "anesthesia")

Exception: In clinical documentation, commas are frequently omitted from the series of demographic descriptors used to identify the patient—most often seen in the opening statements of the history and/or physical examination sections of the report. This string of descriptors, including the patient's age, race, and gender, are generally treated as a single unit, and omitting commas in those instances is acceptable and increasingly preferred.

EXAMPLE

This is a 40-year-old African American male patient with a history of sickle cell anemia.
not:
This is a 40-year-old, African American, male patient with a history of sickle cell anemia.

On examination, she is a 2-year-old white female who is sleeping in her mother's arms.
not:
On examination, she is a 2-year-old, white female who is sleeping in her mother's arms.

When those descriptors include other general adjectives to describe the patient, apply commas to only those items. To omit commas in those instances results in a string of adjectives that becomes too long and visually confusing.

EXAMPLE

This is a well-developed, well-nourished 40-year-old African American male patient with a history of sickle cell anemia.
On examination, she is an adorable, engaging 2-year-old white female.

6.2.2 Items in a Simple Series

Use a comma to separate two or more items in a *simple* series, where none of the items contain internal commas. Do *not* use a comma if all the items are joined by *and* or *or*. Always use a serial comma before the conjunction *preceding* the final item in your series (a, b, and c). It is still acceptable in some sources to omit the serial comma, but both AHDI and the AMA recommend inclusion of that comma for clarity.

EXAMPLE

Dermatologic examination revealed macules, papules, and several small pustules.
The patient is to go home, follow a clear liquid diet for the next 24 hours, transition slowly to a regular diet, and follow up in my office next week.
but:
She complained of nausea and vomiting and some intermittent headache.

Note: To avoid clutter and confusion, use parentheses instead of commas or dashes to set off a series that describes what precedes it.

> The patient had multiple complaints (headache, nausea, vomiting, and fever) and demanded to be seen immediately.
> *preferred to:*
> The patient had multiple complaints—headache, nausea, vomiting, and fever— and demanded to be seen immediately.

6.2.3 Independent Clauses

Use a comma to separate two independent clauses in a compound sentence that are joined by a conjunction (*and, but, or, nor,* or *for*). Each independent clause is underlined below to delineate that each represents a complete thought that is capable of standing alone.

> <u>He was brought to the operating room</u>, and <u>he was prepped and draped in the usual sterile fashion</u>.
>
> <u>She brought her previous films with her to my office today</u>, but <u>I did not find her mammography films to be included in the envelope</u>.

Be careful not to confuse a complex sentence with a compound verb. If no new subject is introduced after the conjunction, you likely have a compound verb, *not* a compound sentence. In those instances, a comma should *not* precede your conjunction.

> He was brought to the operating room and was prepped and draped in the usual sterile fashion.
> *not:*
> He was brought to the operating room, and was prepped and draped in the usual sterile fashion. (This implies that "was prepped and draped in the usual sterile fashion" can stand alone as an independent clause)

6.2.4 Introductory Elements

Use a comma to separate introductory elements (words, phrases, and clauses) from the independent clause that follows it.

EXAMPLE

Yes, I can deliver that message for you. (introductory word)
Under the influence of hallucinogenic drugs, the patient jumped from his second-story window and fractured his leg. (introductory prepositional phrases)
Taking the risks and benefits into consideration, the patient has opted to undergo the procedure. (introductory gerund phrase)
Before she arrived in the emergency room, she told EMS that she was hearing voices. (introductory dependent clause)

Do *not* use a comma after most introductory adverbs or short phrases that answer the questions *when, how often, where,* and *why*.

EXAMPLE

Tomorrow we will admit her to Memorial Hospital for tests.
Every morning the patient walks two miles.
Occasionally he feels short of breath when climbing a flight of stairs.
For that reason we will admit her.

6.2.5 Numbers

Use a comma to separate groups of three numerals in numbers of 5 digits or more, but omit the commas if decimals are used. The comma in 4-digit numbers may be omitted.

EXAMPLE

Platelet count was 345,000.
12345.67
White count was 7100.
or:
White count was 7,100.

Do not place commas between *words* expressing a number.

Four hundred forty-eight
not:
Four hundred, forty-eight.

Trend Note: The *AMA Manual of Style* recommends compliance with SI convention, whereby digits are separated by a "thin space," not a comma, to indicate place values beyond thousands. However, this recommendation pertains primarily to the formal publication of clinical data in periodicals, abstracts, and scientific journals. Transcriptionists who are asked to prepare manuscripts of this nature should be aware of this standard. Due to the compromise of visual clarity that omission of separating commas would create as well as the as-yet lack of widespread adoption of this standard, this recommendation has *not* been made for healthcare records. With the continued movement toward SI convention, however, it is possible that even health records will see a migration to this standard in the future.

4055
13 445
722 654
8 473 308

Use a comma to separate adjacent unrelated numbers if neither can be expressed readily in words. However, it is preferred that the sentence be recast to avoid the confusion of adjacent numerals. The example below represents an instance where both numbers are too large to be readily expressed in words. Recast the sentence, if possible, as below. In a verbatim environment where recasting is prohibited, a separating comma is the only option.

In March of 2002, 2038 patients were seen in the emergency room.
better:
In March of 2002, there were 2038 patients seen in the emergency room.

6.2.6 Dates

Use a comma to separate the day of the month from the year when the full date is expressed.

EXAMPLE

> I last saw her in my office on March 28, 2004.
> He retired from the Navy on April 10, 2007.

Do *not* use a comma when only the month and year are given.

EXAMPLE

> I last saw her in my office in March 2004.
> He retired from the Navy in April 2007.

When the full date (month, day, and year) occur in mid-sentence, use a comma to separate the year from the rest of the sentence.

EXAMPLE

> I last saw her on March 28, 2004, in my office.
> He retired on April 10, 2007, from the Navy.

6.2.7 Titles

Do *not* use commas to separate a person's name from titles such as *Jr* and *Sr* and roman or arabic numerals following a person's name.

EXAMPLE

> She will be referred to Dr. James Baker Jr for further evaluation.
> John Edwards Sr's surgery will be scheduled for tomorrow.

Do *not* use commas to separate *Inc.* or *Ltd.* from a business name unless it is known that the entity in question prefers the separating comma.

EXAMPLE

> Time Inc. has been in the publication business for many years.

6.2.8 Geographic Names and Addresses

Use a comma to separate a city and state, city and country, or state and country. Use a comma to separate the state or country from the rest of the sentence.

> The patient moved to Modesto, California, 14 years ago.
> The patient returned from a business trip to Paris, France, the week prior to admission.

When expressing a complete address as part of a sentence, use a comma to separate the street address from the secondary address information (suite, apartment number, etc.), to separate the secondary address from the city, and to separate the city from the state. Do *not* use a comma to separate the state and zip code. Use a comma to separate the zip code from the remainder of the sentence that follows it.

> We will send the laboratory results to her at 750 East Adams Street, Apt. 401, Pasadena, CA 91104, once we receive them in our office.

In correspondence or other instances where the complete address is displayed in block style, use the following format:

> Ms Susan Smith
> 750 East Adams Street, Apt. 401
> Pasadena, CA 91104

6.2.9 Genetics

Use a comma to separate the chromosome number and sex chromosome in genetic expression. Place the comma without spacing between these numbers.

> The normal human karyotypes are 46,XX (female) and 46,XY (male).
> The test was positive for 47,XX,+21, or Down syndrome.

6.2.10 Units of Measure

Do *not* use a comma to separate two or more measures whose units are the same dimension (weight, volume, time, etc.).

> The patient is 2 years 4 months 3 days old.
> Apgars were normal and weight was 8 pounds 12 ounces.
> She was able to tolerate exercise for 10 minutes 22 seconds.

6.2.11 Dialogue

Use a comma to separate direct dialogue from the rest of the sentence. The comma should precede the opening quotation marks when information introduces the quoted dialogue. The comma should fall *inside* the closing quotation marks when the remainder of the sentence follows the quoted dialogue.

> At the start of the examination, the patient made the point of saying, "I don't want a pelvic exam."
> "I don't want a pelvic exam," the patient made a point of saying.

6.2.12 Omitted Word(s)

Use a comma to separate two parts of an independent clause to indicate the omission of a word or phrase whose meaning is implied. In most instances, this occurs in the second of two sentences to avoid repeating the same word or phrase.

> In test group 1, the duration of treatment was too short; in test group 2, too long. (The comma indicates the omission of "the duration of treatment was.")
>
> She said she was experiencing a drop in blood pressure in the morning; at night, an elevation. (The comma indicates the omission of "she was experiencing.")

6.2.13 Laboratory Values

Use commas to separate values of a single panel or test. Use periods to separate the values of unrelated laboratory tests. In the example below, the CBC values are grouped together in one sentence; the chemistry values in another.

EXAMPLE

LABORATORY DATA: White count 5.2, hemoglobin 15, and hematocrit 39. Sodium 149, potassium 4.2, and chloride 103.

6.3 The Comma—Setting Off

The second function of the comma is to set off nonessential expressions that interrupt the flow of the sentence from subject to verb or verb to complement. Nonessential expressions are words, phrases, and clauses that are not necessary for the grammatical correctness or structural integrity of the sentence.

6.3.1 Basic Rules for Nonessential Expressions

Identifying a nonessential expression can often be confusing to transcriptionists who sometimes misinterpret this to mean that the information contained within a nonessential clause is not important information. The question of whether information is essential or nonessential has very little to do with whether that information is inherently important and more to do with whether it is necessary for the sentence it resides in to have unhindered meaning and structural integrity.

EXAMPLE

We will get the opinion of Dr. Smith, who has expertise in this area, prior to proceeding with surgery. (nonessential)
We will get the opinion of someone who has expertise in this area prior to proceeding with surgery. (essential)

In the examples above, the fact that the individual in question has "expertise" is inarguably important information, *but* it does not have the same impact on the integrity of the sentence around it in each instance. It is nonessential *to the sentence* in the first example, because it merely provides additional information about Dr. Smith, who is specific and *essential* enough to the meaning of the sentence not to require the information that follows it. In the second sentence, the clause in question becomes absolutely essential because it adds specificity that the word "someone" does not adequately provide. Setting off a nonessential word, phrase, or clause implies that it can be removed from the sentence without compromising meaning or structural integrity. To remove the clause in the second sentence would create a compromise of meaning, whereby not enough specific information is given.

EXAMPLE

> The person <u>who drives the patient to all her appointments</u> is her daughter. (essential—tells which person)
> She presents today with her daughter, <u>who drives the patient to all her appointments</u>. (nonessential—further describes "daughter")
>
> The medication <u>that we thought would benefit her most</u> was Protonix. (essential—tells which medication)
> We prescribed Protonix, <u>which we thought would benefit her the most</u>. (nonessential—additional information about "Protonix")

Note: The word "that" most often introduces *essential* clauses, and the word "which" most often introduces *nonessential* clauses.

6.3.2 Interrupting Elements
Use commas to set off words, phrases, and clauses that interrupt the flow of the sentence.

EXAMPLE

> Mary, <u>I believe</u>, has already been seen in the Coumadin clinic.
> She will, <u>if possible</u>, bring her previous films with her on her next visit.
> We could, <u>perhaps</u>, ask Dr. Smith to see her.
> The patient has been told to follow up with me in the office or, <u>if he cannot get to the office</u>, by phone.

6.3.3 Appositives
Use commas to set off an appositive, or expression that provides additional, nonessential information about a noun or pronoun that immediately precedes it.

EXAMPLE

> Jerry Edwards, <u>her husband</u>, has power of attorney for the patient.
> My first suggestion, <u>to start her on steroid treatment</u>, was met with immediate opposition by the patient.
> Open reduction with internal fixation, <u>which is really her only reasonable option at this point</u>, will be scheduled for Thursday.

6.3.4 Afterthoughts

Use commas to set off words, phrases, and clauses that are loosely added onto the end of the sentence, often expressing the opinion or tone of the speaker.

EXAMPLE

This baby is very healthy, isn't he?
The patient was supposed to chart her premenopausal symptoms, if I recall.
Take the patient to outpatient radiology, please.

6.3.5 Transitional Words and Phrases

Transitional expressions are called such because they exist in the second of two related sentences and help the reader transition from the thought or idea expressed in the first sentence to the thought or idea expressed in the second sentence. These transitional expressions can be *complementary* (as with *therefore* and *subsequently*) or *contrasting* (as with *however* and *on the other hand*). Use a comma or commas to set off transitional expressions (*however, therefore, on the other hand, subsequently,* etc.) when they occur in the middle or at the end of the second sentence. When the transitional expression *introduces* the second clause, use a comma to separate the transitional expression from the rest of the sentence.

EXAMPLE

The patient was given D50 in normal saline. Subsequently, she became more responsive.
or:
The patient was given D50 in normal saline; subsequently, she became more responsive.

but:

The patient was given D50 in normal saline. She became, subsequently, more responsive.
or:
The patient was given D50 in normal saline. She became more responsive, subsequently.

The most common misapplication of this rule in transcription occurs with the word *however*, which providers dictate with extreme frequency. It is important to recognize this word as a transitional expression and evaluate its position (introductory, interrupting, or terminating) in the *second* of the two related sentences being expressed. Either a period or semicolon can be used to separate the sentences, but neither terminal punctuation mark has any bearing on the position or role of the transitional word in the second sentence.

EXAMPLE

She was brought to the emergency room in cardiac arrest. Despite all exhaustive efforts, <u>however</u>, we were unable to resuscitate her. (interruptive)

She was brought to the emergency room in cardiac arrest. Despite all exhaustive efforts, we were unable to resuscitate her, <u>however</u>. (terminating)

She was brought to the emergency room in cardiac arrest; <u>however</u>, despite all exhaustive efforts, we were unable to resuscitate her. (introductory)

not:

She was brought to the emergency room in cardiac arrest, however, despite all exhaustive efforts, we were unable to resuscitate her.

In the final example above, setting off the word *however* with commas would result in a faulty construction that would imply that the expression is nonessential and could be removed. Also, do not use transitional words as conjunctions. They do not function in a linking role.

EXAMPLE

She was given Tylenol; however, her headache did not improve.
not:
She was given Tylenol, however her headache did not improve.

6.4 Colons and Semicolons

These major marks of punctuation serve many important roles. Despite how frequently they are used in common communications, they have many critical uses in healthcare documentation.

6.4.1 Colon
The primary function of the colon in punctuation is to introduce a list, series, or enumeration. Place a colon before such expressions as *for example, namely,* and *that is* when they introduce words, phrases, or a series of clauses.
(*see examples next page*)

EXAMPLE

> I have offered the patient several options for treatment: namely, conservative observation, medical management, and surgical intervention.
>
> There are many benefits to association membership: for example, networking opportunities, access to industry news and information, professional resources, and product discounts.

When a sentence uses anticipatory expressions such as *the following, as follows, thus*, and *these*, use a colon to separate the sentence from the list or series that follows it.

EXAMPLE

> The following medications were suggested to the patient to alleviate her symptoms: Tylenol, Bayer, and Aleve.
>
> He is to go home with discharge instructions as follows: (1) Drink clear liquids and advance diet as tolerated, (2) Use Phenergan p.r.n. nausea and vomiting, and (3) Follow up in my office in one week.

Do *not* use a colon to introduce words that fit properly into the grammatical structure of the sentence without the colon: for example, after a verb, between a preposition and its object, or after *because*.

EXAMPLE

> The patient is on Glucophage, furosemide, and Vasotec.
> He came to the emergency room because he was experiencing fever, chills, and nausea.

Use a colon in standard expressions of time. Do *not* use a colon in expressions of military time.

EXAMPLE

> 2:30 p.m.
> 8:00
> 9:45 a.m.
> *but:*
> 1500
> 1435 hours
> 0930

Section 2: General Standards of Style

Use a colon in place of the word *to* in the expression of a ratio. Do *not* use a virgule, dash, hyphen, or other mark for this purpose.

Mycoplasma 1:2
Cold agglutinins 1:4
Zolyse 1:10,000

Use *to* or a hyphen instead of a colon when expressing the ratio using words or letters instead of values; use the colon only when expressing the values associated with the ratio.

I-to-E ratio
Myeloid-to-erythroid ratio
FEV-FVC ratio
but:
Myeloid-to-erythroid ratio was 10:1.
or:
Myeloid-to-erythroid was 10:1.

Use a colon to separate a title and subtitle of an article or publication.

In his article *Premenstrual Syndromes: What Every Clinician Should be Asking,* Dr. Sims discusses the fundamental symptoms associated with PMDD.

David Veillette, FACHE, is the author of *Hospitals in Crisis: A Digital Solution.*

Use a colon to separate volume number and page number in footnotes, end notes, and cited sources.

10:520-595 (meaning Volume 10, pages 520 through 595)

6.4.2 Semicolon

Use a semicolon to separate two independent clauses. While independent clauses are typically separated by periods, a semicolon can be used when the two clauses express closely linked or related concepts or ideas.

She presents today complaining of extreme fatigue; walking from one room to the next can completely exhaust her.

Over half of my patients opt for hormone replacement therapy; the rest prefer alternative treatments.

As stated above in 6.3.5—*Transitional Words and Phrases*, semicolons are most often used to separate two independent clauses that are linked in concept by a transitional expression.

She was prescribed a Z-Pak for her URI; however, she called today because her symptoms have not resolved.

Use a semicolon to separate two independent clauses linked by a transitional expression such as *for example (e.g.), namely,* or *that is*. Do not confuse the use of the semicolon here with the use of the colon outlined in *6.4.1—Colon* when a list or enumeration follows these expressions.

The patient is an ideal candidate for this study; that is, he meets the qualifications for history and risk factors.

Her questions were focused on one area of concern; namely, who is going to perform the procedure?

Use semicolons to separate items in a *complex* series, or a series in which at least one of the items in the series contains internal commas. Separating the items with semicolons provides visual clarity and ease of reading from one item in the series to the next.

The patient received Cerubidine 120 mg daily 3 times on February 26, 27, and 28, 2002; received Cytosar 200 mg IV over 12 hours for 14 doses beginning February 26; and received thioguanine for 14 doses, for a total dose of 200 mg a day, starting February 26.

Section 2: General Standards of Style

6.5 Hyphens

The primary role of hyphens in general language is for word division and in compound expressions, though many other uses in scientific language will be encountered by the medical transcriptionist or editor.

6.5.1 Word Division

Hyphens are used to divide words between syllables when the word does not fully carry to the next line of text. It is important to note that word division is rarely employed in medical transcription anymore since modern word processing programs and transcription platforms function on automatic word wrapping, making it unnecessary for the transcriptionist to bother with word division. However, in those rare instances where an MT may still be working in an environment that requires it, the general rules are outlined below.

- Divide words only between syllables. Consult a reputable dictionary or resource when uncertain of proper syllabic division.
- Do not divide one-syllable words.
- Do not set off a one-letter syllable at the beginning of the word.
- Do not divide a word unless you can leave a syllable of at least three characters on the first line and carry a syllable of at least three characters to the next line.
- Do not divide abbreviations.
- Divide compound words between the words forming the compound.
- Divide a hyphenated compound at the point of hyphenation.
- Divide a word *after*, not *within*, a prefix.
- Divide a word *before*, not *within*, a suffix.
- When possible, divide at the prefix or suffix point rather than in the root.
- When a one-letter syllable occurs in a word, divide *after* that syllable.
- Do not divide words in more than two consecutive lines of text.
- Do not divide at the end of the first line or end of the last full line of a paragraph.
- Do not divide the last word on a page.

6.5.2 Compound Modifiers

Perhaps no other area of language causes greater confusion than the application of hyphens in compound modifiers. The rules for retaining the compounding hyphen when the elements of the compound do *not* precede the nouns they modify depend greatly on (a) a keen understanding of parts of speech, and (b) an ability to determine the role of those compound elements when they are cast away from their nouns.

A *compound modifier*, or compound adjective, consists of two or more words that function as a unit and jointly modify a noun or pronoun. An important reminder is that the words that make up the modifier may or may not be adjectives themselves. It is only when they are combined with other words that the resulting compound becomes a single adjectival expression modifying a noun or pronoun. Compound modifiers are derived from and take the place of adjectival phrases and clauses.

EXAMPLE

Adjective Phrase/Clause	Compound Adjective
window *that is on the second floor*	second-floor window
mass *whose density is high*	high-density mass
a gown *that is as long as the floor*	floor-length gown
display *that catches the eye*	eye-catching display

Hyphenate *all* compound modifiers when they precede and modify a noun or pronoun.

EXAMPLE

scholarly-looking *patient*
second-floor *office*
finger-to-nose *test*
good-natured *female*
well-developed, well-nourished *woman*
fast-acting *medication*
low-frequency *waves*
high-power *field*

In general, *do not hyphenate* these compound expressions when they occur elsewhere in the sentence *if* they no longer function in an adjectival role; in other words, if the expression no longer functions as an adjective modifying a noun and functions instead as some other part of speech, the hyphenation should be dropped. The types of compounds that tend to drop their hyphenation are those formed with adverbs and participles, whereby the participle transitions back to its primary role as a verb.

Before the Noun	Elsewhere in Sentence
an up-to-date history (compound modifier)	We brought her history up to date. (prepositional phrase)
a cause-and-effect relationship (compound modifier)	There is a relationship of cause and effect in this case. (object of the preposition)
an off-the-record comment (compound modifier)	Her comment was off the record. (prepositional phrase)
a well-developed female (compound modifier)	The patient is well developed. ("is developed" is the verb; "well" is the adverb modifying the verb)
a fast-acting medication (compound modifier)	The medication is fast acting. ("is acting" is the verb; "fast" is the adverb modifying the verb)
second-floor office (compound modifier)	The office is on the second floor. (object of the preposition)
random-access memory (compound modifier)	This computer allows random access to stored data. (direct object of the verb)

Do hyphenate compound modifiers that occur elsewhere in the sentence *if* they continue to function as modifying compounds. This almost always occurs when the compound modifier follows a linking verb and functions as a *predicate adjective* modifying the noun or pronoun subject of the sentence.

The patient is good-natured and soft-spoken. (compound predicate adjectives modifying "patient")
The forceps were bone-biting. (compound predicate adjective modifying "forceps")
I found the patient to be panic-stricken. (compound predicate adjective of the infinitive "to be" modifying "patient")
I work part-time. (compound adverb; answers "when")
This commitment will be long-term. (predicate adjective modifying "commitment")

Do not use a hyphen in a compound modifier to link an adverb ending in –*ly* with a participle or adjective. In those instances, the adverb functions to modify the adjective or participle, *not* to serve in a compound role.

recently completed workup
moderately acute pain
financially stable investment

Do not use a hyphen in a compound modifier if the compound modifier is preceded by an adverb.

somewhat well nourished patient
reasonably well articulated history
very well written essay

Some compound modifiers are commonly used together, or are so clear, that they are automatically read as a unit and do not need to be joined with a hyphen.

dark brown lesion
deep tendon reflexes
jugular venous distention
left lower quadrant
low back pain

Do not use hyphens with most disease-entity modifiers even when they precede the noun. Check appropriate medical references for guidance.

cervical disk disease
oat cell carcinoma
pelvic inflammatory disease
sickle cell disease
urinary tract infection
but:
insulin-dependent diabetes mellitus
non-insulin-dependent diabetes mellitus
non-small-cell carcinoma

Section 2: General Standards of Style

Trend Note: The term *non-small-cell carcinoma* is an example of one of those terms that is evolving away from hyphenation. Many sources are beginning to cite *nonsmall-cell carcinoma* as an acceptable expression.

Use a hyphen with two or more eponymic names used as multiple-word modifiers of diseases, operations, procedures, instruments, etc.

EXAMPLE

Osgood-Schlatter disease *(named for US orthopedic surgeon Robert B. Osgood and Swiss surgeon Carl Schlatter)*
but:
Chevalier Jackson forceps *(named for Chevalier Jackson, US pioneer in bronchoesophagology)*

Use a hyphen to join two adjectives that are equal, complementary, or contrasting when they precede or follow the noun they modify.

EXAMPLE

anterior-posterior infarction
physician-patient confidentiality
attorney-client privilege
blue-green eyes

Do *not* hyphenate foreign expressions used in compound adjectives, even when they precede the nouns they modify (unless they are always hyphenated).

EXAMPLE

in vitro experiments
carcinoma in situ
cul-de-sac *(always hyphenated)*
ex officio member

Use a hyphen to form a compound modifier between a number and a word if it precedes and modifies a noun. When the word represents a unit of measure, hyphenate *only* when the unit is an English unit of measure, which is spelled out in full. Do *not* hyphenate compound modifiers if the unit of measure is an abbreviated metric unit, where neither the numeric value nor the unit of measure constitutes an actual *word* with which a compound can be formed. *(see examples next page)*

EXAMPLE

3-week history
2-year-old female
8-pound 5-ounce baby girl
2-inch laceration
but:
3 cm incision
5 mg dosage
5 x 3 x 2 cm mass

Note: This represents a change over previous recommendations in the 2nd edition of this text. Per SI convention and metric standards, no intervening symbols or punctuation should interrupt the flow from numeric value to metric unit, even in a modifying relationship. This is an application that should not have been implied by the standards for compound modifiers. In addition, compound modifiers should be formed by *at least* one complete word, and metric value expressions do not meet that criterion.

Use a hyphen to clarify meaning and to avoid confusion, absurdity, or ambiguity in compound modifiers. The hyphen may not be necessary if the meaning is made clear by surrounding context.

EXAMPLE

large-bowel obstruction *(obstruction of the large bowel)*
large bowel obstruction *(large obstruction of the bowel)*
single-specialty clinic *(facility devoted to one specialty)*
single specialty clinic *(single facility devoted to a specialty)*

Use a hyphen or en dash to hyphenate a compound modifier formed with a one-word modifier or prefix. In these instances the prefix is hyphenated to clearly communicate a modifying relationship with the entire compound and not just the first word.

EXAMPLE

non-disease-entity modifier
not:
nondisease-entity modifier (no such thing as "nondisease")

non-insulin-dependent diabetes mellitus
not:
noninsulin-dependent diabetes mellitus (no such thing as "noninsulin")

6.5.3 Compound Nouns and Verbs

Some compound words are written without hyphenation, some are written separately, and some are joined by hyphens. In the evolution of a newly coined combined word, an expression typically starts out as a hyphenated compound and gradually over time and through widespread usage will evolve into a single entity without hyphenation. Transcriptionists should refer to a reputable dictionary or resource when unsure as to whether a compound word is expressed as a single word or with hyphenation.

EXAMPLE

> attorney at law
> beta-blocker
> chief of staff
> father-in-law
> half-life
> life span
> air bag
> paper clip
> homeowner
> workstation
> crossroad
> free-fall
> money-maker
> school board

Use a hyphen to join two nouns that are equal, complementary, or contrasting.

EXAMPLE

> blood-brain barrier
> fracture-dislocation

Do not hyphenate proper nouns of more than one word, even when they serve as a modifier preceding a noun.

EXAMPLE

> South Dakota residents
> United Airlines pilot

Do not use a hyphen in a combination of proper noun and common noun.

EXAMPLE

Tylenol capsule administration
Bovie cautery hemostasis

Use a hyphen with all compound nouns containing *ex-* when *ex-* means *former* and precedes a noun that can stand on its own.

EXAMPLE

ex-wife
ex-president

Most compound verbs are hyphenated or are one word. Refer to a reputable dictionary or resource for hyphenation. If unable to locate a compound verb in the dictionary, hyphenate the components.

EXAMPLE

to baby-sit	to downgrade
to double-space	to highlight
to test-drive	to troubleshoot
to second-guess	to pinpoint

Do *not* use a hyphen in compound verbs that are formed with a preposition, like *up, in, down,* etc.

EXAMPLE

I am going to <u>make up</u> that test next week.
He will <u>slow down</u> his exercise for the next few weeks.
She will <u>follow up</u> with me on Monday.

When the compounds above are used as nouns, they drop their hyphenation and become joined compounds. When they function as adjectives, they should be hyphenated. In some instances, as with *followup* and *followthrough*, both the adjective and noun forms have dropped their hyphenation and have become single compounds, though the hyphenated form (*follow-up*) is still acceptable when used as an adjective.

> She has a <u>followup</u> (or <u>follow-up</u>) appointment with me on Tuesday.
> She will be seen in <u>followup</u> on Tuesday.
>
> I am going to take a <u>make-up</u> test next week.

6.5.4 Numbers Spelled Out

When expressing numbers in words, hyphenate all compound numbers between 21 and 99 (or 21st and 99th), whether they stand alone or are part of a number over 100. Of note, the only instance where numbers would be spelled out like this in healthcare documentation would be when a number occurs at the beginning of a sentence that cannot be recast.

> twenty-one
> forty-three million
> seven hundred thirty-five

When there is more than one acceptable expression, choose the simplest form for clarity of communication.

> fifteen hundred
> *not:*
> one thousand five hundred

6.5.5 Serial Numbers

Use hyphens in the expression of serial numbers (medical record numbers, social security numbers, etc.).

> MR#: 05-38-9964
> SSN: 111-22-3333

6.5.6 Fractions

Use hyphens to express fractional numbers that are combined with whole numbers, whether spelled out or expressed with numerals.

2-1/2 inches
3-3/4 hours
three-fourths of the bottle
two-thirds majority

6.5.7 Ranges

Use a hyphen in place of the word *to* in range expressions if all of the following five conditions have been met: (1) the phrases *from...to, from...through,* and *between...and* are *not* used, (2) decimals and/or commas do not appear in the numeric values, (3) neither value contains four or more digits, (4) neither value is a negative, and (5) neither value is accompanied by a symbol.

Our new office hours will be 1-4 p.m. Tuesdays and Thursdays.
Systolic blood pressures were in the 150-180 range.
BP was 120-130 over 80-90.
There were 8-12 wbc's per high-power field.

See 6.7.2—*Meaning "Per" or "Over"* for ranges that are combined with *over* expressions.

6.5.8 Prefixes and Suffixes

Do *not* use a hyphen after common prefixes except when they precede a proper noun, a capitalized word, or an abbreviation: *ante-, anti-, bi-, co-, contra-, counter-, de-, extra-, infra-, intra-, micro-, mid-, non-, over-, peri-, pre-, post-, pro-, pseudo-, re-, semi-, sub-, super-, supra-, trans-, tri-, ultra-, un-,* and *under-.*

antimicrobial
posttraumatic
overproduction
comorbidity
preoperative
perimenopausal

Use a hyphen after a prefix when the unhyphenated word would have a different meaning.

re-creation, recreation
re-treat, retreat
un-ionized, unionized

Use a hyphen after a prefix or before a suffix to avoid an unusual or awkward combination of letters, as in repetitive vowels or three of the same consonants sequentially.

anti-inflammatory
bell-like
de-emphasize

Note: Be careful to check a reputable dictionary or resource when using words like those above. Again, as language evolves, many of these words drop their hyphenation. A number of industry resources already cite *antiinflammatory* without hyphenation, though the hyphenated form is still acceptable.

6.5.9 Suspensive Hyphens

Use a *suspensive* hyphen after each incomplete modifier when there is a series of two or more hyphenated compounds that have a common last word, or base.

10- to 12-year history
3- to 4-inch incision
full- and split-thickness grafts
1st-, 2nd-, and 3rd-trimester symptoms

Do *not* use a suspensive hyphen with a stand-alone prefix that precedes an unhyphenated prefix compound.

We will perform a preoperative and postoperative evaluation.
not:
We will perform a pre- and postoperative evaluation.

This test will usually determine if a patient is hypertensive or hypotensive.
not:
This test will usually determine if a patient is hyper- or hypotensive.

6.5.10 Single Numbers, Symbols, or Letter Compounds

Some terms with a single letter or symbol followed by a word are hyphenated; others are not. Check appropriate references for guidance, and consider the use of hyphens in such terms as optional if you are unable to document. Even if such terms are not hyphenated in their noun forms, they should be hyphenated in their adjectival forms.

B-complex vitamins
T wave, T-wave abnormality
B-cell helper
J curve
Z-plasty
T-shirt
I beam

Do *not* hyphenate modifiers in which a letter or number is the second element.

grade A eggs
study 1 protocol
type 1 diabetes mellitus

6.6 Parentheses, Braces, and Brackets

These marks are most often used to set off parenthetical expressions that are supplemental, but not essential, to the sentence. They are rarely used in transcription and should only be included in those instances where specifically directed to do so by the dictator.

6.6.1 Parentheses

Parentheses are used to provide parenthetical (incidental or supplementary) information that is not closely related to the rest of the sentence. They may or may not be dictated, and the transcriptionist should avoid using them unless they are dictated or they are the best choice for ensuring clarity of communication. It is better to use commas to set this information off.

EXAMPLE

> A great deal of swelling was present (more so on the left than the right).
> *better:*
> A great deal of swelling was present, more so on the left than the right.

Punctuation should not precede or follow the parenthetical expression unless the sentence requires it.

EXAMPLE

> The patient is improving (despite her repeated insistence that she is dying), and we plan to discharge her to an assisted living facility next week.

Punctuation should not be included *within* the parenthetical expression unless the expression requires it.

EXAMPLE

> The regimen we started her on (atenolol, enalapril, and HCTZ) seems to be doing an adequate job of controlling her blood pressure.

Use parentheses to enumerate items within a sentence, separating the enumerated items by commas or semicolons.

EXAMPLE

> He has a long history of known diagnoses, including (1) chronic silicosis, (2) status post left thoracotomy, and (3) arteriosclerotic cardiovascular disease.

6.6.2 Braces and Brackets

Brackets may be used around a parenthetical insertion within a parenthetical insertion. Follow the rules for parentheses.

EXAMPLE

> The patient had had multiple complaints (headache, nausea, vomiting, and [he thought] fever) and demanded to be seen immediately.

Note: An author will often dictate "brackets" instead of "parentheses" in error.

Use brackets to express chemical concentration. When concentrations are expressed as percentages, use the percent sign rather than the spelled-out form and do not use brackets.

EXAMPLE

> [HCO3-] *or* [HCO$_3$-]
> 15% HNO3 or HNO$_3$

When expressing chemical formulas, use parentheses for innermost units, adding brackets and then braces, if necessary.

EXAMPLE

> chlorphenoxamine hydrochloride
> 2-[1-(4-chlorophenyl)-1-phenylethoxy]-N,N-dimethylethanamine hydrochloride
>
> hydroxychloroquine sulfate
> 7-chloro-4-{4-[ethyl(2-hydroxyethyl)amino]-1-methylbutylamino}-quinoline sulfate

6.7 Virgule or Forward Slash (/)

The virgule, also known as *diagonal, slant line, slash,* or *solidus,* is used for a variety of purposes, particularly in the reporting of clinical data and scientific values. When dictated, the author will usually say "slash" or "forward slash." However, there are many instances, as outlined below, where the virgule is indicated even when not dictated.

6.7.1 Equivalence/Duality

Virgules are often used to express equivalence—an instance where two terms are of equal weight in an expression. When the word *and* is implied between the expressions, a virgule (/) can be retained.

> Her treatment/diagnostic planning was discussed with the therapist.
> I had a long discussion with his sister/caregiver about home intervention.

When it comes to duality, or an instance where the word *or* is implied between the expressions, do *not* use a virgule.

> Each patient was given <u>his or her</u> test results by phone.

Trend Note: The preference in these instances is increasingly to recast the sentence to use the plural in order to avoid sexist language.

> The treatment regimen is one that any patient can follow on <u>his or her</u> own.
> *better:*
> The treatment regimen is one that patients can follow on <u>their</u> own.

6.7.2 Meaning *Per* or *Over*

Use a virgule for the word *per* when the following conditions have been met: (1) The construction involves at least one *metric* unit of measure, and (2) at least one element includes a specific numeric quantity.

> The CD4+ cell count was 200/mcL.
> Blood volume was 70 mL/kg of body weight.
>
> Hemoglobin level was 14 g/dL.
> *but:*
> Hemoglobin levels are reported in grams per deciliter.

When these expressions involve *nonmetric* units of measure, spell out the word *per* and do not use the virgule, since the virgule implies an abbreviated expression and nonmetric units are abbreviated in the record. *Exception:* Use a virgule when the expression combines a metric unit with a nonmetric unit.

EXAMPLE

Heart rate was 120 beats per minute.
She takes 5 mg of Valium per day.
She weighs in 3 days per week.
but:
Her IV was set to run at 10 mcg/min while she was in the ER.

Do *not* use the virgule in place of *per* when a prepositional phrase intervenes between the two units of measure.

EXAMPLE

She was given 4.5 mEq of potassium per liter.
He was advised to take 81 mg of aspirin per day.

Do *not* use the virgule in place of *per* when neither element in the expression represents a unit of measure (when both elements are numeric) or when there are two numeric values accompanying different units of measure, particularly in drug concentration expressions. When the units differ or the units and/or elements are unknown, a virgule should not be used to imply direct relationship. *Exception*: If it can be confirmed that such an expression is part of the legally registered trademark for a medication, express the concentration with a virgule as indicated by the manufacturer.

EXAMPLE

The patient was prescribed Advair 250 per 50 b.i.d.
I called in a prescription for Hydro-Tussin HD 200 mg per 10 mL.
but:
I will start her on Nortrel 0.5/35 for pregnancy prevention and management of her PMS. (legally trademarked name)

Use a virgule to express *over* in certain relational expressions.

EXAMPLE

Blood pressure is 160/100.
There is a grade 1/4 murmur heard over the left sternal border.

Section 2: General Standards of Style

When a range is combined with an *over* or *out of* expression, spell out the expression to avoid being misread as a fraction. Do not use a virgule to express the relationship.

EXAMPLE

Strength in the right extremity is 4 to 4+ over 5.
not:
Strength in the right extremity is 4-4+/5.

She described her pain as a 5 to 6 out of 10.
not:
She described her pain as a 5-6/10.

When a hyphen is used to express a range of two large numbers, express both numbers in their entirety, even if dictated in shortened expression, to avoid confusion or lack of clarity.

EXAMPLE

D: Platelet counts were 300 to 450 thousand.
T: Platelet counts were 300,000-450,000.
not:
T: Platelet counts were 300-450,000.

6.7.3 Dates

Virgules may be used to separate numerals representing the month, day, and year in tables and figures. This form may also be used for the date of service, operation, admission, or discharge when capturing patient demographic data as well as for dates dictated and transcribed at the bottom of the report.

EXAMPLE

DATE OF ADMISSION: 05/02/2007
DATE OF DISCHARGE: 05/04/2007

As above, the trend in most formal documentation is to reflect an 8-digit date when using virgule constructions (MM/DD/YYYY), but transcriptionists should defer to facility preference and user interface requirements.

In text, it is preferable to spell out dates in full, writing out the name of the month. However, if dates are used repeatedly and become cumbersome in the record, dates may be expressed using virgule constructions for visual clarity.

Likewise, some facilities have a strong preference for virgule construction in the record and do not want dates spelled out in full. In formal correspondence, they should always be spelled out. In narrative records, follow the guideline above where facility preference is unknown.

When only the month and day are dictated, it is preferable for the medical transcriptionist to add the year, *if known*.

> D: The patient was seen on April 4th.
> T: The patient was seen on April 4, 2000. (if date is known)

6.7.4 Fractions

Use a virgule to separate the numerator from the denominator in fractions.

> 4/5
> 2/3
> 1/2

Do *not* use a virgule to separate these elements when they are expressed as words, not numerals. Use a hyphen instead.

> four-fifths
> two-thirds
> one-half

6.7.5 Visual Acuity

Express visual acuity with arabic numerals separated by a virgule.

> Visual acuity is 20/200, corrected to 20/40.

6.8 Quotation Marks

Quotation marks are used most often in clinical documentation to capture a direct statement or comment from the patient or others involved in the patient's history. Place quotation marks at the beginning and end of each quotation, being careful to capture only those elements that represent a direct quote.

6.8.1 Capitalization

Begin a complete quotation with a capital letter if the quoted material represents an independent clause.

EXAMPLE

> The pathology report reads, "Specimen is consistent with microadenoma."
> Despite my concern that she needed to be admitted, the patient adamantly refused admission, stating, "I don't trust hospitals, and I want to go home."

Do not capitalize the first word of a quotation if it represents a word, phrase, or dependent clause that has a grammatical relationship with the rest of the sentence.

EXAMPLE

> She says that she has "bad blood."
> The patient repeatedly mumbled the words "no needles" throughout the entire examination.

6.8.2 Punctuation

Punctuation marks typically fall inside the closing quotation marks to facilitate the unhindered punctuation of the sentence in which those quotations reside.

EXAMPLE

> The patient stated that "the itching is driving me crazy," and she scratched her arms throughout our meeting.
> The consultant's report reads, "The patient is a 21-year-old male referred to me by Dr. Wilson."
> Despite previously being told she has "sugar diabetes," the patient's glucose levels continue to be within the normal range.

The exceptions to the rule above apply to the use of question marks, exclamation points, and semicolons. Semicolons should always fall outside the quotation marks. However, to avoid this visually questionable construction, it is better to use other terminal punctuation, such as a period.

The patient clearly stated "no allergies"; however, his medical record states he is allergic to penicillin.
better:
The patient clearly stated "no allergies." However, his medical record states he is allergic to penicillin.

With question marks and exclamation points, their inclusion within the quoted material is dependent on meaning. Place the exclamation point or question mark inside the ending quotation mark if the material being quoted is being expressed as an exclamation or question. Place the exclamation point or question mark outside the ending quotation mark if the entire sentence, not the quoted material, represents the exclamation or question.

Patients frequently ask, "How long will I be out of work?"
She greeted me with "What's up?" when I entered her room.
Did she just say "help me"?
The patient yelled "No!" every time we came near him.
I want to walk into his office and say, "I quit!"
Stop saying "no"!

6.8.3 Feet and Inches

Do not use single or double quotation marks to represent feet and inches in dimensional expressions. Use the English units spelled out in full.

The patient is 5 feet 10 inches tall.
not:
The patient is 5'10" tall.

CHAPTER

7

Capitalization

Introduction

Capital letters serve many purposes. They serve to indicate the beginning of sentences and are an integral aid to the reader. They distinguish names, titles, and proper nouns from the rest of the sentence. Some, however, are merely conventions. They are usages adopted by people of formal education for no other reason than that they are customary. Conventional usage of capitalization sets the standard of expectation in formal writing.

The fundamental role of capitalization is to give distinction, importance or emphasis to words. A word is capitalized at the beginning of a sentence, for example, to clearly delineate that a new sentence has begun. In that role, capital letters serve as visual markers that assist the reader in transitioning from one concept to the next. Most words, however, are capitalized primarily to emphasize their identities as entities of significance. The medical transcriptionist who is expected to recognize those myriad entities will need to be knowledgeable and possess excellent referencing skills in order to ensure their accurate inclusion. Some terms (like *board of directors*) may function either as proper nouns or as common nouns, and an interpretive eye that understands the significance of those terms in context will be necessary in determining their application. Given the debate over the use of capitalization in formal writing (some experts feel that overusing capitalization results in the reality that when too many words stand out, none stand out), it is always important to let the need for clarity guide you in the use of capitalization for emphasis.

As in all other areas of language usage, inconsistencies can be found in the application of rules related to capitalization. In standard usage, for example, the names of seasons are not capitalized, but many print publications choose to capitalize them. Many of the rules outlined below will caution you to verify that the entity in question customarily capitalizes any or all of the words that refer to that entity. For example, it is important to know that "3M" is trademarked that way, with the arabic numeral and capital M without a space in between. This is where knowledge about proper names and/or the ability to verify them will be essential.

7.1 First Words

First words, or opening words, in a variety of expressions require capitalization to set them off from text around them, often to indicate the introduction of a new thought or concept.

7.1.1 Sentences
Capitalize the first word of every sentence.

EXAMPLE

> She comes in today complaining of worsening sinusitis.
> Why would he need this procedure?

Capitalize an independent question within a sentence.

EXAMPLE

> The question is, Do the benefits of this procedure outweigh the risks?
> The patient found herself wondering, How long can I live with this pain?

7.1.2 Quotations
Capitalize the first word of a quoted sentence. Capitalize the first word only when the quoted material represents an independent clause, or complete sentence. Do not capitalize the first word of quoted material when it represents a phrase or subordinate clause.

EXAMPLE

> When I asked her to explain her hesitation about the procedure, she said, "I hate anesthesia."
> The patient presented to the emergency room complaining of "pounding headaches" off and on for the last 4 days.

Note: Listen carefully when an author dictates quoted material to ensure that the quoted material accurately reflects what was stated.

EXAMPLE

> D: The patient stated he was quote just minding <u>his</u> own business unquote when another guy in the bar threw the first punch.
> T: The patient stated he was "just minding <u>my</u> own business" when another guy in the bar threw the first punch.

7.1.3 Following a Colon

Do *not* capitalize the first word after a colon if the material that follows is subordinate and cannot stand alone as a sentence.

EXAMPLE

> Two antibiotics are used in this case: <u>a</u>mpicillin and gentamycin.
> She was told to follow these guidelines: <u>r</u>est, ice, and elevate.

Do capitalize the first word after a colon if it is a proper noun or other word that is automatically capitalized.

EXAMPLE

> We will prescribe the appropriate protocol for her breast cancer: <u>T</u>axotere and carboplatin.

Capitalize the first word of an independent clause after a colon to express special emphasis or a formal rule/instruction.

EXAMPLE

> Let me say this: <u>T</u>he patient should not attempt to ambulate until her sutures are removed.
> Here is the key consideration: <u>C</u>esarean patients who did not have low-transverse incisions are poor candidates for VBAC due to risk of uterine rupture.

Capitalize the first word after a colon when the material following the colon consists of two or more sentences.

There are several risks to the procedure: First, there is the potential that her chronic pain will actually be made worse, not better. Second, she could have improvement in her pain but significant loss of mobility as a result.

Capitalize the first word after a colon when the material preceding the colon is a short introductory word such as *Note, Caution,* or *Wanted.*

Note: The patient denies any allergy to adhesives.

7.1.4 Lists and Outlines

Capitalize each item in a list or an outline, even when items in the list represent single words, phrases, or clauses.

The patient will be discharged home to:
1. Rest and elevate the arm.
2. Call for fevers over 101.5 or red streaks of infection running up the arm.
3. Return to my office in 2 days for wound check and bandage change.

7.1.5 Parenthetical Expressions

When a sentence, or independent clause, is set off by *dashes* or *parentheses* within another sentence, do not capitalize the first word following the opening dash or parenthesis (unless it is a proper noun or other word that is automatically capitalized).

She is a candidate for VBAC (she tells me she would like to attempt vaginal delivery, if possible), so we have noted that on her chart.

She complained today of some recurring ulcers in her mouth, and I have recommended she use one of the over-the-counter products for that (Orajel will work well for this).

When the information within parentheses or dashes represents a word, phrase, or subordinate clause, do not capitalize the first word.

EXAMPLE

> Given her risk factors (smoking and BCPs), I have told her that thrombotic events are much more of a concern.
> She will pick up her films–both the mammography and sonography reports from February–and bring them with her when she returns next week.

7.2 Titles and Designations

Capitalize major words in titles and designations. Be sure to consult a reputable source to verify the spelling and capitalization preferences for all titles and designations.

7.2.1 Titles with Personal Names

Capitalize all personal, executive, professional, civic, military, and religious titles when they precede personal names. *(See 6.1.1—Period)*.

EXAMPLE

> Mrs Mary Smith, Mrs. Mary Smith
> Ms Ashley Brooks, Ms. Ashley Brooks
> Vice President William Jones
> Professor David Taylor
> Dr Edward A. Washington, Dr. Edward A. Washington
> Mayor-elect Anita Wallace
> Colonel Walter C. Banks
> Reverend Andrew Howard

Do *not* capitalize such titles when the personal name that follows is an appositive, set off by commas.

EXAMPLE

> She was given the assignment by her professor, David Taylor.
> After each service, the reverend, Andrew Howard, meets with visitors in the main lobby.
> The patient was referred by his doctor, Edward Washington, for consultation.

Do *not* capitalize general occupational titles when they precede personal names. These can be readily distinguished from official titles by remembering that official titles can be used with a personal name when it stands alone; occupational titles cannot.

> I am fascinated by the books of author Robin Cook.
> She will be transferred to the care of surgeon Adam Winters.

Do *not* capitalize official titles when they follow a personal name or are used in its place. *Exceptions:* Retain capitalization for all high-ranking national officials, state officials, foreign dignitaries, and international figures.

> During his two terms as president, he worked tirelessly toward change in the organization.
> David Taylor, professor of chemistry at the university, will be honored at the banquet.
> She was appointed Secretary of State by the President.
> While in Rome, he had the honor of meeting the Pope.

Capitalize all official titles when used in direct address.

> Can you tell me, Reverend, what time your service starts?
> What I need to know, Doctor, is how long I will be out of work after the procedure.

7.2.2 Family Titles

Capitalize family titles such as *mother, sister, father, mom, dad,* etc., when they are followed by a personal name and when they stand alone.

> At the time of discharge, Mom and Dad were told their son is now at greater risk for febrile seizures and were instructed to watch this closely.
> I counseled Mom about the need to monitor her son's diet and exercise.
> The patient says she was brought to my office by Aunt Mary.

Do *not* capitalize family titles when they are preceded by a possessive pronoun or when they are preceded by an article, such as *the*.

I spoke to <u>her</u> <u>m</u>other and <u>f</u>ather about my concern for long-term disability as a result of her injury.
The patient said <u>his</u> <u>b</u>rother Steven would be coordinating his care.
The mom and dad were informed of the risks and benefits of the procedure.

7.2.3 Titles of Publications and Articles

Capitalize all words in literary and artistic titles except articles, short conjunctions, and short prepositions unless they occur as the first or last word of the title.

<u>T</u>he <u>P</u>ower of <u>P</u>ositive <u>T</u>hinking
<u>W</u>ho <u>M</u>oved <u>M</u>y <u>C</u>heese?
<u>H</u>ealth <u>D</u>ata <u>M</u>atrix
<u>A</u>utonomic <u>R</u>esponse in <u>D</u>epersonalization <u>D</u>isorder

Note: Do *not* capitalize the word *the* when it precedes a title unless it is part of the title.

the <u>N</u>ew <u>E</u>ngland <u>J</u>ournal of <u>M</u>edicine
the <u>J</u>ournal of the <u>A</u>merican <u>M</u>edical <u>A</u>ssociation
<u>T</u>he <u>N</u>ew <u>Y</u>ork <u>T</u>imes

Titles of articles take *initial capitals* only when they are used in a reference or source citation.

Sierra M, Senior C, Dalton J. <u>A</u>utonomic response in depersonalization disorder. *Arch Gen Psychiatry.* 2002;59(8):100-103.

Treat unique documents and forms within a medical facility as you would an article. Generic references would not be capitalized. However, a document or form uniquely created and named by a facility should be capitalized when it is referenced within the document. Likewise, when a reference to a specific form or document could be confused for a common noun or phrase, it is best to use initial capitals for the name of the form being referenced.

sign-in sheet
admission form
anesthesia permission form

but:

Dermatology Patient Intake Questionnaire
Permission to Use Anesthesia form

7.2.4 Credentials

Capitalize the abbreviated forms of professional credentials, especially when they follow a personal name. Do *not* capitalize credentials that are spelled out when they are generally referenced in a sentence unless they follow a personal name as a formal title.

She is a CMT.
Lisa Johnson, CMT
She became a certified medical transcriptionist in 1995.
James A. Smith, MD
James A. Smith, Doctor of Medicine

7.2.5 Academic Degrees and References

Do *not* capitalize academic degrees used in general description or classification. Do capitalize academic degrees that follow a personal name as a formal title.

She has a bachelor of arts in education from the University of Florida.
He is working on his master's degree in science.
Robert Adler, Doctor of Sociology

Do *not* capitalize the words *freshman, sophomore, junior,* and *senior.* Capitalize the word *grade* when referring to grade levels only when a number follows it but not when a number precedes it.

> She is a freshman in college this year.
> The patient is spending his junior year up North with his mother.
> The patient lives at home with her parents and is in Grade 6.
> The patient lives at home with her parents and is in the sixth grade.

7.2.6 Legal References

Do *not* capitalize general references to legal terms, such as *power of attorney, living will,* etc., unless the full formal name of the law or document is referenced.

EXAMPLE

> The patient's husband has power of attorney for her care decisions.
> We requested a copy of her Durable Medical Power of Attorney.

7.3 Proper Nouns

Capitalize all proper nouns or official names of a person, place, or thing. Do *not* capitalize these nouns when they function as common nouns.

7.3.1 Personal Names

Capitalize a person's name with careful attention to that person's preference for expression. Likewise, you should verify personal preference for spelling and inclusive punctuation.

EXAMPLE

> George H. W. Bush
> Sara Beth *or* Sarah Beth
> Steven L. Smith, Jr. *or* Stephen L. Smith Jr

Capitalize the *O'* prefix in names that contain it as well as the letter that follows the apostrophe.

EXAMPLE

> O'Keefe
> O'Brian
> *not:*
> O'brian

7.3.2 Organizational Designations

Express *business names*—companies, unions, associations, societies, independent committees/boards, schools, political parties, conventions, foundations, fraternities, sororities, clubs, and religious organizations—according to the business's style and usage. Use the full name before using the abbreviated form to avoid confusion among similar abbreviations except for businesses (such as IBM) that are better known by their abbreviations than by their full names. Retain inclusive symbols only when it is known that to do so is the organization's preference.

EXAMPLE

AT&T
the University of Florida
St. John's United Methodist Church
the Committee for Economic Development
Wal-Mart
Alpha Delta Pi Sorority
Association for Healthcare Documentation Integrity
Campbell Soup Company

When the common noun (*company, association, society,* etc.) is used in place of the full name, do *not* capitalize the short form unless special emphasis is required (legal documents, meeting minutes, bylaws, formal communications, etc.) or when the common noun is personified (*See 7.4.2—Personification*).

EXAMPLE

The association was founded in 1978 in Modesto, California.
The company has been suffering from a 3-year downward trend in sales.
The Association announced today that it will be conducting a yearlong research study on salary trends.

Capitalize the abbreviated forms of *company, corporation, incorporated,* and *limited* when the business name incorporates those abbreviations in its formal name or title. Do not precede these abbreviations with a comma.

EXAMPLE

Ford Motor Co.
Apple Inc.
Target Corp.

7.3.3 Eponyms

Capitalize eponyms, or words named after a person. Eponyms are extremely common in medical language, where many diseases, signs, syndromes, tests, procedures, instruments, and surgical equipment names are named after the person(s) who invented, created, or discovered those things. Some eponyms are named after patients in whom a new sign, syndrome, or disease was identified.

EXAMPLE

Homans sign
Lyme disease
Down syndrome
Lou Gehrig disease
Wolff-Parkinson-White syndrome

Do *not* capitalize the adjectival or verbal forms derived from eponyms.

EXAMPLE

parkinsonism (from Parkinson disease)
cushingoid (from Cushing syndrome)
bovied (from Bovie cautery)
gram-negative (from Gram stain)
brussels sprouts (from Brussels)
arabic numerals (from Arabia)

Do capitalize the adjectival forms of words derived from proper nouns that are *not* eponyms, most of which represent geographic designations.

EXAMPLE

American (from America)
Norwegian (from Norway)
Spanish (from Spain)

7.3.4 Departments, Divisions, and Specialties

Departments and Divisions: Do *not* capitalize common organizational terms such as *department, division,* or *committee* when they are expressed as general reference. This includes organizational terms unique to the clinic or acute care setting such as *clinic, laboratory, emergency room, intensive care unit,* etc. Because these terms represent areas, departments, or divisions that are common to many or all facilities, they should be treated as common nouns and not capitalized in general reference. *(see examples next page)*

He works as an OR tech in the department of surgery at St. Mary's Hospital.
She was transferred to the floor from the emergency room.
The patient will have her tests performed in the laboratory of Baptist Hospital.
The procedure will be done down in the outpatient surgery center.
He will follow up in the eye clinic next week.

Capitalize the common organizational terms above when they are part of the formal name, including part of a federal government agency name.

He works for the State Department in Washington, DC.
I am referring the patient to Anderson-Evans Surgery Center.
The patient presents with his previous records from The Mayo Clinic in Jacksonville.
Her insurance requires her to have her blood work done at Quest Labs.
The Division of Blind Services will be contacting her to assess her new needs in the workplace.

Specialties: Much confusion exists with certain words that can function as both common nouns *and* organizational entities. Certain common nouns like *anesthesia, pathology, surgery, radiology, housekeeping, cardiology, dialysis,* etc., have unique meanings that have nothing to do with an organizational term. The word *anesthesia*, when used as a common noun, refers to "loss of sensation" or a drug that produces the same. The words *pathology, radiology, cardiology,* and other similar terms refer to medical specialties or "the study of" something. However, each of these common nouns is frequently referred to as an organizational entity, given personifying characteristics or used to substitute for the departments or individuals involved in the application of those common terms. When they are functioning in the sentence as an organizational entity, they should be capitalized. When it is their primary or common meaning that is being referred to in the sentence, they should *not* be capitalized. In most cases, when these words function as organizational entities, you will be able to identify them either by their obvious personification or by determining whether they are functioning as a departmental entity. It is usually helpful to substitute both the definition of the word and the full departmental entity in place of the word to see which makes sense in context.

> She will be given general induction <u>a</u>nesthesia prior to the procedure.
> *Substitute:* She will be given general induction "drug for loss of sensation" prior to the procedure. (correct)
> *Substitute:* She will be given general induction "the anesthesia department" prior to the procedure. (incorrect)
>
> She was referred to <u>A</u>nesthesia for presurgical consult this morning.
> *Substitute:* She was referred to "the anesthesia department" for presurgical consult this morning. (correct)
> *Substitute:* She was referred to "loss of sensation" prior to the procedure. (incorrect)
>
> The specimen was sent for <u>p</u>athology.
> *Substitute:* The specimen was sent for "study or evaluation of disease." (correct)
> *Substitute:* The specimen was sent for "the pathology department." (incorrect)
>
> The specimen was sent to <u>P</u>athology.
> *Substitute:* The specimen was sent to "the pathology department." (correct)
> *Substitute:* The specimen was sent to "study or evaluation of disease." (incorrect)

Note: In the last two examples, the words *for* and *to* determine the function of the word.

7.3.5 Drug Terminology

Brand Names: The brand name is the manufacturer's name for a drug; it is the same as the trade name, trademark, or proprietary name. It may suggest a use or indication, and it often incorporates the manufacturer's name. Capitalize brand names, trade names, and trademark names. Refer to a reputable pharmacology reference or resource to confirm brand status.

> <u>T</u>agamet
> <u>T</u>ylenol
> <u>V</u>incristine
> <u>A</u>ugmentin

Many brand names use idiosyncratic, or mixed, capitalization in their names. Defer to facility preference for the retention of idiosyncratic capitalization, as both are generally acceptable.

EXAMPLE

> pHisoHex *or* Phisohex
> GlycoLax *or* Glycolax
> PediaCare *or* Pediacare
> NyQuil *or* Nyquil

Exception: Chemotherapy protocols and investigational agents that use idiosyncratic capitalization should be transcribed that way. In many instances the capitalized portions of those terms represent acronyms that identify specific protocol components.

EXAMPLE

> CyHOP
> m-BACOD
> DCVax-Brain
> COBARTin

Generic Names: The generic name, also known as the nonproprietary name, is the established, official name for a drug. In the United States, it is created by the US Adopted Names (USAN) Council. International nomenclature is coordinated by the World Health Organization. Generic names are in the public domain; their use is unrestricted. Do *not* capitalize generic names. When the generic name and brand names of a medication sound alike, use the generic spelling unless it is certain the brand name is being referenced. Refer to a reputable pharmacology reference or resource to confirm generic status.

EXAMPLE

> aminophylline
> penicillin
> epinephrine
> lithium
> polymyxin
> prednisone

Do *not* capitalize illegal/illicit drug names or their street references.

marijuana
cocaine
crack
heroin

Do *not* capitalize medicinal herb names used in alternative medicine.
Do capitalize the proper nouns that accompany them.

mugwort
saffron
ginkgo biloba
ginseng

St. John's wort
St. James weed

Do not confuse the medicinal herb names with their genus/species names.
When these are used, capitalize the genus, but not the species, name.
(See 7.3.6—Organisms—below)

Crocus sativus (saffron)
Zingiber officinale (ginger)
Hypericum perforatum (St. John's wort)

7.3.6 Organisms
Always capitalize genus names and their abbreviated forms when they are
accompanied by a species name.

Haemophilus influenzae, H influenzae
Escherichia coli, E coli
Staphylococcus aureus, S aureus

Do *not* capitalize genus names used in plural and adjectival forms or when used in the vernacular or when they stand alone (without a species name).

staphylococcus
group B streptococcus
staphylococci
staphylococcal infection
staph infection
strep throat

The suffixes *–osis* and *–iasis* indicate disease caused by a particular class of infectious agents or types of infection. Do *not* capitalize terms formed with these suffixes.

amebiasis
dermatophytosis

7.3.7 Geographic Names

Capitalize the names of places—countries, cities, towns, counties, continents, islands, streets, buildings, parks, airports, peninsulas, bodies of water, monuments, forests, canyons, dams, mountains, and regions—when they name a specific location by proper name. Do *not* capitalize the names of places described by common nouns in general reference.

the Antarctic
Persian Gulf
Central America
Duval County
Hoover Dam
LaGuardia International Airport
The Bronx
555 W. State Street
Upstate New York

The common geographical name is *not* capitalized in compound expressions.

> Indian and Pacific oceans
> Jefferson and Adams streets
> Mississippi and Missouri rivers

Some common geographic names are capitalized purely because of their clear association with a particular place but only when that association is unambiguous in context.

> the Hill (Capitol Hill)
> the Continent (Europe)
> the Village (Greenwich Village)
> the Big Apple (New York)
> the Twin Cities

Capitalize the word *city* only when it is part of the name of the city, or in the nickname of that city.

> Carson City
> the Windy City (Chicago)

7.3.8 Sociocultural Designations

Capitalize the names of races, languages, nationalities, ethnicities, tribes, political parties, religions, and religious denominations. Do *not* capitalize *white* or *black* as a designation of race. *(see examples next page)*

EXAMPLE

African American
Chinese woman
English language
Native Americans
Hispanics
Latina female
the French
Methodist
Hindi
Republican
Democrat
single white female

Do *not* capitalize references to general religious observances unless they are formed from proper nouns.

EXAMPLE

baptism
bar mitzvah
seder
communion

7.3.9 Events, Awards, and Legislation

Capitalize the names of special and historical events, but not the common nouns that may accompany them.

EXAMPLE

the Great Depression
Revolutionary War
Civil War era
D-day

Capitalize the names of awards, medals, and honors.

EXAMPLE

Nobel Peace Prize
Congressional Medal of Honor
Academy Award

Capitalize the formal titles of acts, laws, bills, and treaties, but do not capitalize the common nouns that are used in place of them.

Americans with Disabilities Act
the Treaty of Versailles
Family and Medical Leave Act of 1993
Public Law 89-74

but:

the act
the law
the treaty
the amendment

7.3.10 Computer Terms

Refer to a reputable resource for programming languages and operating systems that are written in all capitals.

BASIC
COBOL
FORTRAN
MS-DOS
OS/2

Refer to a reputable resource for software applications that are expressed as compound nouns requiring a capital letter at the beginning of each element.

WordPerfect
PageMaker
PowerPoint

Use initial caps with computer *commands, functions,* or *features.*

Use the Back button on your browser to return to the home page.
Put a word or phrase in the box and click Search.
You will find that email in my Saved Items folder.

7.3.11 Compass Points

Capitalize *north, south, east,* and *west* and words derived from these terms (*eastern, southeastern,* etc.) when they identify a specific region or are part of a proper name.

out West
in the North
the Midwest
the North Pole
the East Coast
Southern hospitality

Do *not* capitalize these words when they are expressed as general direction or location.

Travel west on the interstate until you reach exit 20.
She lives on the east side of town.
The forecast indicated easterly winds.

7.3.12 Times, Seasons, and Holidays

Capitalize the days, months, holidays, and religious days.

Tuesday
March
Christmas
Hanukkah
Ramadan
Martin Luther King Day
Good Friday

Do not capitalize the names of seasons unless they are personified.

The AHDI annual convention is in late summer.
Every fall, she comes to stay with her sister here in Florida.
I have always found Winter to be an unwelcome friend.

7.3.13 Programs and Concepts

Do not capitalize the names of *programs*, *movements*, or *concepts* when they are used as general reference and are not part of a proper name.

social security check	Social Security Administration
civil rights activist	Civil Rights Act
libertarian ideas	Libertarian Party

7.3.14 Referenced Report Headings

When a heading is referred to in the body of the report, use *initial capitals* for each word in the heading (except articles and prepositions) to clearly delineate the reference as a proper heading and not a common noun or phrase. Though the heading itself may have been formatted in all capitals, reference to that heading elsewhere in the report should *not* be expressed in all capitals.

For further information, please refer to the Past Medical History.
REVIEW OF SYSTEMS: Normal, except as noted in the History of Present Illness.

However, when it is clear in context that the physician is not referencing a specific section of the report but is, instead, using the phrase as a general reference, do *not* capitalize or delineate as a formal title.

EXAMPLE

Her past medical history includes an allergy to penicillin.
The patient presented to the emergency room with a chief complaint of protracted nausea and vomiting.

7.4 Special Rules

There are some capitalization rules that fall outside of the titles and proper nouns outlined above and must be categorized separately.

7.4.1 Acronyms and Initialisms

Do *not* capitalize the words from which an acronym or initialism is derived (*See Chapter 9—Abbreviations*) unless the words from which the acronym is an official name, title, or proper noun.

EXAMPLE

coronary artery bypass grafting (CABG)
peripheral vascular disease (PVD)
New York Heart Association (NYHA)

Be aware that some case studies, protocols, and clinical trials are given acronyms that do not always represent initialisms, where the abbreviation is formed by the first letters of each word. They are given their acronyms to facilitate ease of identification and reference. Do *not* use unusual capitalization to indicate how the study name was derived. Refer to a reputable resource to verify both the name of the study and its derived acronym. These should be in all capitals when used in their acronym forms. When spelled out, follow the guidelines for formal titles outlined above. (*See 7.2—Titles and Designations*)

EXAMPLE

Evaluation of Platelet IIb/IIa Inhibitor for Stenting (EPISTENT)
Clopidogrel as Adjunctive Reperfusion Therapy (CLARITY)
C7E3 Fab AntiPlatelet Therapy in Unstable Refractory Angina (CAPTURE)

7.4.2 Personification

Places or things that are assigned the *qualities, actions,* or *characteristics* of a person are called *personified* nouns. Nouns functioning in a personified role in a sentence should be capitalized. Some nouns are capitalized whether personified or not because they already represent proper nouns. They are said to be personified, however, when they are assigned human qualities.

EXAMPLE

> She has been a member of the association for 10 years. (common)
> The Association announced today that it would be increasing member dues. (personified)
> The patient spends much of his time outdoors enjoying nature and wildlife. (common)
> There is no one more unpredictable than Mother Nature. (personified)
> She went on a White House tour while visiting Washington, DC. (proper)
> The White House issued a statement regarding the tragic events. (personified)

Personification refers to the concept of giving an inanimate object human, or animated, qualities. In the example above, *Association* is capitalized and personified in the instance of "the Association announced." Obviously an association does not have a human mouth and cannot literally announce anything. In those instances, the common noun takes on the role of a human, and thus is capitalized to differentiate it from its common noun usage.

7.4.3 Hyphenated Compounds

Capitalize only those elements of a hyphenated word that are proper nouns or proper adjectives when they occur *within a sentence*. Capitalize only the first element of a hyphenated word when it occurs *at the beginning of a sentence*.

EXAMPLE

> We watched a documentary about ex-President Gerald Ford.
> Ex-President Gerald Ford was featured in a documentary I watched this weekend.
> I told the patient to follow up with me in mid-September.
> Mid-September surgeries will be rescheduled.

When hyphenated compounds occur in *headings, titles, subtitles* or *tables*, do *not* capitalize the second part of a hyphenated compound if either part is a hyphenated prefix or suffix or if the compound is commonly read as a unit (consult a reputable medical dictionary for verification).

Long-term Treatment of Rheumatoid Arthritis
Full-time Respiratory Therapist

Some compounds represent words that are not commonly read as a unit and carry equal weight in the compound. When that is the case, both parts should be capitalized when used in headings, titles, etc.

B-Cell Lymphoma
Drug-Resistant Bacteria

Section 2: General Standards of Style

CHAPTER

8

Plurals and Possessives

Introduction

The rules for pluralizing and expressing possession are pretty straightforward but critical for the detailed transcriptionist to pay close attention to, particularly as they apply to eponyms, foreign terms, and unusual formations, since authors will not always dictate these accurately.

8.1 Plurals

The basic rules for pluralization are outlined below. When you are unsure about the plural form of a word, consult a dictionary or reputable resource. When the dictionary lists more than one plural form, the first is usually the preferred one.

8.1.1 Basic Rules

Follow general rules for forming noun plurals based on the noun ending. Add *s* to most nouns in the singular form to form the plural.

EXAMPLE

    cats
    dogs
    patients
    checks
    ideas

Form the plural by adding *es* to words ending in *s*, *x*, *ch*, *sh*, or *z*.

taxes
lunches
sashes
quartzes

Form the plural by adding *s* or *es* to nouns ending in *y* depending on whether the *y* is preceded by a consonant or vowel. When preceded by a consonant, change *y* to *i* and add *es*. When preceded by a vowel, add *s*.

copy	copies
family	families
party	parties
delay	delays
pray	prays
key	keys
toy	toys

Form the plural by adding *s* to nouns ending in *o* when preceded by a vowel.

stereo	stereos
ratio	ratios
tattoo	tattoos

Singular nouns ending in *o* preceded by a consonant can take variable plural forms. Some add *s* and some add *es*. Consult a dictionary for confirmation.

ego	egos
banjo	banjos
potato	potatoes
echo	echoes

Singular nouns ending in *f, ef,* or *ff* form their plurals either by adding *s* or by changing the *f* or *ef* to *ve* and adding *s*.

EXAMPLE

cliff	cliffs
belief	beliefs
bailiff	bailiffs
roof	roofs
but:	
half	halves
hoof	hooves
leaf	leaves
knife	knives

8.1.2 Irregular Forms

Nouns whose plurals are formed in unusual ways are considered irregular forms. Consult a dictionary for confirmation of these irregular plurals.

EXAMPLE

woman	women
mouse	mice
moose	moose
child	children

Some words are always singular in usage.

EXAMPLE

ascites
herpes
lues

Some words are always plural in usage.

EXAMPLE

adnexa
genitalia

Some words retain the same form, whether singular or plural.

biceps, triceps, quadriceps
facies
series
forceps
scissors

Some words are dictated incorrectly as nouns but are actually adjectives. Recast the sentence by using the modifying form with its noun.

D: She had multiple decubiti on her back and buttocks.
T: She had multiple decubitus ulcers on her back and buttocks.

8.1.3 Compound Nouns

Compounds are expressed as separate spaced words, single words, or hyphenated words. For single-word compounds, pluralize the final element of the word as though it stands alone.

birthday	birthdays
backpack	backpacks
doghouse	doghouses
strawberry	strawberries

For spaced words or hyphenated compounds, pluralize the chief noun of the compound.

father-in-law	fathers-in-law
leave of absence	leaves of absence
runner-up	runners-up
passerby	passersby

Section 2: General Standards of Style

If the compound does *not* contain a noun, pluralize the final element.

EXAMPLE

know-it-all	know-it-alls (*not* knows-it-all)
run-through	run-throughs (*not* runs-through)
hang-up	hang-ups (*not* hangs-up)

Form the plural of compounds ending in *ful* by adding *s*.

EXAMPLE

teaspoonfuls (*not* teaspoonsful)
cupfuls (*not* cupsful)

8.1.4 Proper Nouns

Pluralize surnames by adding *s* unless they end in *s*, *x*, *ch*, *sh*, or *z*, in which case you should add *es* to pluralize.

EXAMPLE

the Smiths
the Maxwells
the Bushes
the Joneses

Pluralize proper names by adding *s* or *es* based on word ending, but be careful to retain original spelling.

EXAMPLE

Marys
Johns
Texans
Christmases
Februarys
Rolexes

8.1.5 Personal Titles

Pluralized personal titles are rarely ever encountered in the health record, and when they are dictated, it is best to list the titles separately than to use plural titles, which are used only in rare and extremely formal situations, such as on event invitations.

> Messrs Smith and Wesson (formal usage)
> Mr Smith and Mr Wesson (ordinary usage)
> Misses Jones and Abernathy (formal usage)
> Miss Jones and Miss Abernathy (ordinary usage)

It is not uncommon for an author to refer to more than one physician using a pluralized personal title. Again, list the titles separately.

> D: She will be referred to doctors Lewis and Kendrick.
> T: She will be referred to Dr Lewis and Dr Kendrick.
> *not:*
> T: She will be referred to Drs Lewis and Kendrick.
>
> D: Dear doctors Lewis and Kendrick:
> T: Dear Dr Lewis and Dr Kendrick:

8.1.6 Diagnoses

When multiple diagnoses are dictated, express pluralization in the heading to reflect the same, even if the singular form of the heading is dictated.

> *Dictated:*
> Diagnosis...status post motor vehicle accident, laceration to right eyebrow, and neck strain.
>
> *Transcribed:*
> DIAGNOSES
> 1. Status post motor vehicle accident.
> 2. Laceration to right eyebrow.
> 3. Neck strain.

When a patient presents with a group of symptoms and the diagnosis is unclear, the clinician may refer in the medical report to the *differential diagnosis* in order to compare and contrast the clinical findings of each. Although it consists of two or more possible diagnoses, the term is singular and always takes a singular verb.

EXAMPLE

The differential <u>diagnosis is</u> myocardial infarction versus costochondritis versus gastrointestinal etiology.

not:

The differential <u>diagnoses are</u> myocardial infarction versus costochondritis versus gastrointestinal etiology.

8.1.7 Abbreviations

Form the plural of most abbreviations, except for units of measure, by adding *s* to the singular form.

EXAMPLE

bldg.	bldgs.
No.	Nos.
but:	
mm	mm
mcg	mcg
dL	dL
cc	cc (carbon copies)
mL	mL
mg	mg

Form the plural of uppercase abbreviations by adding *s*.

EXAMPLE

ABGs
WBCs
EEGs
CMTs
PhDs
VIPs

Form the plural of lowercase abbreviations by adding an apostrophe plus *s*.

wbc's
rbc's
c.o.d.'s

Form the plural of brief forms by adding *s*.

exams
segs
polys
lymphs
labs

8.1.8 Numbers and Letters

Double-digit numbers expressed as figures are pluralized by adding *s*. Single-digit numbers are pluralized by adding an apostrophe plus *s*.

She retired in the early 1990s.
Diastolic pressures were in the 110s.
She is in her 20s.
She scored four 5's on the questionnaire.

Numbers expressed in words are pluralized by adding *s* or *es*.

ones
tens
twenty-ones

Single letters are pluralized by adding an apostrophe plus *s*.

> flipped T's
> inverted Q's
> three A's and two B's

8.1.9 Microorganisms

When referring to the common plural of a genus, use lowercase letters. For organisms that do not have a common plural, add the word *species* or *organisms* to the genus name to indicate a plural use. Consult a dictionary to confirm the existence of a widely accepted plural form.

Chlamydia	chlamydiae
Escherichia	Escherichia organisms
Mycobacterium	mycobacteria
Proteus	Proteus species
Pseudomonas	pseudomonads
Salmonella	salmonellae
Staphylococcus	staphylococci
Streptococcus	streptococci

8.1.10 False Singulars

Be careful of nouns that sound plural but are, in fact, singular in their usage.

> measles
> mumps
> mathematics
> genetics

8.1.11 Foreign Terms

The current lexicography of medical language is vast and complex. This living and constantly evolving language has been profoundly influenced over time by a diverse number of cultural and linguistic sources, many of which are still evident in the language today. While certainly the English medical terms with which we are familiar can be etymologically traced to earlier language forms, there are quite a few foreign terms that remain unaltered in circular usage today.

The influence of foreign language is evident throughout medical terminology. Most anatomical terms are either derived from the Latin or Greek (*abdomen* from *abdominis*) or still referred to by their Latin or Greek names (*rectus abdominis, flexor digitorum profundus,* etc.). Medical language is also peppered with other terms of international origin, such as French (*torsade de pointes, curettage, cerclage,* etc.) and German (*blitz, ersatz, mittelschmerz,* etc.). When encountered in dictation, they should be transcribed as dictated, with the exception that providers are not always accurate in the dictation of singular and plural forms of Latin and Greek terms. This section will provide insight into the standards as they relate to foreign terms, but pay particular attention to the rules for singular and plural forms of these terms. As a medical transcriptionist, you will be expected to recognize the context of these terms and determine if the singular or plural form is appropriate, regardless of how the term may be dictated.

Do not italicize foreign abbreviations, words, and phrases used in medical reports. Capitalize, punctuate, and space according to the standards of the language of origin. Omit accent marks except in proper names or where current usage retains them. In electronic environments where accent marks are restricted, drop them to prevent document formatting and conversion problems.

EXAMPLE

cul-de-sac
en masse
facade
i.e.
in vivo
naive
peau d'orange
resumé

Do not translate foreign words or abbreviations unless the originator translates them.

Greek Letters: Spell out the English translation when the word stands alone. Do not capitalize English translations. Use the Greek letter or spell it out when it is part of an extended term, according to the preferred form; consult appropriate references for guidance.

EXAMPLE

alpha	α
beta	β
gamma	γ

In extended terms, use of a hyphen after the Greek letter is optional, but the hyphen is not used after the English translation.

EXAMPLE

β-globulin or B globulin
beta globulin

Medical terms derived from Latin or Greek: General rules for pluralizing these foreign terms follow. Consult appropriate medical dictionaries for additional guidance.

Form the plural of words ending in *–en* by changing *–en* to *–ina.*

EXAMPLE

foramen	foramina

Form the plural of words ending in *–a* by adding *–e.*

EXAMPLE

conjunctiva	conjunctivae
urethra	urethrae
vertebra	vertebrae
fossa	fossae

Form the plural of words ending in –us by changing –us to –i.

meniscus	menisci
embolus	emboli
monticulus	monticuli
staphylococcus	staphylococci
exceptions:	
meatus	meatus
processus	processus

Form the plural of words ending in –on by changing –on to –a .

ganglion	ganglia
criterion	criteria
encephalon	encephala

Form the plural of words ending in –is by changing –is to –es.

diagnosis	diagnoses
prognosis	prognoses
epiphysis	epiphyses
crisis	crises
exceptions:	
arthritis	arthritides
epididymis	epididymides

Form the plural of words ending in –um by changing –um to –a.

diverticulum	diverticula
folium	folia
epithelium	epithelia
endocardium	endocardia

Form the plural of words ending in *–ix* or *–ex* by changing those endings to *–ices*.

index	indices
appendix	appendices
fornix	fornices
cortex	cortices

The plural forms of Latin terms that consist of a noun-adjective combination are often difficult to determine. (In Latin, the adjective must agree in number, gender, and case with the noun it modifies.) In the following list we show such terms in their singular and plural forms; they are all in the nominative case.

singular	plural
processus vaginalis	processus vaginales
chorda tendinea	chordae tendineae
verruca vulgaris	verrucae vulgares
nucleus pulposus	nuclei pulposi
pars interarticularis	partes interarticulares
placenta previa	placentae previae
musculus trapezius	musculi trapezii

Sometimes the genitive case (used in Latin to show possession) is misread as a plural, causing confusion. The following terms consist, for the most part, of a noun in the nominative case plus a noun in the genitive case.

Latin term	English translation
abruptio placentae	rupture of the placenta
bulbus urethrae	bulb of the urethra, bulbous urethra
cervix uteri	neck of uterus, uterine cervix
chondromalacia patellae	chondromalacia of the patella
corpus uteri	body of uterus, uterine corpus
os calcis	bone(s) of the heel(s); (plural: ossa calcium)
os coxae	bone(s) of the hip(s); (plural: ossa coxae)
pars uterina placentae	part of the placenta derived from uterine tissue
pruritus vulvae	itching of the vulva
muscularis mucosa	muscular (layer) of mucosa
lamina muscularis mucosae	muscular (layer) of mucosa associated with the lamina

Note: Transcriptionists should be particularly careful when erroneously combined forms of Latin terms are dictated. Consult a reputable dictionary or resource to confirm the correct expressions of these terms.

EXAMPLE

> D: neuroforaminal narrowing
> T: neural foraminal narrowing

8.1.12 Use of *Bilateral*

Bilateral is an adjective that may modify either a plural or a singular noun, depending upon the meaning.

EXAMPLE

> bilateral decision (a decision made by people on both sides of an issue acting together)
> bilateral pneumonia (one condition that is present in both lungs at the same time)
> bilateral mastectomies (two breasts, both removed separately)
> bilateral tympanostomies (separate tubes placed in both ears)
> bilateral tube insertions (separate tube insertions)

Sometimes authors use the word *bilateral* when they mean *both*. When this happens, the MT should substitute the word *both* or recast the sentence.

EXAMPLE

> D: There were lesions on bilateral hands.
> T: There were lesions on both hands.
> *or:*
> T: There were bilateral hand lesions.

8.2 Possessives

There are general and specialized rules for showing possession, as well as exceptions to these rules. Some of these rules and exceptions follow. Consult appropriate resources when in doubt about the formation of a possessive.

8.2.1 Singular Nouns

Express possession of singular nouns *not* ending in s by adding an apostrophe plus s to the noun.

EXAMPLE

patient's medication
children's hospital
Mary's admission
New York's football team

The expression of possession for singular nouns that end in s is determined by pronunciation. If a new syllable is formed in the pronunciation of the possessive, add an apostrophe plus s to the noun.

EXAMPLE

boss's instructions
witness's testimony
Congress's role
Dallas's transportation system
Mr Fernandez's decision

If a new syllable is not formed (or would be awkwardly formed) in the pronunciation of the possessive, add an apostrophe only.

EXAMPLE

Moses' flight to Egypt
Mr Cummings' office
goodness' sake
Dr Hodges' schedule

8.2.2 Plural Nouns

Express possession for nouns that end in s or es by adding only an apostrophe.

EXAMPLE

coaches' decision
patients' preferences
attorneys' fees
the Jones' address

Pay particular attention to meaning to ensure the appropriate use of a singular versus a plural noun when forming possession.

EXAMPLE

witness's or witnesses'?
patient's or patients'?

In some cases, a resource will be the only guide for determing the singular or plural status of a common possessive term.

EXAMPLE

deacon's bench
not:
deacons' bench

Parsons table
not:
Parson's table
not:
Parsons' table

Express possession of irregular plural nouns, those that do not end in s or es, by adding an apostrophe plus s.

EXAMPLE

women's clothing
mice's cage
children's books

8.2.3 Organizational Names

Express possession of a personal or organizational name that ends in an abbreviation, number, or prepositional phrase by adding an apostrophe plus *s*.

> Apple Inc.'s new product
> Bank of America's interest rates
> Edward Smith Jr's business address

When an organizational name or title contains words that can be interpreted as either possessive or descriptive, follow these guidelines: (a) use an apostrophe plus *s* if the term is a singular possessive noun or an irregular plural noun, *or* (b) do not use an apostrophe if the term is a descriptive plural that does not imply ownership or possession.

> Children's Hospital (irregular plural noun)
> Wendy's hamburgers (singular possessive noun)
> Harper's Bazaar (singular possessive noun)
> Women's Birthing Center (irregular plural noun)
> *but:*
> educators conference (regular plural)
> teachers lounge (regular plural)
> American Bankers Association (regular plural)
> US Department of Veterans Affairs (regular plural)

When contemplating the guidelines above, always defer to the organization's preference, when known.

> Boys' Clubs of America
> Diners Club
> Mrs Paul's fish sticks
> Mrs Fields cookies

8.2.4 Compounds

Express possession of *singular* compound nouns (whether one word, separate words, or hyphenated) by adding an apostrophe plus *s*.

daughter-in-law's opinion
owner-operator's license
attorney general's decision
living will's stipulations
notary public's signature
backpack's contents

Express possession of *plural* compounds (whether one word, separate words, or hyphenated) by first forming the plural. Add only an apostrophe if the plural form ends in *s*. Add an apostrophe plus *s* if the plural form does not already end in *s*.

assistant principal	assistant principals	assistant principals'
stockbroker	stockbrokers	stockbrokers'
follicle-stimulator	follicle-stimulators	follicle-stimulators'
but:		
editor in chief	editors in chief	editors in chief's
mother-in-law	mothers-in-law	mothers-in-law's
notary public	notaries public	notaries public's

Note: Consider recasting the sentence to avoid the use of possessive plural forms that do not end in *s*.

D: She got two notaries public's signatures on the form.
T: She got the signature of two notaries public on the form.

8.2.5 Pronouns

Express possession of *personal pronouns* by selecting the possessive form for each.

mine
hers
yours
its
ours
theirs

Express possession of the relative pronoun *who* by selecting the possessive form *whose*.

Do not confuse personal possessive pronouns with similarly spelled contractions. Since contractions are to be avoided in clinical records, there should be no instance where these personal pronouns contain an apostrophe.

Each kit comes with its own instructions. (*not* it's)
I know it is only a matter of time until I have to have surgery. (*not* it's)

Express possession of *indefinite pronouns* by adding an apostrophe and s with the exception of those pronouns that do not have possessive forms.

anyone else's opinion
somebody's problem
each other's needs
no one's responsibility

but:
needs of each
not:
each's needs

8.2.6 Abbreviations
Express possession of *singular* abbreviations by adding an apostrophe plus *s*.

MD's diagnosis
CMT's test scores
the AMA's recommendation

Express possession of *plural* abbreviations by adding an *s* plus an apostrophe.

MDs' diagnoses
CMTs' test scores
CPAs' meeting

8.2.7 Eponyms
AHDI first advocated dropping the possessive form for eponyms in 1990. We adopted this standard because it promotes consistency and clarity. Likewise, *The AMA Manual of Style* and other industry resources have acknowledged this trend away from the possessive form. It is important to note, however, that use of the possessive form is acceptable in environments where client or facility preference prevails.

Apgar score
Babinski sign
Down syndrome
Gram stain
Hodgkin lymphoma
Alzheimer disease
Lou Gehrig disease

When the noun following the eponym is omitted, the possessive form is preferred (*See 8.2.9—Solitary Possessives below*).

The patient reports a great deal of stress associated with caring for a parent with Alzheimer's.
She was diagnosed with Hodgkin's in early 2002.

8.2.8 Separate/Joint Possession

When two or more individuals are used to show *separate* possession (or ownership), express possession separately with each individual. Usually, the use of the word *the* with each individual stresses separate possession.

EXAMPLE

> the doctor's and the patient's signatures
> *not:*
> the doctor and the patient's signatures
>
> the Williams' and the Smith's houses
> *not:*
> the Williams and the Smith's houses

When one of the individuals is expressed with a possessive pronoun, avoid awkward phrasing and recast the sentence.

EXAMPLE

> D: my and the patient's signatures
> T: the patient's and my signatures
> *better:*
> T: the patient's signature and mine

Express *joint* possession (or common ownership) by two or more individuals by adding the apostrophe plus s to the final name alone.

EXAMPLE

> the doctor and the patient's discussion
> the Williams and the Smith's property line

8.2.9 Solitary Possessives

When the noun that is modified by the possessive is *implied* but not expressed, express the possessive as though the noun were included. For the examples below, the implied noun is provided in brackets.

EXAMPLE

> We're attending a party at the Smith's [house].
> You can probably get a prescription at your doctor's [office].

In many instances, the implied phrases above should be inserted or the sentence recast to avoid an awkward construction.

You can probably get a prescription at your doctor's office.
or:
You can probably get a prescription from your doctor.

8.2.10 Inanimate Possessives

Do not express possession with inanimate objects. Use a prepositional phrase to express relationship instead.

the balance of power (*not* the power's balance)
the second chapter of the book (*not* the book's second chapter)

However, for inanimate possessive phrases that have become expressive phrases in the vernacular, retain the possessive expression.

cat's meow
bee's knees
stone's throw
for heaven's sake

In addition, possessive phrases that refer to time, measurement, or money should likewise retain their possessive expressions.

one day's notice
two dollars' worth
five dollars' change
30 degrees' flexion
20 weeks' gestation

8.2.11 Preceding Verbal Nouns

Use the possessive form of a noun or pronoun modifying a gerund (*See 4.3.2—Verbal Phrases*).

EXAMPLE

D: I discussed with the patient <u>him</u> wanting to be sent back to work.
T: I discussed with the patient <u>his</u> wanting to be sent back to work.

D: We are concerned about the <u>patient</u> taking so long to respond to treatment.
T: We are concerned about the <u>patient's</u> taking so long to respond to treatment.

8.2.12 With *Of* Phrases

Recast prepositional phrases beginning with *of* that contain possessive nouns or pronouns to avoid awkward phrasing.

EXAMPLE

D: I referred her to a colleague of mine's clinic for treatment.
T: I referred her to the clinic of a colleague of mine for treatment.

D: She was brought here by one of her friend's daughter.
T: She was brought here by the daughter of one of her friends.

It is acceptable to retain the possessive object of the preposition *of* when it is someone's name.

EXAMPLE

He is a friend of John's.
Susan is a business associate of Adam's.

CHAPTER

9

Abbreviations

Introduction

Abbreviations, acronyms, and brief forms are often used in medical dictation to speed up communication, but they frequently create confusion instead. While the originator may think that dictating the abbreviation *AML* is the fastest way to communicate *acute myelocytic leukemia*, medical transcriptionists know better. They face the dilemma: Does *AML* mean acute monocytic leukemia, acute myeloblastic leukemia, acute myelocytic leukemia, acute myelogenous leukemia, acute myeloid leukemia, or perhaps even some less common alternative? In the numerous publications devoted to translating medical abbreviations, abbreviations with single meaning appear to be in the minority.

There is no nationally recognized list of approved abbreviations for use in medical reports, nor does AHDI propose such a list. However, it is important to note that The Joint Commission (formerly JCAHO) mandates that in order to be accredited as an acute care facility, a hospital should use uniform data definitions whenever possible; they note that an abbreviation list (which might be interpreted as a list of abbreviations to avoid) is one way to meet this requirement. Furthermore, The Joint Commission has put forth its own list of dangerous abbreviations as well as guidelines for their adoption (*See 9.3—Dangerous Abbreviations*).

9.1 General Rules

The use of abbreviations in health encounter documentation is widely prevalent. There are many factors and considerations that have to be taken into account when establishing practices and policies governing their use in transcription. The primary consideration for the expansion or retention of a dictated abbreviation should be the promotion of clarity. Attention must be paid to the potential for misinterpretation when encountering abbreviations in dictation.

Note: It must be stated clearly that transcriptionists should be vigilant and thorough in their research of acceptable abbreviations, their appropriate expressions, and the meanings associated with them. Locating an abbreviation in a reference book or online is not necessarily sufficient justification for its inclusion or expansion in the record. Transcriptionists should confirm that research against the information in the record to ensure contextual accuracy.

9.1.1 Definitions

The word *abbreviation* has become synonymous with any short expression that is perceived to represent a longer word or group of words, but there are three distinct types of abbreviations typically encountered in speech and writing:

- *Acronym*: An abbreviation formed from the initial letters of each of the successive words or major parts of a compound term or of selected letters of a word or phrase that is pronounced as a word (e.g., *AIDS, GERD,* and *LASIK*).

- *Initialism*: An abbreviation formed from the initial letters of each of the successive words or major parts of a compound term or of selected letters of a word or phrase that is not pronounced as a word but by each letter (e.g., *ALS, CPK,* and *HIV*).

- *Brief Form*: An abbreviation that results in a shortened form of a single word rather than the initial letters of a series of words (e.g., *phone, exam, Pap smear,* and *labs*).

9.1.2 General Use

Clarity of communication is essential. Avoid the use of abbreviations, acronyms, and brief forms except for internationally recognized and accepted units of measure and for widely recognized terms and symbols. Do not use any that readers will not immediately recognize. Unless the abbreviation, acronym, or brief form is so widely used that it has in essence become a term in its own right, use the expanded form first, followed by its abbreviated form in parentheses. Then use the abbreviated form throughout the remainder of the document.

9.1.3 Facility Policy

As with other points of style and standards, provider/client preference will often be the final word on this issue. A healthcare provider or facility that is concerned about transcription costs, particularly in a per-unit billing environment, may restrict the expansion of many abbreviations despite the standards outlined here. Other providers and facilities may be more risk-management-minded and may require the expansion of all abbreviations. It is important for the MT to be aware that variability in the application of these standards may exist in the job setting.

It is also important to note that interoperability between disparate healthcare systems will require facilities to be contemplative and careful about the abbreviations they deem acceptable within their health systems since those records will be used outside of those systems by other providers and facilities.

9.1.4 Productivity

The decision to expand an abbreviation should never be made on the basis of its impact on productivity or potential wages, even in the absence of a company policy or provider preference. Transcribing a dictated abbreviation in abbreviated or expanded form should be based on the rules and exceptions outlined in this text with consideration for facility policies. The utilization of word-expansion software to increase productivity often facilitates the quick and easy expansion of any and all abbreviations encountered in dictation; however, their expansion or retention should be judiciously considered on the basis of these principles and not on productivity goals.

9.1.5 Terms Dictated in Full

Do *not* use an abbreviation when a term is dictated in full. *Exception:* Units of measure *(See 9.1.8—Multiple/Uncertain Meanings—below).*

EXAMPLE

> D: The patient has a history of shortness of breath.
> T: The patient has a history of shortness of breath.
> *not:*
> T: The patient has a history of SOB.

Some facilities allow for the abbreviation of dosage instructions when dictated in full. AHDI does not recommend doing this arbitrarily unless the provider/facility clearly has a preference for this practice. If facility preference is unknown, transcribe in full as dictated. If facility preference dictates abbreviation of these terms, even if dictated in full, be careful *not* to use any of the dosage abbreviations that appear on the dangerous abbreviations list *(See 9.3—Dangerous Abbreviations—below)*.

EXAMPLE

> D: The patient is to take Tylenol three times a day as needed for pain.
> T: The patient is to take Tylenol t.i.d. p.r.n. pain. (when facility preference
>   is known)
> *or:*
> T: The patient is to take Tylenol three times a day as needed for pain.
>   (in all other instances)

9.1.6 First-Time Reference

When common abbreviations, or those that are universally recognized and understood within health care, are used within the medical record, they do not require expansion, even the first time they are referenced in a report (except in titles; *See 9.1.7—Report Section Titles—below*). However, when an abbreviation is uncommon or rarely encountered or it represents an organizational name, it is customary to spell out the reference in full the first time it is used. The abbreviation is then included in parentheses after the full expression to indicate that from that point forward, only the abbreviation will be used. Once the expanded form has been provided the first time, it does not require further expansion throughout the record (unless dictated).

EXAMPLE

> D: The patient will be referred to SPC for consultation.
> T: The patient will be referred to Southside Prosthetics Center (SPC) for
>   consultation.
>
> D: I had a long discussion with the patient's family about her HRQOL.
> T: I had a long discussion with the patient's family about her health-related
>   quality of life (HRQOL).

9.1.7 Report Section Titles

Write out an abbreviation in full if it is used in the admission, discharge, preoperative, or postoperative diagnosis; consultative conclusion; or operative title. These are critical points of information, and their meanings must be clearly communicated to ensure informed clinical decision-making, continuity of patient care, correct reimbursement, and accurate statistical data-gathering. Transcribe the diagnosis in full and include the dictated abbreviation in parentheses immediately following.

EXAMPLE

Dictated
Diagnosis CAD.

Transcribed
DIAGNOSIS
Coronary artery disease (CAD).

There are two common exceptions to this rule. The first involves the dictation of non-disease-entity abbreviations (like laboratory tests, units of measure, etc.) as part of these titles. When these accompany diagnostic and procedure statements, they may be used if dictated.

EXAMPLE

Dictated
Diagnosis status post altercation with a three centimeter laceration to the right eyebrow.

Transcribed
DIAGNOSIS
Status post altercation with a 3 cm laceration to the right eyebrow.

Dictated
Discharge diagnosis kidney failure with elevated BUN.

Transcribed
DISCHARGE DIAGNOSIS
Kidney failure with elevated BUN.
not:
DISCHARGE DIAGNOSIS
Kidney failure with elevated blood urea nitrogen.

The second exception involves those rare disease-entity abbreviations that are better known by their abbreviations than by the full delineation (like HIV, AIDS, etc.). Remember that the goal is always clarity of communication. In instances where a transcriptionist can confidently assess that a disease entity is better known by its abbreviation, it is best to leave it abbreviated, even in diagnostic and operative titles. When in doubt, transcribe in full.

EXAMPLE

Dictated
Diagnosis acute oral thrush secondary to AIDS.

Transcribed
DIAGNOSIS
Acute oral thrush secondary to AIDS.

9.1.8 Multiple/Uncertain Meanings

When an abbreviated diagnosis, conclusion, or operative title is dictated and the abbreviation used is not familiar or has multiple meanings, the meaning may be discerned if the originator uses the extended term elsewhere in the dictation or if the content of the report somehow makes the meaning obvious. If the extended form cannot be determined in this way and there is easy and immediate access to the patient's record or to the person who dictated the report, the MT should use these as resources to determine the meaning. If these attempts are unsuccessful, the abbreviated form should be transcribed as dictated and the report flagged with a request for the originator to provide the extended form.

EXAMPLE

Dictated
Diagnosis AML.

Transcribed
DIAGNOSIS
AML.

Flag report for verification.

9.1.9 Units of Measure

Abbreviate *metric* units of measure that accompany numeric values and/or are part of virgule constructions. Use the same abbreviation for singular and plural forms. Do not use periods with abbreviated units of measure. Use these abbreviations only when a numeric quantity precedes the unit of measure.

EXAMPLE

> She was put on 2 L of oxygen.
> An approximately 2.5 cm incision was made.
> *but:*
> The wound measured several centimeters.

Spell out common *nonmetric* units of measure to express weight, depth, distance, height, length, and width, except in tables. Do not abbreviate most nonmetric units of measure, except in tables. Do *not* abbreviate nonmetric units in virgule constructions except when the expression combines a metric unit with a nonmetric unit *(See 6.7.2—Virgule, Meaning Per or Over).*

EXAMPLE

> The baby weighed 8 pounds 9 ounces.
> She gave the child 2 tablespoons of Motrin.
> She weighs in 3 days per week.
> Her IV was set to run at 10 mcg/min while she was in the ER.

9.1.10 Business Names

Some businesses are readily recognized by their abbreviations or acronyms and may be referred to by the same if dictated and if there is reasonable assurance the business will be accurately identified by the reader. Most abbreviated forms use all capitals and do not use periods, but be guided by the entity's designated abbreviated form.

EXAMPLE

> IBM equipment
> He is an ACLU attorney.
> She found the item on eBay.

9.1.11 Geographic Names

Abbreviate state and territory names when they are preceded by a city, state, or territory name. Do not abbreviate names of states, territories, countries, or similar units within reports when they stand alone. Use abbreviations in state names in an address (such as in a letter or on an envelope).

> She was seen in an ER in Orlando, FL, a month ago.
> The patient moved here 3 years ago from Canada.

9.1.12 Contractions

Avoid the use of contractions in the record, even if dictated, except in direct quotations. When possible, extend abbreviations that contain contractions, particularly when they represent slang or coined terms.

> D: The patient can't recall when she last had a Pap smear.
> T: The patient cannot recall when she last had a Pap smear.
>
> D: The patient OD'd on heroin and alcohol.
> T: The patient overdosed on heroin and alcohol.
>
> D: Stool was guaiac'd.
> T: Stool was guaiac tested.

When using contractions in a direct quote, take care to place the apostrophe correctly.

> The mother reported, "He's been hysterical."

9.2 Grammar and Punctuation

Abbreviations, because they represent words or phrases, fall within certain guidelines for placement, capitalization, and punctuation.

9.2.1 Placement

A sentence may begin with a dictated abbreviation, or such abbreviated forms may be expanded.

EXAMPLE

> D: WBC was 9200.
> T: WBC was 9200.
> *or:*
> White blood count was 9200.

Avoid separating a numeral from its associated unit of measure or accompanying abbreviation; that is, keep the numeral and unit of measure together at line breaks. When automatic word wrapping brings the unit of measure to the second line, carry the numeric value to the next line with it or, for those in a Microsoft Word environment, consider using the Ctrl+Shift+Space feature to keep the numeral and unit of measure together.

EXAMPLE

> ....The specimen measured
> 4 cm in diameter.
> *not:*
> ....The specimen measured 4
> cm in diameter.

When expanding a *dictated* abbreviation in the diagnosis or operative title sections of the report, place the abbreviation in parentheses following the expanded expression. This documents in the record that the abbreviation was dictated by the author and expanded by the transcriptionist. If the term is dictated in full, there is no need to include the abbreviation reference *(See 9.1.7—Report Section Titles—above)*.

EXAMPLE

> D: DIAGNOSIS: Status post MI with CABG x4.
> T: DIAGNOSIS: Status post myocardial infarction (MI) with coronary artery
>   bypass grafting (CABG) x4.

9.2.2 Capitalization

Capitalize all letters of most acronyms, but when they are expanded, do not capitalize the words from which they are formed unless they are proper names.

AIDS (acquired immunodeficiency syndrome)
BiPAP (bilateral positive airway pressure)
TURP (transurethral resection of prostate)

Do not capitalize abbreviations derived from Latin terms. The use of periods within or at the end of these Latin abbreviations remains the preferred style, although it is also acceptable to drop the periods for general Latin terms *(See 6.6.1—Period)*.

Use lowercase abbreviations with periods for Latin abbreviations that are related to doses and dosages. Avoid using all capitals because they emphasize the abbreviation rather than the drug name. Avoid lowercase abbreviations without periods because some may be misread as words.

e.g.	*exempli gratia*	for example
et al.	*et alii*	and others
etc.	*et cetera*	and so forth
a.c.	*ante cibum*	before food
b.i.d.	*bis in die*	twice a day

Do not capitalize a brief form unless the extended form is routinely capitalized.

segmented neutrophils	segs
examination	exam
Papanicolaou smear	Pap smear
Kirschner wire	K-wire

Do not capitalize most units of measure or their abbreviations. Learn the obvious exceptions, and consult appropriate references for guidance.

meter	m
kilogram	kg
mole	mol
centimeter	cm
exceptions:	
liter	L
kelvin	K
milliliter	mL
ampere	A
decibel	dB
hertz	Hz
joule	J
milliequivalent	mEq

Always capitalize genus name abbreviations when they are accompanied by the species name. The use of a period after the genus name abbreviation is acceptable, but both AHDI and the AMA recommend dropping it.

H influenzae
E coli
C difficile

Do not abbreviate the *species* name even if the genus name is abbreviated.

H influenzae
not:
H flu

9.2.3 Punctuation/Possession

Do not use periods within or at the end of most abbreviations, including acronyms, abbreviated metric units of measure, and brief forms. Use a period at the end of abbreviated nonmetric units of measure if they may be misread without the period (only in virgule constructions and tables).

EXAMPLE

wbc	WBC	mg	cm
exam	prep	mEq	mL
but:			
inches	feet	pounds	yards

in. (misread as "in" without the period in virgule constructions and tables)

Do not use periods with abbreviated academic degrees and professional credentials.

EXAMPLE

John Smith, MD
Mary Jones, CMT
Robert Williams, PhD

Use periods in lowercase drug-related abbreviations derived from Latin terms.

EXAMPLE

b.i.d.	t.i.d.	a.c.
p.r.n.	p.o.	q.4 h.

Note: AHDI continues to discourage dropping periods in lowercase abbreviations that might be misread as words (*bid* and *tid*).

Do *not* use periods with abbreviated personal and courtesy titles unless it is known that the person in question prefers the inclusion of a period or periods. While the use of periods in these instances is still acceptable, there continues to be a strong trend toward dropping them and their omission is now preferred. Defer to facility preference.

EXAMPLE

John A. Smith Jr
Ms Emily Williams
Dr Edward Jones
Walter W. Adams III

Use a lowercase s without an apostrophe to form the plural of a capitalized abbreviation, acronym, or brief form.

EXAMPLE

EKGs	PVCs	exams
labs	monos	CABGs

Use 's to form the plural of lowercase abbreviations.

EXAMPLE

rbc's	wbc's

Use 's to form the plural of single-letter abbreviations.

EXAMPLE

X's	K's	flipped T's

Add 's to most abbreviations or acronyms to show possession.

EXAMPLE

The AMA's address is...
AHDI's position paper on full disclosure states...

9.3 Dangerous Abbreviations

Some abbreviations, particularly with respect to medication orders, have proven to be dangerous. For example, the *U* in *insulin 6 U* could possibly be misread as a zero, or a medication that is given once a day may mistakenly be given four times a day if *q.d.* were misread as *q.i.d.* These types of errors can and do happen and have at times caused fatalities.

Organizations involved in identifying and preventing such problems include the United States Pharmacopeia (USP), the Institute for Safe Medication Practices (ISMP), the US Food and Drug Administration (FDA), and the National Coordinating Council for Medication Error Reporting and Prevention (NCC MERP). ISMP has published a list of dangerous abbreviations and dose designations as reported to the USP-ISMP Medication Errors Reporting Program, and AHDI promotes the adoption of this list.

9.3.1 The Joint Commission Standards

Almost 50% of Joint Commission standards is directly related to patient safety in some way. In July of 2002, The Joint Commission approved its first six (6) National Patient Safety Goals (NPSGs), designed to improve safety measures in identified key areas of patient management and care. In 2004, The Joint Commission began developing program-specific NPSGs for each of its accreditation and certification programs. Goal 2, "Improve the effectiveness of communication among caregivers," speaks specifically to the quality of communication among members of the healthcare team.

The second directive of Goal 2 addresses the subject of abbreviations: "Standardize a list of abbreviations, acronyms, and symbols that are *not* to be used throughout the organization."

This directive generated quite a response from the healthcare community, because The Joint Commission included as part of this goal a list of abbreviations considered so dangerous that their use would be prohibited in the healthcare setting and would be part of future standards by which healthcare organizations would be measured. The original list recommended by the ISMP was quite extensive. The prospect of changing and/or upgrading pharmaceutical processes, programs, and software systems to reflect these new abbreviation standards has been daunting, and the cost associated with those changes has in many cases been prohibitive. According to The Joint Commission's NPSG website frequently asked questions list,

The long-term objective of this requirement continues to be 100 percent compliance, in all forms of clinical documentation, with a reasonably comprehensive list of

prohibited "dangerous" abbreviations, acronyms, and symbols. However, recognizing that this type of change will take time, the survey and scoring of this requirement has been modified, effective immediately, for surveys conducted through the end of 2004, as follows:

If, on survey, the organization has not yet achieved 100 percent compliance as evidenced by open and closed medical record review, a score of "In compliance" will be recorded if the following conditions are met:
- *Use of any item on the list is "sporadic" (less than 10 percent of the instances of the intended term are abbreviated or symbolized); AND*
- *Whenever any prohibited item has been used in an order, there is written evidence of confirmation of the intended meaning before the order is carried out; AND*
- *The organization has implemented a plan for continued improvement to achieve 100 percent compliance by the end of 2004.*

In other words, The Joint Commission is allowing for the fact that transition to this new standard will take time. A facility will have to demonstrate that it has made reasonable efforts to ensure that the abbreviations on the never use list have been eliminated from all patient care documentation as the facility transitions to full compliance.

As a transcriptionist in that environment, it will be important to understand the evolution of this standard and how strictly it may be applied by your employer. AHDI recommends learning and memorizing all of the abbreviations considered dangerous and editing those abbreviations appropriately when you encounter them in dictation since, out of habit, many dictators will still continue to use those abbreviations.

Given the fact that transition to a full and comprehensive list of dangerous abbreviations, such as those outlined by ISMP, has been deemed to be unreasonable in the short term, The Joint Commission has released a "minimum list" of abbreviations that "must be included on each accredited organization's *Do Not Use* list. These are as follows:

Abbreviation	Potential Problem	Preferred Term
U (for unit)	Mistaken as zero, four or cc	Write "unit"
IU (for international unit)	Mistaken as IV (intravenous) or 10 (ten)	Write "international unit"

continued next page

q.d. or Q.D. q.o.d. or Q.O.D. (Latin abbreviation for once daily and every other day)	Mistaken for each other. The period after the Q can be mistaken for an "I" and the "O" can be mistaken for "I".	Write "daily" and "every other day"
Trailing zero (X.0 mg) [Note: Prohibited only for medication-related notations]; Lack of leading zero (.X mg)	Decimal point is missed.	Never write a zero by itself after a decimal point (X mg), and always use a zero before a decimal point (0.X mg)
MS MSO$_4$ MgSO$_4$	Confused for one another. Can mean morphine sulfate or magnesium sulfate.	Write "morphine sulfate" or "magnesium sulfate"

Note: The rule above for omitting trailing zeros only pertains to medication dosages. However, this rule does *not* apply to measurements outside of the medication domain. When an author chooses to dictate a trailing zero on any other measurement (i.e., to describe a mass, lesion, wound, specimen, organ, etc.), this should be transcribed *as dictated*. The use of the trailing zero after the decimal can be an intentional inclusion on the part of the physician/dictator to ensure a reflection of exact, or precise, measurement versus an approximate measurement. The transcriptionist should *not* assume a precise measurement where none is indicated, however. The trailing zero should only be included *if dictated*.

Transcriptionists should also be aware that while *U* for *unit* is now prohibited as above, it is still acceptable to use it when referring to certain types of insulin.

EXAMPLE

U100
U40
U500
but:
500 units of insulin
not:
500 U insulin

In addition to this minimum list, The Joint Commission requires any organization that did not already have a banned list of abbreviations in place to identify and apply at least another three *Do Not Use* abbreviations, acronyms, or symbols of its choosing (effective April 1, 2004). The Joint Commission recommends selecting those additional *Do Not Use* items from the following list of additional abbreviations considered to be dangerous:

Abbreviation	Potential Problem	Preferred Term
µg (for microgram)	Mistaken for mg (milligrams) resulting in one thousand-fold dosing overdose.	Write "mcg"
h.s. or H.S. (for half-strength or Latin abbreviation for bedtime)	Mistaken for either half-strength or hour of sleep (at bedtime). Likewise, q.h.s. or q.H.S. mistaken for every hour. All can result in a dosing error.	Write out "half-strength" or "at bedtime"
t.i.w. or T.I.W. (for three times a week)	Mistaken for three times a day or twice weekly resulting in an overdose.	Write "3 times weekly" or "three times weekly"
s.c. or S.C. s.q. or S.Q. (for subcutaneous)	Mistaken as SL for sublingual, or "5 every" and the Q mistaken for "every"	Write "subcutaneous" or "subcutaneously"
D/C (for discharge)	Interpreted as discontinue whatever medications follow (typically discharge meds).	Write "discharge"
cc (for cubic centimeter; pertains to *liquid* measurements only, not mass)	Mistaken for U (units) when poorly written.	Write "mL" for milliliters
A.S., A.D., A.U. (Latin abbreviation for left, right, or both ears)	Mistaken for OS, OD, and OU, etc.).	Write: "left ear," "right ear" or "both ears"

Note: The rule for changing *cc* to *mL* above only pertains to liquid volume. MTs should continue to transcribe cubic centimeter references to *mass* as *cc*, as are encountered in measuring organs, tissues, and specimens of solid volume. In addition, when *cc* is used to describe other non-liquid volumes, such as gas, this should be retained and *not* changed to mL.

EXAMPLE

D: Ultrasound revealed a 25 cc prostate.
T: Ultrasound revealed a 25 cc prostate.
not:
T: Ultrasound revealed a 25 mL prostate.

D: There was a 150 cc difference on spirometry from last measurement.
T: There was a 150 cc difference on spirometry from last measurement.
not:
T: There was a 150 mL difference on spirometry from last measurement.

Note: AHDI is aware that The Joint Commission has published a statement about the role of the medical transcriptionist in editing erroneously dictated dangerous abbreviations as follows:

The primary responsibility for compliance rests with the author of the documentation. "Author," in this context, includes a person who dictates documentation to be transcribed. We would consider it inappropriate for a transcriptionist to interpret or speculate on the intended meaning of any dictation that is not clear. If a "do not use" term is used in the dictation and the dictation is clear, that term should be transcribed as spoken; not translated or edited into its presumed meaning. If the dictation is not clear, then there must be a mechanism by which the originator can clarify it. [Joint Commission Patient Safety Goals, New, 1/07]

AHDI asserts that, despite the recommendation above, the statement does not prohibit MTs from being deployed in a risk management role in identifying and correcting erroneously dictated dangerous abbreviations, and facilities should consider the risk of assuming that the author will recognize the error at the point of authentication. A physician who has dictated a dangerous abbreviation is highly unlikely to recognize that error when signing off on the report; thus, restricting MTs from engaging in informed judgment to correct these abbreviations will likely result in these errors being perpetuated in the record. Likewise, flagging these inclusions to the attention of the dictator unnecessarily burdens the author with frequent minor corrections to the record that could have easily been made by the transcriptionist – thus restricting the forward progress of the record in the system. Given the debate over this issue, MTs should defer to facility policy and practice when approaching the potential for editing these abbreviations.

9.3.2 ISMP Recommendations

As indicated above, the original list of dangerous abbreviations was generated by the ISMP, a nonprofit organization of pharmacists, nurses, and physicians who work collaboratively with government agencies to promote safe medication practices. Although The Joint Commission has pulled from this list its standards for NPSG 2 as outlined previously, it still strongly recommends the adoption of policies related to all the abbreviations on the ISMP list below. AHDI recommends that transcriptionists adopt the corrections recommended for the full ISMP list even if ultimately their facilities and/or employers require adoption of only the minimum list indicated by The Joint Commission. In other words, it is better to err on the side of caution by knowing and applying all corrections for dangerous abbreviations. Thus, in addition to The Joint Commission list of abbreviations provided in the previous section, the remaining entries recommended by ISMP are provided below:

Abbreviation/ Dose Expression	Intended Meaning	Misinterpretation	Correction
Apothecary symbols	dram minim	Misunderstood or misread (symbol for dram misread for "3" and minim misread as "mL").	Use the metric system.
ARA◦A	vidarabine	cytarabineARA◦C	
AZT	zidovudine (Retrovir)	azathioprine	
CPZ	Compazine (prochlorperazine)	chlorpromazine	Use the complete spelling for all drug names
DPT	Demerol-Phenergan-Thorazine	diphtheria-pertussis-tetanus (vaccine)	
HCl	hydrochloric acid	potassium chloride (The *"H"* is misinterpreted as *"K."*)	

continued next page

HCT	hydrocortisone	hydrochlorothiazide	
HCTZ	hydrochlorothiazide	hydrocortisone (seen as HCT250 mg)	
MTX	methotrexate	mitoxantrone	
TAC	triamcinolone	tetracaine, Adrenalin,cocaine	Use the complete spelling for all drug names
ZnSO$_4$	zinc sulfate	morphine sulfate	
"Nitro" drip	nitroglycerin infusion	sodium nitroprusside infusion	
"Norflox"	norfloxacin	Norflex	
per os	orally	The "os" can be mistaken for "left eye."	Use "p.o.," "by mouth," or "orally."
qn	nightly or at bedtime	Misinterpreted as "qh" (every hour).	Use "nightly."
qhs	nightly at bedtime	Misread as every hour.	Use "nightly."
q6PM, etc.	every evening at 6 PM	Misread as every six hours.	Use 6 PM "nightly."
U or u	unit	Read as a zero (0) or a four (4), causing a 10-fold overdose or greater (4U seen as "40" or 4u seen as 44").	"Unit" has no acceptable abbreviation. Use "unit."
x3d	for three days	Mistaken for "three doses."	Use "for three days."
BT	bedtime	Mistaken as "BID" (twice daily).	Use "at bedtime"
ss	sliding scale (insulin) or ½ (apothecary)	Mistaken for "55."	Spell out "sliding scale." Use "one-half" or use "½."

> and <	greater than and less than	Mistakenly used opposite of intended.	Use "greater than" or "less than."
/ (slash mark)	separates two doses or indicates "per"	Misunderstood as the number 1 ("25 unit/10 units" read as "110" units.)	Do not use a slash mark to separate doses. Use "per."
Name letters and dose numbers run together (e.g., Inderal 40 mg)	Inderal 40 mg	Misread as Inderal 140 mg.	Always use space between drug name, dose and unit of measure.

9.4 Acceptable Forms/Symbols

One of the inevitable questions that arises when addressing the rules and exceptions for abbreviations is, *How will I know if an abbreviation or brief form is acceptable?* Certainly, it can be difficult to get a handle on the rules for expanding or retaining, capitalizing, and punctuating these abbreviated terms if you are unfamiliar with the terms themselves and their general use and adoption in the healthcare setting.

Medical language, like all languages, is a living, evolving entity. The point at which an abbreviation, term, or phrase becomes "acceptable" is difficult to pinpoint, and references and resources will not always agree on the status of that new abbreviation, term, or phrase. Fundamentally, it is *usage* that determines the adoption and evolution of newly coined terms and/or abbreviations derived from those terms. This can be frustrating to anyone trying to master the language, because a slang term or unacceptable abbreviation at a given point in time will likely evolve through usage to an acceptable status and then finally to formal inclusion in medical lexicography.

In the healthcare setting, a transcriptionist will begin to recognize over time whether a term or abbreviation he or she is hearing in dictation is one commonly used by others or is an obvious shortcut or faulty word construction on the part of that particular dictator. Many providers, in an effort to document quickly, will coin new terms, insert back formations, or abbreviate sections of the report that are not typically abbreviated. Again, the ultimate goal in evaluating these scenarios is to promote clarity, and experience and informed interpretive judgment will assist you in making the right decisions when those situations arise.

Refer to the guidelines in Chapter 2 (*2.1.4—Slang, Jargon, and Brief Forms* and *2.1.5—Back Formations*) for specific guidelines on how to edit *unacceptable* abbreviations and brief forms.

9.4.1 Abbreviations and Short Forms

The examples provided in this section are by no means exhaustive, and you should always consult appropriate references when in doubt. An up-to-date abbreviations/acronyms text can help guide you.

a.k.a.: Abbreviation meaning *also known as*. Use lowercase letters with periods to distinguish from *AKA*, meaning *above-knee amputation*.

EXAMPLE

> The report was published by the National Academies, a.k.a. National Academy of Sciences, National Academy of Engineering, National Research Council, Institute of Medicine.

a.m, AM, p.m., PM: Acceptable abbreviations for *ante meridiem* (before noon) and *post meridiem* (after noon), with the lowercase forms being preferred. Formal publications use small capitals, which, if available, may also be used in transcription.

EXAMPLE

> 8:15 a.m. *or* 8:15 AM

Do not use these abbreviations with a phrase such as *in the morning, in the evening, tonight, o'clock*.

EXAMPLE

> 8:15 a.m. *not* 8:15 a.m. o'clock
> 10:30 PM *not* 10:30 PM in the evening

Use periods with *a.m.* and *p.m.* so that *a.m.* won't be misread as the word *am*. Do not use periods with the uppercase *AM* and *PM*. Insert a space between the numerals preceding these abbreviations and the abbreviations themselves, but do not use spaces within the abbreviations.

> 11 a.m. *or* 11 AM
> *not:*
> 11a.m. *or* 11AM
> 11 a. m. *or* 11 A M

BPM, bpm: Abbreviation for *beats per minute*.

> Pulse: 70 beats per minute.
> *or:*
> Pulse: 70 BPM.
> *or:*
> Pulse: 70 bpm.

BP: Abbreviation for *blood pressure*.

> D: Blood pressure 110/80.
> T: Blood pressure 110/80.
> *or:*
> T: BP 110/80.

Blood types: Write out *negative* and *positive* rather than – or + because the minus or plus sign is easily overlooked.

> B positive
> O negative

DNR: A DNR or "do not resuscitate" order is placed in a patient's chart when either the patient or the family has indicated that no emergency resuscitative measures are to be employed.

> His status was changed to DNR yesterday.

Dr, Dr.: Courtesy title for doctors. Use only for earned doctorates (medical or other), not honorary doctorates. While the use of periods in these instances is still acceptable, there continues to be a strong trend toward dropping them and their omission is now preferred. Defer to facility preference.

EXAMPLE

John A. Smith Jr
Ms Emily Williams
Dr Edward Jones
not:
Dr. George W. Bush

Use *Dr* not *Doctor* in salutations unless the salutation is directed to more than one doctor. Do not use *Drs* as a plural form in salutations; write out *Doctors* instead.

EXAMPLE

Dear Dr Watson:
Dear Doctors Watson and Crick:

Do not use *Dr* or *Doctor* when credentials are given.

EXAMPLE

John Brown, MD
not:
Dr John Brown, MD

Drug terminology: Use lowercase abbreviations with periods for Latin abbreviations that are related to doses and dosages. Do not use abbreviations found on the "Dangerous Abbreviations" list from ISMP *(See 9.3.2—ISMP Recommendations—above)*. Avoid using all capitals because they emphasize the abbreviation rather than the drug name. Avoid lowercase abbreviations without periods because some may be misread as words. Do not translate. *(see next page)*

Abbreviation	Latin Phrase	English Translation
a.c.	ante cibum	before food
b.i.d.	bis in die	twice a day
gtt.	guttae	drops (spell out)
n.p.o.	nil per os	nothing by mouth
n.r.	non repetatur	do not repeat
p.c.	post cibum	after food
p.o.	per os	by mouth
p.r.n.	pro re nata	as needed
q.4 h.	quaque 4 hora	every 4 hours
q.h.	quaque hora	every hour
q.i.d.	quarter in die	four times a day
t.i.d.	ter in die	three times a day
u.d.	ut dictum	as directed

Note: We have inserted a space after the numeral *4* in *q.4 h.* on the advice of ISMP so that the number is more easily and clearly read. Invalid Latin abbreviations such as *q.a.m.* (*every morning*) and mixed Latin and English abbreviations such as *q.4 hours* (*every 4 hours*) have become commonplace. However, as with all abbreviations, avoid those that are obscure (like *a.c.b.* for *before breakfast*) or dangerous. For example, *b.i.w.* is both obscure *and* dangerous. It is intended to mean *twice weekly* but it could be mistaken for *twice daily* resulting in a dosage frequency seven times that intended.

AHDI continues to discourage the dropping of periods in lowercase abbreviations that might be misread as words (for example, *bid* and *tid*).

Exam: Acceptable brief form for *examination* when dictated, except as a heading.

The physical exam was negative.

PHYSICAL EXAMINATION
HEENT: Head normal.
NECK: Supple.

Jr, Jr.; Sr, Sr.: Abbreviations for *junior* and *senior* in names. While the use of periods and commas in these instances is still acceptable, there continues to be a strong trend toward dropping them and their omission is now preferred. Defer to facility preference.

Do not use all capitals (JR, SR).

Dr Martin Luther King Jr
or:
Dr. Martin Luther King, Jr.

MD: Abbreviation for *Doctor of Medicine*. Preferred style is without periods. If periods are used, do not space within the abbreviation (M.D., not M. D.).

mEq: Abbreviation for *milliequivalent*. Use with numerals. Do not use periods. Do not add *s* for plural.

20 mEq

mg%: Abbreviation for *milligrams percent*. Equivalent to milligrams per deciliter (mg/dL), which is the preferred nomenclature, but transcribe as dictated. Do not use periods. Do not space between *mg* and *%*.

mmHg: Abbreviation for *millimeters of mercury*. Use with pressure readings (blood pressure, tourniquet pressure, etc.). Need not use if not dictated.

subcu: Abbreviated form for *subcutaneous* or *subcuticular*. When "subcu" is dictated and you are unsure which term is intended, spell *subcu* or *subcut*. Do not use the abbreviation *sub q* because the *q* can be mistaken for a medication dosage.

EXAMPLE

> D: The wound was closed with running subcu stitches of 5-0 Prolene.
> T: The wound was closed with running subcu stitches of 5-0 Prolene.

9.4.2 Symbols

Often symbols serve as abbreviated forms of words or phrases in language. Given the trend to avoid symbols in health data capture in order to promote interoperability and electronic exchange, defer to facility preference when deploying some of these symbols.

Ampersand (*&*): Symbol meaning *and*. Use with certain single-letter abbreviations separated by *and*. Do not space before or after the ampersand. Do not use ampersand forms in operative titles or diagnoses. Check appropriate references to identify other acceptable uses.

EXAMPLE

> D&C
> T&A

Degrees (°): In expressing angles in orthopedics, write out *degrees* or use the degree sign (°).

EXAMPLE

> The patient was able to straight leg raise to 40 degrees.
> *or:*
> The patient was able to straight leg raise to 40°.

Use the degree sign (°) in imaging studies and temperature expressions.

EXAMPLE

> Positioning the patient's head at a 90° angle allowed for efficient acquisition of data over a 180° arc.
> Temperature was 99.1°F.

If the symbol is not available, spell out *degree* or *degrees*.

Ditto marks ("): Do not use ditto marks (") to indicate *the same*; instead, repeat the term or phrase. Do not use ditto marks as a symbol for *inches*, except in tables as a space-saving device.

> The infant was 22 inches long.
> *not:*
> The infant was 22" long.

Division symbol (÷): Do not use the division symbol (÷) except in tables and mathematical expressions.

Equal, equal to (=): Do not use the equal symbol (=) except in tables and mathematical presentations.

Greater, greater than, less than (< >): The word *greater* is overused in medical parlance and is often dictated inappropriately when *more, longer,* or *over* would be a better choice of words. As so often happens, shorthand is used in a handwritten patient chart, and a dictating physician will read the chart while dictating and will use the words that go with the shorthand symbol, when that may not be the best translation of the symbol.

> D: The pain persisted greater than 24 hours.
> T: The pain persisted longer than 24 hours.

The greater than (>) and less than (<) symbols are often mistaken for their opposite sign in meaning, and ISMP advises against their use.

> The patient's performance on the trial is in the impaired range (289 seconds, less than the 1st percentile).
> She weighed less than 100 pounds.
> The patient exhibited greater lung capacity following treatments.

Section 2: General Standards of Style

Greek letters: Spell out the English translation when the word stands alone. Do not capitalize English translations. Use the Greek letter or spell it out when it is part of an extended term, according to the preferred form; consult appropriate references for guidance.

alpha	α
beta	β
gamma	γ

In extended terms, use of a hyphen after the Greek letter is optional, but the hyphen is not used after the English translation.

β-globulin *or* B globulin
beta globulin

Minus, minus sign (–): Write out the word *minus* if you are not certain the symbol will be noticeable or clear. Write out *minus* to indicate below-zero temperatures.

minus 40, –40
but:
minus 38 degrees
not:
-38 degrees

Negative sign (–): Do not use except in tables or special applications, e.g., blood nomenclature. Also avoid if its usage may cause the reader to overlook it.

blood type O negative
preferred to:
blood type O–

Number (#), No.: Use *No.* or # before an apartment, suite, or room number only when the words *apartment, suite,* and *room* (or their abbreviations) are not used.

100 Adams Street, No. 228
100 Adams Street, #228
not:
100 Adams Street, Apt. #228.

Do not use *No.* or # before a house number in the street address.

1400 Magnolia Avenue
not:
#1400 Magnolia Avenue

Do *not* use the # sign to represent the words *pound* or *pounds.*

Percent (%): Note that *percent* is a single word. Do not use the abbreviation *pct.* except in tables. Instead, use % or *percent.* Use the symbol % after a numeral. Do not space between the numeral and the symbol.

13% monos, 1% bands
She has had a 10% increase in weight since her last visit.
MCHC 34%
10% solution

Use numerals for the number preceding %. When the number is written out, as at the beginning of a sentence, write out *percent.*

The discount was 50%.
Fifty percent of the patients in the study reported mild side-effects.
not:
Fifty % of the patients in the study reported mild side-effects.

Plus, plus sign (+): Do not use the plus sign without a numeral.

EXAMPLE

> +1, +2, +3
> *or:*
> 1+, 2+, 3+
> *not:*
> +, ++, +++

In laboratory or technical readings, use the symbol unless it will not be noticeable or clear.

EXAMPLE

> 3+ gram-positive cocci

X, x: Use only with numerals. Use a lowercase *x* in expressions of area and volume, as a multiplication symbol, and when it takes the place of the word *times*. A capital *X* is generally used to express magnification. Use a lowercase *x* to express *by* in dimensions. When the word "times" is dictated and can be translated as *for*, it should be transcribed as *for* rather than *times* or *x*. When the word "times" is dictated and means the number of times a thing was done, the letter *x* can be used.

EXAMPLE

> X30 magnification
> 13 x 2 cm
>
> D: The patient was given antibiotics to take times 2 weeks.
> T: The patient was given antibiotics to take for 2 weeks.
>
> Blood cultures were negative x3.

Section 3
Measurement and Quantitation

CHAPTER

10

Numbers

Introduction

At the heart of patient encounter documentation is the quantifying information that enables the healthcare team to diagnose, treat, and manage patients. There is arguably no more critical information recorded and relied upon than the numeric values that represent a wide variety of indicators for both cause and effect in managing disease. Whether it is the patient's age, vital signs, duration of symptoms, wound measurements, laboratory values, drug dosages, length of stay, indication of pain, or classification of disease, numbers are a critical part of the patient record. They need to be communicated clearly and accurately in all areas of the report, and they represent an area of tremendous potential error in the record.

10.1 Cardinal and Ordinal Numbers

Numerals, or figures, stand out from the surrounding text and serve a functional purpose in medical reports, where they should be used almost exclusively as opposed to spelled-out numbers. As with other points of style and standards, provider/client preference will often be the final word on this issue, though it is not likely that an employer or client will ask that you spell out numerals in vital areas of the report. You may, however, encounter providers who are well published or are particularly formal in the letters they dictate. They might require you to use the old rule of spelling out numbers under 10 in their correspondence, but again, any numeric values (such as vital signs, laboratory values, or drug dosages) should still be expressed with numerals, even in correspondence.

10.1.1 Arabic Numerals

Most numerals used in medicine are expressed as arabic numerals. Therefore, a general rule is to use arabic numerals unless roman numerals are specified or unless there is strong documentation that the preferred form is roman. The arabic numerals are 0, 1, 2, 3, 4, 5, 6, 7, 8, 9.

She was seen in the emergency room 1 hour after the accident.
He tried 3 different medications without success.
The specimen weighed less than 2 pounds.

Keep in mind that the rules for numbers specified by formal grammar do not apply in this setting. Many were taught to spell out all numbers under the number 10 and to use arabic numerals for all numbers greater than 9. However, in the clinical setting, numbers need to be read and communicated quickly and clearly. Spelling out numeric values, even under the number 10, is not considered the most efficient way to communicate them to the many care providers who may ultimately read and/or quickly seek information from the record. While the patient record is a formal, legal document, its primary function in the healthcare setting is to communicate information that contributes to the ongoing treatment and care of the patient. Numeric values that stand out on the page are less likely to be overlooked or misinterpreted, so the standard is to use them in transcription.

10.1.2 Roman Numerals

Do not use periods with roman numerals. Seven letters make up the roman numeral system. Capital letters are used except in special circumstances; e.g., lowercase letters (i, v, x, etc.) are used as page numbers for preliminary material (contents pages, preface, etc.) in a book and for formal outlining in publication.

I = 1
V = 5
X = 10
L = 50
C = 100
D = 500
M = 1000

When a letter follows a letter of greater value, it increases the value of the preceding letter.

VI (5 + 1 = 6)

When a letter precedes a letter of greater value, it diminishes the value of the following letter.

IV (5 - 1 = 4)

A bar over a letter indicates multiplication by 1000.

$\overline{X}$ = 10,000

The following is a list of the most common uses for roman numerals in the health record. It is by no means exhaustive, and MTs should refer to a reputable dictionary or reference for confirmation of expression for any classification system.

- Axis designations for psychiatric diagnoses
- Billroth anastomosis
- Blood factors
- Cancer stages
- Catterall hip score for Legg-Perthes disease
- Clark levels for malignant melanoma
- Cranial nerves (*though arabic numerals are acceptable*)
- Crowe classification for hip dysplasia
- Decubitus ulcers
- EKG standard bipolar leads
- LeFort classification of facial fractures
- Mallampati-Samsoon airway assessment
- Mayo classification of olecranon fractures
- Neer staging for shoulder impingement
- Neer-Horowitz classification of fractures
- New York Heart Association (NYHA) classification of heart failure
- Ranchos Los Amigos cognitive function scale
- Salter and Salter-Harris classifications of fractures
- Schatzker classification of tibial plateau fractures
- Wars, people, and animals

10.1.3 Ordinal Numbers

Ordinal numbers are used to indicate order or position in a series rather than quantity. As outlined in 10.1 above, for formal publication and correspondence, the preference for all numbers, including ordinals, is to spell them out (*first* through *ninth*) and use numerals for numbers 10 and above (*10th, 11th,* and so on). In the health record, however, all ordinals should be expressed with numerals (*1st, 2nd,* etc.) to promote clarity of communication. Word processors will typically automatically format the ordinal suffixes (*-st, -nd, -rd,* and *-th*) so that they are superscripted. In electronic environments where superscripting is not supported, these should be expressed in regular type. Do not use a period with ordinal numbers.

EXAMPLE

> 3rd rib (*or* third)
> 5th finger (*or* fifth)
> She is to return for her 3rd (*or* third) visit in 2 days.
> She was in her 9th (*or* ninth) month of pregnancy.
> His return visits are scheduled for the 15th and 25th of next month.
> 4th cranial nerve...

10.2 Rules and Exceptions

The rules and exceptions outlined in this section should be learned and applied well. Like the dangerous abbreviations indicated in Chapter 9, the erroneous transcription of a number can lead to potential risk management and continuity of care issues that must be carefully addressed. As in other areas of style and standards, when determining how a particular dictated value should be transcribed, clarity of expression will always be the single driving factor.

10.2.1 Punctuation

This section provides general guidelines for the use of punctuation when expressing numeric values in the record. For detailed information about punctuation and relevant examples, refer to *Chapter 6—Punctuation*. For information about specific usage scenarios, refer to section *10.3 Numeric Referents* later in this chapter.

Periods: Use a period with numeric values in the following instances:

- To separate a whole number from a decimal fraction.
- After the numbers used to enumerate items in a list *unless* the numbers are enclosed in parentheses.

Commas: Use a comma with numeric values in the following instances:

- To separate groups of 3 numerals in numbers of 5 digits or more unless decimals are used. The comma in 4-digit numbers may be omitted. *(See the trend note in 10.2.3—Multiple Digits below.)*
- To separate adjacent unrelated numbers if neither can be expressed readily in words.
- To separate the day of the month from the year when the full date is expressed.
- To separate the year from the rest of the sentence when the full date (month, day, and year) occurs in mid-sentence.
- To separate the chromosome number and sex chromosome in genetic expression.
- To separate values of a single panel or test in the laboratory data section of the report.

Do *not* use a comma with numeric values in the following instances:

- Between *words* expressing a number.
- When only the month and year are given.

Colons: Use a colon with numeric values in the following instances:

- In standard expressions of time.
- In place of the word *to* in the expression of a ratio.
- To separate volume number and page number in footnotes, endnotes, and cited sources.

Do *not* use a colon in expressions of military time.

Hyphens: Use hyphens with numeric expressions in the following instances:

- To form a compound modifier between a number and an English word or *nonmetric* unit if it precedes and modifies a noun.
- When expressing numbers in words—for compound numbers between 21 and 99 (or 21st and 99th), whether they stand alone or are part of a number over 100.
- In the expression of serial numbers (medical record numbers, social security numbers, etc.).
- To express fractional numbers that are combined with whole numbers, whether spelled out or expressed with numerals.
- In place of the word *to* in range expressions if all five conditions for ranges have been met. *(See 6.5.7—Ranges.)*

- To express a compound word formed by a single number and a word or letter.

Do *not* use hyphens with numeric expressions in the following instances:

- To form a compound modifier between a number and a *metric* unit (*See Note below*).
- To form a compound expression where the number is the *second* element in the expression.

Note: This represents a change over previous recommendations in the 2nd edition of this text. Per SI convention and metric standards, no intervening symbols or punctuation should interrupt the flow from numeric value to metric unit, even in a modifying relationship. This is an application that should not have been implied by the standards for compound modifiers. In addition, compound modifiers should be formed by *at least* one complete word, and metric value expressions do not meet that criterion.

10.2.2 Plurals
Use 's to form the plural of single-digit numerals.

EXAMPLE

> We dressed the wound with 4 x 4's.
> We like to see newborns with 4's and 5's on Apgar assessment.

Add s without an apostrophe to form the plural of multiple-digit numbers, including years.

EXAMPLE

> She is in her 20s.
> She was born in the 1940s.

10.2.3 Multiple Digits
Express numerals of 5 digits or more by using commas to separate numerals in groups of threes, but omit the commas if decimals are used. The comma in 4-digit numbers may be omitted.

Platelet count was 345,000.

White count was 7100.
or:
White count was 7,100.

12345.67

Do not place commas between *words* expressing a number.

Four hundred forty-eight
not:
Four hundred, forty-eight.

Trend Note: The *AMA Manual of Style* recommends compliance with SI convention, whereby digits are separated by a "thin space," not a comma, to indicate place values beyond thousands. However, this recommendation pertains primarily to the formal publication of clinical data in periodicals, abstracts, and scientific journals. Transcriptionists who are asked to prepare manuscripts of this nature should be aware of this standard. Due to the compromise of visual clarity that omission of separating commas would create as well as the as-yet lack of widespread adoption of this standard, this recommendation has *not* been made for healthcare records. With the continued movement toward SI convention, however, it is possible that even health records will see a migration to this standard in the future.

4055
13 445
722 654
8 473 308

10.2.4 Proper Names

Use words or figures for numbers in proper names, according to the entity's preference.

> 20th Century Insurance
> Three Dollar Cafe

10.2.5 End of Line

Avoid separating a numeral from its associated unit of measure or accompanying abbreviation; that is, keep the numeral and unit of measure together at line breaks. When automatic word wrapping brings the unit of measure to the second line, carry the numeric value to the next line with it.

> ....The specimen measured
> 4 cm in diameter.
> *not:*
> ....The specimen measured 4
> cm in diameter.

10.2.6 Combining Numerals with Words

Use a combination of numerals and words to express rounded large numbers and consecutive numerical expressions.

When a large number is rounded by use of the words *million* or *billion*, the number should be expressed with a combination of numerals and words. When used in a range expression, the unit should be repeated to avoid ambiguity.

> There are approximately 6.7 billion people worldwide, according to current population statistics.
>
> The disease affects 4 million to 6 million people.
> *not:*
> The disease affects 4 to 6 million people.

　　　　　　　　　　　　　　　　　　Section 3: Measurement and Quantitation

When decimal expressions are combined with the words *hundred, thousand, million* or *billion,* such as "four point two thousand" or "five point eight million," numerals may be transcribed in one of two ways:

4.2 thousand
or:
4200

5.8 million
or:
5,800,000

When two numbers are consecutive, spell out one of them to avoid confusion.

The patient was instructed to drink four 8-ounce glasses of water a day.
Discharge Medication: Os-Cal 500 one daily.
two 8-inch drains

Use a comma to separate adjacent unrelated numerals if neither can be readily expressed in words and the sentence cannot be readily reworded.

In March 2002, 2038 patients were seen in the emergency room.

10.2.7 Beginning of Sentence
Spell out numbers that begin a sentence, or recast the sentence.

D: Fourteen days ago she started having severe cramping.
T: Fourteen days ago she started having severe cramping.
or:
T: She started having severe cramping 14 days ago.

Exception: A complete year that begins a sentence need not be spelled out, but it is better to recast the sentence, if possible.

> D: 1995 was when her symptoms began.
> T: 1995 was when her symptoms began.
> *better:*
> T: Her symptoms began in 1995.

10.2.8 *One* Used as a Noun or Pronoun

Spell out the number *one* when it is used as a noun or pronoun.

> The radiologist compared the previous x-rays with the most recent <u>one</u>.
> She is the <u>one</u> who is electing to have this surgery performed.
> If <u>one</u> looks closely, a hairline fracture can be seen at the epiphyseal line.

10.2.9 Nonspecific Numbers

Spell out nonspecific (indefinite) numeric expressions.

> She described hundreds of symptoms. *(not 100s)*
> Several thousand people were tested.

10.2.10 The Number *Zero*

Zero is always spelled out when it stands alone as a general expression. When combined with a classification description or unit of measure, the numeral should be used to express the value.

> The patient had zero response to the treatment.
> Her symptoms usually appear when the outside temperature drops below zero.
> *but:*
> gravida 1, para 0
> pain of 0/5
> 0 °F

       Section 3: Measurement and Quantitation

10.3 Numeric Referents

This section outlines the rules and exceptions as they apply to different numeric values commonly encountered in the health record and about which transcriptionists often have questions and/or need clarification.

10.3.1 Age
Use numerals to express ages, except at the beginning of a sentence.

EXAMPLE

37 years old
3-year-old child
3-year 7-month-old girl

When the author dictates in clipped format and begins a sentence with a reference to the patient's age, recast the sentence or write out the number.

EXAMPLE

D: 7-year-old patient who comes in today for...
T: A 7-year-old patient who comes in today for...
or:
T: This 7-year-old patient comes in today for...
or:
T: Seven-year-old patient who comes in today for...

Use hyphens to form a compound modifier when the patient's age is expressed as a modifier, whether the noun following it is expressed or implied.

EXAMPLE

This is a 15-year-old boy who presents with a laceration to the right eyebrow.
or:
This is a 15-year-old who presents with a laceration to the right eyebrow.

13-year-olds
not:
13 year olds

Do not hyphenate the patient's age when it is used as a general descriptor and not as a compound modifier.

> The patient, who is 15 years old, presents with a laceration to the right eyebrow.
> *not:*
> The patient, who is 15-years-old, presents with a laceration to the right eyebrow.

Use numerals plus *s* in general reference to the patient's age by decade. Do not use an apostrophe.

> The patient is in her 50s.
> *not:*
> The patient is in her 50's.
> *not:*
> The patient is in her fifties.

10.3.2 Caliber (Weapons)

Caliber is a term used to indicate the diameter of a bullet in hundredths of an inch. A bullet that is 30 hundredths of an inch (.30) in diameter is called a "30 caliber" bullet and is expressed in writing as *.30 caliber*. The term *caliber* is of English origin and is used by ammunition and firearm manufacturers throughout the world. Firearms and ammunition of European origin use the metric system and would refer to a .30-caliber bullet as a 7.62 mm bullet. The term *caliber* is also used to describe the weapon or firearm that uses a particular size of bullet. Express calibers with a decimal point followed by arabic numerals and a hyphen when preceding and modifying a noun. Do not place a leading zero before the decimal point.

> .38-caliber pistol
> .22-caliber bullet

10.3.3 Classification Terms

Consult a reputable dictionary or resource to confirm the use of appropriate numerals (arabic or roman) when referencing classification systems. For a more specific breakdown of classification systems and their guidelines, refer to the specialty chapters found in section 4 of this text.

10.3.4 Clock Referents

When an anatomic position is described in terms of clock-face orientation as seen by the viewer, use *o'clock*. Do *not* transcribe as an expression of *time*. Hyphenate the expression since it forms a compound modifier preceding and modifying the word "position." If the word "position" is not dictated but position, and not time, is clearly implied, transcribe the full expression to avoid confusion.

EXAMPLE

The incision was made at the 3-o'clock position.
not:
The incision was made at the 3:00 position.

D: The incision was made at 3-o'clock.
T: The incision was made at the 3-o'clock position.

When the clock-face orientation is expressed as a partial hour, omit the word *o'clock*, even if dictated.

EXAMPLE

D: The cyst was found at the 2:30 o'clock position.
T: The cyst was found at the 2:30 position.

10.3.5 Dates

When the month, day, and year are given in this sequence, set off the year by commas. Do not use ordinals.

EXAMPLE

She was admitted on December 14, 2001, and discharged on January 4, 2002.
not:
...January 4th, 2002 *(4th is an ordinal)*

Do not use commas when the month and year are given without the day, or when the military date sequence (day, month, year) is used.

> She was admitted in December 2001 and discharged in January 2002.
> She was admitted on 14 December 2001 and discharged on 4 January 2002.

Do not use punctuation after the year if the date stands alone, as in admission and discharge dates on reports.

> Admission date: April 4, 2000
> Discharge date: April 5, 2000

Use ordinals when the day of the month precedes the month and is preceded by *the*; do not use commas. Do not use ordinals in month/day/year format.

> the 4th of April 2001 *not* April 4th, 2001

When the military style is used, the day precedes the month. Use numerals; do not use commas. Write out or abbreviate the month (without periods) and use arabic figures for day and year.

> 4 April 2001
> 4 Apr 2001

It is preferable to spell out dates used in the body of a report, writing out the name of the month and using four digits for the year. However, this is preferred only when an occasional date is referenced. When dates are used repeatedly throughout the report, as in a long history or hospital course, they should be expressed as numerals separated by virgules to promote visual clarity and ease of identification in the record.

Section 3: Measurement and Quantitation

> The patient was previously seen on April 4, 2001.
>
> Electrolytes on 4/24/2001 revealed a sodium of 135, potassium 4.3, bicarbonate 25, chloride 102. Repeated on 4/25/2001 and again on 4/26/2001, electrolytes remained within normal limits.

Though it is acceptable and may be facility preference to express only the last two digits of the year in a virgule expression, the preference is to express the full year so there is no ambiguity. This is particularly important when expressing birth dates and historical dates that represent years that could have occurred in either the 20th or 21st centuries.

> D: This elderly patient with a birth date of 12/22/06 presents today for consultation.
> T: This elderly patient with a birth date of 12/22/1906 presents today for consultation.

When only the month and day are dictated, and not the year, add the year only if you are certain what year is being referred to.

> D: The patient was last seen on April 4th.
> T: The patient was last seen on April 4, 2001. (if certain of year)

Divide dates at the end of a line of text between the day and the year. Avoid dividing between the month and the day.

> ....February 17,
> 2001
> *not:*
> ....February
> 17, 2001

10.3.6 Decimals

Use numerals to express decimal amounts. Use the period as a decimal point or indicator. Always use the decimal form with metric units of measure, even when they are dictated as a fraction. Do *not* use the decimal form when *non-metric* units are used; use fractions instead.

EXAMPLE

D: The mass was two and a half centimeters in diameter.
T: The mass was 2.5 cm in diameter.

D: The scar measured 2.5 inches.
T: The scar measured 2-1/2 inches.

Exception: When the originator uses a fraction that cannot be exactly translated into decimals, transcribe as dictated. Likewise, use the decimal form with *nonmetric* forms of measure when a precise measurement is intended and the fraction form would be both cumbersome and inexact. Two or more places may follow the decimal.

EXAMPLE

D: one third centimeter
T: 1/3 cm

The 0.1816-inch screw was inserted.

When whole numbers are dictated, do not add a decimal point and trailing zero, especially with drug dosage references, because of their potential to be misread (*See 9.3.1—The Joint Commission Standards*). It also indicates a degree of specificity that, if not dictated, was not intended by the originator.

EXAMPLE

2 mg
not 2.0 mg

However, when the decimal point and zero following a whole number are dictated to emphasize the preciseness of a measurement, e.g., of a pathology specimen or a laboratory value, transcribe them as dictated. Do not, however, insert the decimal point and zero if they are not dictated.

EXAMPLE

D: The specimen measured 4.8 x 2.0 x 3.4 mm.
T: The specimen measured 4.8 x 2.0 x 3.4 mm.
but:
D: The specimen measured 4.8 x 2 x 3.4 mm.
T: The specimen measured 4.8 x 2 x 3.4 mm.

For quantities less than 1, place a zero before the decimal point, except when the number could never equal 1 (e.g., in bullet calibers and in certain statistical expressions such as correlation coefficients and statistical probability).

EXAMPLE

0.75 mg
.22-caliber rifle

Do not exceed two places following the decimal except in special circumstances, e.g., specific gravity values, or when a precise measurement is intended.

EXAMPLE

0.0624 K-wire
specific gravity 1.030

10.3.7 Fractions

Express precise fractions, those used to describe an exact value followed by a *nonmetric* unit of measure, by using numerals.

EXAMPLE

The laceration measured 2-1/2 inches.
There was a 3/4-inch scar on the outer left thigh.
Approximately 1-1/2 hours prior to admission, the patient had onset of gradually worsening chest pain.

Spell out general fractions, those used to describe a general or rounded value *not* followed by a unit of measure.

Nearly three-fourths of my patients participate in a managed care plan.
There was about a half-second delay before we saw a response on the monitor.
The test was concluded after half an hour.
About an hour and a half prior to admission, the patient had onset of gradually worsening chest pain.

Use numerals for fractional measurements forming compound modifiers preceding a noun.

A 3/4-pound tumor was removed.
The abdomen shows a 4-1/4-inch scar.

Spell out fractional measurements that are less than one when they do not precede a noun.

The tumor weighed three quarters of a pound. (precedes a prepositional phrase)

Place a hyphen between numerator and denominator when neither contains a hyphen of its own.

one-fourth empty
two-thirds full
but:
one forty-eighth *or* 1/48
twenty-three thirty-eighths *or* 23/38

Hyphenate fractions when they are written out and used as adjectives; do not hyphenate when they are written out and are used as nouns or as objects of a prepositional phrase.

one-half normal saline (adjective)
one third of the calf (noun phrase)
The patient cut the medication in half because she did not tolerate it well.
(object of preposition "in")

When the author dictates an expanded expression to represent a precise measurement, this should still be expressed as a precise fraction with numerals so that the measured value is clearly communicated in the record.

D: The patient smokes a pack and a half a day.
T: The patient smokes 1-1/2 packs a day.
or:
T: The patient smokes 1-1/2 packs of cigarettes a day.

10.3.8 Lab Values

Use arabic numerals and decimals to express lab values.

WBC 5.2, hemoglobin 14, and hematocrit 33.
Sodium 139, potassium 4.6, chloride 106, and bicarb 28.

Use commas to separate values of a single panel or test. Use periods to separate the values of unrelated laboratory tests. In the example below, the CBC values are grouped together in one sentence; the chemistry values, in another.

LABORATORY DATA: White count 5.2, hemoglobin 15, and hematocrit 39.
Sodium 149, potassium 4.2, and chloride 103.

Do not use a comma to separate a lab value from the test it describes.

White count 5300.
not:
White count, 5300.

When a lab value is expressed as a percentage, use whatever form is dictated.

D: Polys 58%.
T: Polys 58%.

D: Polys 0.58.
T: Polys 0.58.

D: Polys 58.
T: Polys 58.

For more information about the expression of a specific laboratory test or value, refer to the specialty chapters found in section 4 of this text.

10.3.9 Money

Express exact amounts of dollars and cents with numerals, using a decimal point to separate dollars from cents.

$4.56

When written out, lowercase all terms.

a million dollars

For numbers less than one dollar, use numerals; spell out and lowercase *cents*. Do not use the decimal form. Do not use the dollar sign ($). Do not use the cent sign (¢) except in tables.

8 cents
not:
$.08 *or* 8¢

20 cents
not:
20¢ *or* $.20

However, in tables that include amounts over $1, those amounts that are less than $1 should include a zero preceding the decimal so that entries are consistent.

$4.20
$0.80

For amounts over one dollar, use the dollar sign ($) preceding the dollar amount, and separate dollars and cents by a decimal point. Do not use a decimal following the dollar amount if cents are not included.

$1.08
$1.20

$40
not:
$40.00 (unless listed in a column with other amounts that include cents.)

For ranges, repeat the dollar sign or cent sign but do not repeat the word forms. Use *to* instead of a hyphen with dollar-sign or cent-sign forms.

$4 to $5
not:
$4-$5

10¢ to 15¢
not:
10¢-15¢

Use *to* with word forms.

4 to 5 dollars
not:
4-5 dollars

10 to 15 cents
not:
10-15 cents

Use *'s* or *s'*, whichever is appropriate, with units of money used as possessive adjectives.

1 dollar's worth
2 cents' worth

Do not use the possessive form with compound adjectives.

a 2-dollar bill

Sometimes it is important to distinguish US dollars from other currencies, such as Canadian dollars. There is no space between the letters and the $ symbol.

US$4.56
Can$4.56

The euro is the established (2002) currency for the European Union. Only time and usage will tell what the accepted plural forms will be. However, the official dossier from the European Union calls for the English plural of euro to be the same as the singular forms: *euro* and *cent*.

200 euro equal 200 cent

The official abbreviation for the *euro* is EUR.

Section 3: Measurement and Quantitation

10.3.10 Number of, No.,

A collective noun that may be singular or plural. If preceded by *the*, it takes a singular verb. If preceded by *a*, it takes a plural verb.

EXAMPLE

> *The* number of adhesions *was* minimal.
> *A* number of adhesions *were* present.

Use *number* to refer to persons or things that can be counted. *Number* tells how many; *amount* tells how much (mass).

EXAMPLE

> There was a small amount of bleeding, given the large number of wounds.
> A large number of people were present.
> *not:*
> A large amount of people were present.

Use *No.* or # as an abbreviation for *number*. Note that the abbreviation capitalizes the initial letter and has an ending period: *No.* When the symbol # is used, the numeral follows it with no space between. Consult a reputable resource or dictionary for appropriate use of the abbreviation versus the symbol in any given case.

EXAMPLE

> No. 4 blade
> #4 blade
> Tylenol No. 3

Use the abbreviation or symbol with a figure to indicate position or rank.

EXAMPLE

> He is No. 4 on the appointment list.
> *or:*
> He is #4 on the appointment list.

Use the symbol with arabic numerals for model and serial numbers.

> model #8546
> serial #185043

Use *No.* or # before an apartment, suite, or room number only when the words *apartment, suite,* and *room* (or their abbreviations) are not used.

> 100 Adams Street, No. 228
> 100 Adams Street, #228
> *not:*
> 100 Adams Street, Apt. #228.

Do not use *No.* or # before a house number in the street address.

> 1400 Magnolia Avenue
> *not:*
> #1400 Magnolia Avenue

Do not use the abbreviation or symbol in names of schools, fire companies, lodges, or similar numbered units.

> Public School 4
> Engine Company 3

See 10.3.12—Sutures, Catheters, Needles, and Wires below for use of the # symbol or *No.* when referencing catheters.

Section 3: Measurement and Quantitation

10.3.11 Patient-Identifying Numbers

Use arabic numerals to express numbers used to identify the patient, such as social security numbers, birth dates, telephone numbers, medical record numbers, account numbers, insurance numbers (unless they also contain alpha characters), etc.

EXAMPLE

SSN: 555-99-0101
MRN: 9999999
DOB: 12/12/1979

We will call the patient (555-932-8473) when her lab results return.

10.3.12 Sutures, Catheters, Needles, and Wires

Sutures: The United States Pharmacopeia (USP) system sizes, among other things, steel sutures and sutures of other materials. The sizes range from 11-0 (smallest) to 7 (largest). Thus, a size 7 suture is different from and larger than a size 7-0 suture. Use *0* or *1-0* for single-aught sutures; use the "digit hyphen zero" style to express sizes 2-0 through 11-0. Express sizes 1 through 7 with whole numbers. Place the # symbol before the size if "number" is dictated.

EXAMPLE

1-0 nylon or 0 nylon
but:
2-0 nylon
not:
00 nylon

4-0 Vicryl
not:
0000 Vicryl

The Brown and Sharp (B&S) gauge system sizes stainless steel sutures. Use whole arabic numerals ranging from 40 (smallest) to 20 (largest). Thus, a size 30 suture is smaller than a size 25.

EXAMPLE

size 30 stainless steel suture

Catheters: The French scale is commonly used for sizing catheters, sounds, and other cylindrical instruments. A #1-French is equivalent to 0.33 mm or 1/77 inches of diameter. Thus the size in French units is roughly equal to the circumference of the catheter in millimeters. Precede by # or *No.* if the word "number" is dictated. Since the word "French" is linked directly to the diameter size (and is not an eponym), the number should be correlated to the word "French" with a hyphen. In other words, French does not describe "catheter," but instead partners with the numeral to designate size.

EXAMPLE

5-French catheter
#5-French catheter
not:
size 5 French catheter
not:
catheter, size 5 French

Needles: The diameter of hypodermic needles is indicated by the needle gauge. Various needle lengths are available for any given gauge. There are a number of systems for gauging needles, including the Stubs Needle Gauge and the French Catheter Scale. Needles in common medical use range from 7 (the largest) to 33 (the smallest) on the Stubs scale. Generally speaking, odd-numbered gauges are used for needles, and even-numbered gauges correlate to IV catheters. A 21-gauge needle is the most commonly used to draw blood. For IV catheter placement, 18- to 22-gauge lines are started depending on the condition of the patient's available vessel. The phrase "large bore" refers to catheters of 14-gauge, 16-gauge, or 18-gauge size, when rapid infusion is needed. Needle gauge is inversely proportional to its diameter, so the larger the gauge number, the narrower the diameter. Express using arabic numerals and hyphenate with "gauge" as a compound modifier when preceding the word "needle."

EXAMPLE

21-gauge needle
18-gauge IV line
23-gauge butterfly

Wires, pins, and screws: These materials, typically used in orthopedics, are generally measured in portions of an inch, though frequently metric equivalents are used instead. In the case of pins and screws, typically the size expressed represents the *thread diameter*, which is not the same as the *head diameter*. Transcribe as dictated. When a number alone is given to identify this surgical hardware, it cannot be assumed that the number represents a measurement and could instead represent a numbering system of identification for that particular product. Again, transcribe as dictated; do not add a unit of measure or express as a decimal/fraction when this information is unknown.

EXAMPLE

D: a three thirty two Steinmann pin
T: a 3/32-inch Steinmann pin

D: a four point five cortex screw
T: a 4.5 cortex screw
or:
T: a 4.5 mm cortex screw

D: a number sixteen pin
T: a #16 pin
not:
T: a 16 mm pin
not:
T: a 16-inch pin

When more than one dimension is used to identify a screw or pin (i.e., thread diameter and thread length), express these dimensions fractionally, being careful to express thread diameters as decimals when indicated.

EXAMPLE

D: a six five sixteen cancellous bone screw
T: a 6.5/16 cancellous bone screw
or:
T: a 6.5/16 mm cancellous bone screw

Note: In the example above, it should be assumed that since the author dictated "six five" and not "sixty-five," the expression is intended to represent the phrase "six point five," the most common expression of thread diameters.

Kirschner wires, or K-wires, are measured in portions of an inch but are written using decimals and expressed in thousandths. Be careful to include the zero *after* the decimal point, as physicians do not typically remember to dictate it.

EXAMPLE

D: a four five K wire and a six two K wire
T: a 0.045 K-wire and a 0.062 K-wire

10.3.13 Time Referents

Do not abbreviate English units of time except in virgule constructions and tables. Do not use periods with such abbreviations.

> The patient is 5 days old.
> He will return in 3 weeks for followup.
> The patient describes 2 hours of worsening headache prior to arrival in the ER.

For on-the-hour expressions, it is preferable not to add the colon and 00. (*See military time below.*)

> 8:15 a.m.
> *but:*
> 8 a.m. *or* 8 o'clock in the morning
> *not:*
> 8:00 a.m. *or* 8:00 o'clock
> *not:*
> 8 a.m. o'clock, 8 o'clock a.m., *or* eight o'clock

Noon: Refers to the middle of the day and end of the morning, so it is equivalent to 12 p.m. Do not capitalize. Do not use *12* with it.

> The infant was born at noon, January 14, 2006.

Midnight: Refers to the end of a day in terms of dates, *but* it is equivalent to 12 a.m. Do not capitalize. Do not use *12* with it.

> Twin A was born at midnight, December 31, 2006; twin B at 12:14 a.m., January 1, 2007.

Military time: Identifies the day's 24 hours by numerals 0100 through 2400, rather than 1 a.m. through noon and 1 p.m. through midnight. Hours 0100 through 1200 are consistent with a.m. hours 1 through noon, while hours 1300 through 2400 correlate with p.m. hours 1 through midnight, respectively. This form always takes four numerals, so insert the preceding or following zeros as necessary. Do not separate hours from minutes with a colon. Do not use *a.m.* or *p.m.* If the word *hours* is not dictated it may be added for clarity, but this is not absolutely necessary.

EXAMPLE

1300 hours
0845 hours

Use *'s* or *s'*, whichever is appropriate, with units of time used as possessive adjectives.

EXAMPLE

1 year's experience
2 months' history
3 days' time

Sequence: Give hours, minutes, seconds, tenths, and hundredths, in that sequence, using figures and colons as follows.

EXAMPLE

8:45:4.78

Time Span: Use a hyphen to express time spans as compound modifiers preceding a noun.

EXAMPLE

1-month course
3-day period

Do not separate related time-span units by punctuation.

EXAMPLE

Labor lasted 8 hours 15 minutes.

Time Zones: In extended forms, capitalize only those terms that are always capitalized, e.g., *Atlantic, Pacific.* Note: Some references capitalize *Eastern,* but some do not; be consistent. Lowercase *standard time* and *daylight time. Daylight time* is also known as *daylight-saving time.* Either form is correct, except that when linking the term to the name of a time zone, use *daylight time*, not *daylight-saving time*. Do not capitalize. Do not hyphenate.

Pacific daylight time

Use the abbreviation only when it accompanies a clock reading. Use all capitals in abbreviated forms, with no periods. Do not use commas before or after the abbreviation.

10 a.m. EST
Eastern standard time is...

The time in the zone where an event occurs determines the date (and time) of the event.

Tonight/Yesterday: Be specific when referring to dates. When *tonight* is dictated, include the date to which it refers except in direct quotations. Similarly, when *yesterday* is dictated, include the date to which it refers except in direct quotations.

The following was dictated on March 5, 2002:
D: The patient will be admitted to the hospital tonight.
T: The patient will be admitted to the hospital tonight, March 5, 2002.

To avoid redundancy, do not combine the word *tonight* with the abbreviation *p.m.*

8 tonight *or* 8 o'clock tonight *or* 8:00 tonight *or* 8 p.m.
not:
8 p.m. tonight

Years/Decades/Centuries/Years: Use numerals to express specific years. When referring to a single year without the century, precede it by an apostrophe.

EXAMPLE

> 2001
> '99

Decades: Express with numerals except in special circumstances. Add *s* (without an apostrophe) to form the numeric plural.

EXAMPLE

> The patient was well until the 1990s.

Use a preceding apostrophe in shortened numeric expressions relating to decades of the century ('90s), but omit the preceding apostrophe in expressions relating to decades of age (80s).

EXAMPLE

> He grew up in the '70s.
> He is in his 50s.

Spell out and capitalize special references for decades.

EXAMPLE

> the Roaring Twenties, the Gay Nineties

Spell out and lowercase century numbers *first* through *ninth*; use numerals for 10th and higher.

EXAMPLE

> third century
> 21st century

Use a hyphen when *century* is part of a compound modifier.

EXAMPLE

> 20th-century music

For proper names, use the form preferred by the organization.

> The Twenty-First Century Foundation
> 20th Century Fox

10.3.14 IV Fluids

There are myriad IV fluids that can be encountered in the health record, but the most commonly confused IV fluid references are those that relate to dextrose and normal saline. Dextrose is typically referred to by its percentage in water:

- D5W = 5% dextrose
- D10W = 10% dextrose
- D50W = 50% dextrose

Normal saline (NS) solutions are comprised of sodium chloride, or NaCl, and water:

- Normal saline = 0.9% NaCl in water
- Half normal saline = 0.45% NaCl (half of 0.9%) in water
- Quarter normal saline = 0.23% (a quarter of 0.9%) in water

Do *not* express quarter and half values for normal saline using 0.5 or 0.75 because these would not accurately reflect the concentration. When combined with each other in dictation, transcribe as shown below:

> D: D5 normal saline
> T: D5/NS
>
> D: D10 and a half
> T: D10/0.45 NaCl
> *or:*
> T: D10 and half normal saline
> *not:*
> T: D10-1/2 NS or D10.5 NS
>
> D: D5 and a quarter
> T: D5/0.23 NaCl
> *or:*
> T: D5 and quarter normal saline

Do *not* hyphenate partial values for normal saline. These do not represent compound modifiers. To hyphenate would create an erroneous implication. It is the unit "normal saline" to which the concentration "half" or "quarter" refers.

EXAMPLE

half normal saline
not:
half-normal saline

CHAPTER

11

Percents, Proportions, Ratios, and Ranges

Introduction

The diagnosis and management of disease is predicated upon scientific testing and measurement, the findings of which are expressed not only as singular values but often in contrast, comparison, or relationship to other closely related values. Examples of such expressions would be percents, proportions, ratios, and ranges. How does the MT determine the most appropriate way to represent this information in the record? This chapter will focus on special circumstances where numeric values might be expressed in terms of relationship to other values.

For some determinations, a single value or finding is not as revealing or diagnostically helpful as the relationship between two or more values. In those instances, the significant finding may be derived from determining a proportion, ratio, or range. For example, high levels of low-density lipoprotein cholesterol (LDL-C) and low levels of high-density lipoprotein cholesterol (HDL-C) are significant independent positive risk factors for coronary artery disease and carotid artery atherosclerosis. Conversely, a high level of HDL-C is a significant independent negative risk factor. However, it is the total cholesterol (TC) to high-density lipoprotein cholesterol ratio that is a more valuable measure of coronary artery disease risk than TC or LDL-C levels alone. Similarly, the ratio of protein to creatinine in urine can be used to estimate the magnitude of proteinuria.

Significant laboratory values and many medication dosages often involve expressions of proportion. References to the liquid delivery form of a medication will often include a reference to the strength of that medication per usual dose—per milliliter (mL) for injectables and drops and per 5 mL or 15 mL for oral liquids and syrups. It is thus not uncommon to hear a physician dictate an ear drop, for example, by both strength and dosage: "Otomycin 10,000 units per milliliter, one drop in each ear twice a day."

These numeric expressions, like others covered to this point, represent areas of critical content in a patient record and potential for misinterpretation and clinical error. Knowledge of the clinical context will help guide you in applying these standards. Knowing whether the dictated phrase "two to three" should be expressed as *2 to 3, 2-3,* or *2:3* will depend entirely on the MT's awareness of the context in which this phrase is dictated and whether a range or ratio is being referenced. Thus, care will need to be taken to ensure that they are expressed accurately and without ambiguity.

11.1 Percents

Percent is used to express a ratio or fraction that literally means "per one hundred." It expresses the fractional relationship between a value and 100.

11.1.1 Abbreviated

Keep in mind that *percent* is a single word and should not be expressed as *per cent*, nor should it be expressed as *pct.* except in tables. When abbreviated in the record, use the *percent* symbol, %. Use the symbol % after a numeral. Do not space between the numeral and the symbol.

EXAMPLE

> 13% monos, 1% bands
> She has had a 10% increase in weight since her last visit.
> MCHC 34%
> 10% solution

Use numerals for the number preceding %.

EXAMPLE

> 50% *not* fifty %

According to the SI (International System of Units), it is common and acceptable for percents to be expressed as a fraction of one. MT experience would indicate that it is more common and acceptable for *percent* to be dropped in dictation (and thus in transcription). Use the expression dictated; do not convert.

EXAMPLE

> polys 58% *or* polys 0.58 *or* polys 58
> MCHC 34% *or* MCHC 0.34 *or* MCHC 34

11.1.2 Spelled Out

When the number is written out, as at the beginning of a sentence, write out *percent*.

EXAMPLE

Fifty percent of the patients were given a placebo.

11.1.3 In Ranges

In a range of values, repeat % (or *percent*) with each quantity. See *11.4—Ranges* below for the specific criteria outlined for use of hyphens in range expressions.

EXAMPLE

Values ranged from 13% to 18%.
not:
Values ranged from 13 to 18%.
not:
Values ranged from 13-18%.

Fifty percent to eighty percent...
not:
Fifty to eighty percent...

11.1.4 Percentages Less Than Zero

When the amount is less than 1 percent, place a zero before the decimal.

EXAMPLE

0.5% *not* .5%

With whole numbers, avoid following the number by a decimal point and a zero, since such forms are easily misread. The decimal point and zero may be used if it is important to express exactness. Use it if dictated. *Note:* Keep in mind the dangerous abbreviations recommendations about leading and trailing zeros.

EXAMPLE

5% *not* 5.0%

Use decimals, not fractions, with percents.

0.5% *not* 1/2%

11.2 Proportions

A *proportion* is a special type of ratio expressing a relationship between the part and the whole. When expressed as a fraction, the numerator represents a portion of the total; the denominator is the total.

11.2.1 Numeric Expressions
Always use numerals in expressions of proportions.

5 parts dextrose to 1 part water
The CD4+ cell count was 200/mcL.
Pain was 4/5.
4 out of 5 physicians

11.2.2 With *Per*
Use a virgule for the word *per* when the following conditions have been met: (1) The construction involves at least one *metric* unit of measure, and (2) at least one element includes a specific numeric quantity.

Blood volume was 70 mL/kg of body weight.
Hemoglobin level was 14 g/dL.
but:
Hemoglobin levels are reported in grams per deciliter.

When these expressions involve *nonmetric* units of measure, spell out the word *per* and do not use the virgule, since the virgule implies an abbreviated expression and nonmetric units are abbreviated in the record. *Exception:* Use a virgule when the expression combines a metric unit with a nonmetric unit.

EXAMPLE

> Heart rate was 120 beats per minute.
> She takes 5 mg of Valium per day.
> She weighs in 3 days per week.
> *but:*
> Her IV was set to run at 10 mcg/min while she was in the ER.

Do *not* use the virgule in place of *per* when a prepositional phrase intervenes between the two units of measure.

EXAMPLE

> She was given 4.5 mEq of potassium per liter.
> He was advised to take 81 mg of aspirin per day.

Do *not* use the virgule in place of *per* when neither element in the expression represents a unit of measure (when both elements are numeric) or when there are two numeric values accompanying different units of measure, particularly in drug concentration expressions. When the units differ or the units and/or elements are unknown, a virgule should not be used to imply direct relationship. *Exception:* If it can be confirmed that such an expression is part of the legally registered trademark for a medication, express the concentration with a virgule as indicated by the manufacturer.

EXAMPLE

> Kantrex 0.5 g per 2 mL
> phenobarbital 20 mg per 5 mL
>
> The patient was prescribed Advair 250 per 50 b.i.d.
> I called in a prescription for Hydro-Tussin HD 200 mg per 10 mL.
> *but:*
> I will start her on Nortrel 0.5/35 for pregnancy prevention and management of her PMS. (legally trademarked name)

11.3 Ratios

Ratio refers to the fractional expression of *relationship* between one quantity and another whose value is determined by dividing the numerator by the denominator.

11.3.1 Expressed with Colons
Use a colon in place of the word *to* in the expression of a ratio. Do *not* use a virgule, dash, hyphen, or other mark for this purpose.

EXAMPLE

Mycoplasma 1:2
Cold agglutinins 1:4
Zolyse 1:10,000

11.3.2 Expressed with *To* or a Hyphen
Use *to* or a hyphen instead of a colon when expressing the ratio using words or letters instead of values; use the colon only when expressing the values associated with the ratio.

EXAMPLE

I-to-E ratio
Myeloid-to-erythroid ratio
FEV-FVC ratio
but:
Myeloid-to-erythroid ratio was 10:1.
or:
Myeloid-to-erythroid was 10:1.

11.4 Ranges

An MT will also encounter references to the range between two values. Where ranges are concerned, there is often confusion about when to use the word *to* and when to use a hyphen between two numbers that describe a range of values.

11.4.1 Use of Hyphen versus *To*

Use a hyphen in place of the word *to* in range expressions if all of the following five conditions have been met:

1. The phrases *from…to*, *from…through*, and *between…and* are *not* used.
2. Decimals and/or commas do not appear in the numeric values.
3. Neither value contains four or more digits.
4. Neither value is a negative.
5. Neither value is accompanied by a symbol.

EXAMPLE

Our new office hours will be 1-4 p.m. Tuesdays and Thursdays.
Systolic blood pressures were in the 150-180 range.
BP was 120-130 over 80-90.
There were 8-12 wbc's per high-power field.

When any of the five above conditions is *not* met, use *to* (or other appropriate wording) in place of a hyphen.

EXAMPLE

3+ to 4+ edema *not* 3-4+ edema
$4 to $5 million
-25 to +48
Weight fluctuated between 120 and 130 pounds

Do not use a *colon* between the limits of a range. Colons are used to express ratios, not ranges.

EXAMPLE

80-125
not:
80:125

11.4.2 With *Over* or *Out Of*

When a range is combined with an *over* or *out of* expression, spell out the expression to avoid being misread as a fraction. Do not use a virgule to express the relationship.

Strength in the right extremity is 4 to 4+ over 5.
not:
Strength in the right extremity is 4-4+/5.

She described her pain as a 5 to 6 out of 10.
not:
She described her pain as a 5-6/10.

11.4.3 With Large Numbers

When a hyphen is used to express a range of two large numbers, express both numbers in their entirety, even if dictated in shortened expression, to avoid confusion or lack of clarity.

D: Platelet counts were 300 to 450 thousand.
T: Platelet counts were 300,000 to 450,000.
not:
T: Platelet counts were 300-450,000.

11.4.4 Blood Pressure

Blood pressure ranges should be expressed consistently, using *to* or a hyphen between the ranges of the diastolic pressures and systolic pressures, but these should not be combined in a virgule (/) construction as they may be misunderstood.

D: Blood pressure was 100 to 120 over 70 to 80.
T: Blood pressure was 100-120 over 70-80.
or:
T: Blood pressure was 100 to 120 over 70 to 80.
or:
T: Blood pressure was in the 100-120 over 70-80 range.

Not acceptable because they may be misunderstood are:

> 100-120/70-80
> *or:*
> 100/70 to 120/80.

11.4.5 EKG Leads

For EKG sequential leads, repeat the *V*. Do not use a hyphen or dash.

> leads V1 through V5
> *or:*
> leads V_1 through V_5
> *not:*
> V1 through 5 *or* V_1 through $_5$
> *not:*
> V1-V5 *or* V_1-V_5
> *not:*
> V1-5 *or* V_{1-5}

11.4.6 Money

For ranges related to money, repeat the dollar sign or cent sign but do not repeat the word forms. Use *to* instead of a hyphen with dollar-sign or cent-sign forms.

> $4 to $5
> *not:*
> $4-$5
>
> 10¢ to 15¢
> *not:*
> 10¢-15¢

11.4.7 Intervertebral Disk Spaces

Use a hyphen to express the space between two vertebrae (the intervertebral space). It is not necessary to repeat the same letter before the second vertebra, but it may be transcribed if dictated.

EXAMPLE

C1-2 *or* C1-C2
L5-S1

When expressing a range between two *nonadjacent* vertebrae where the word *through*, not *to*, is used, spell out and do not hyphenate. To hyphenate, especially in reference to fusions, would imply an erroneous construction.

EXAMPLE

D: We performed a fusion of T10 through T12.
T: We performed a fusion of T10 through T12.
not:
T: We performed a fusion of T10-T12.

Note: In the example above, to express this as *T10-T12* would imply that T10 was fused to T12 rather than a procedure that involved fusion of T10 to T11 and T11 to T12.

CHAPTER

12

Units of Measure

Introduction

Chapters 10 and 11 focused on the delineation of *quantity* in the medical record, those critical value areas of a report where numbers, or fractions thereof, are used to quantify certain measurements in a patient's diagnosis, treatment, and care. This chapter, however, will focus on those common terms that *qualify*, or provided definitive value to, that information. This chapter will outline the most common and significant qualifiers in the medical record—*units of measure*. These two sides of the same coin are equally important in providing a full diagnostic picture. In order for a patient's diagnostic information to be meaningful, it must be quantified *and* qualified. A numeric value alone will be of little significance without an understanding of the method or measurement from which that value is derived or the system by which it is being measured. If I tell you that a patient's wound measurement was an 8, that information alone would be insufficient. *Is it 8 inches? 8 cm? 8 fingerbreadths?* The value must be qualified. Likewise, a general measurement of "a few inches" does not provide the diagnostic context that is often critical to care. The value must be more clearly quantified. A quantified numeric value and a qualified unit of measure will provide the greatest level of detail, and it is this kind of data that is extracted for patient care and for statistical warehousing.

Most values in the record must be qualified for them to have meaning, although quite often the qualifier is implied. While it will be important for you to memorize and recognize the myriad units of measure that are commonly encountered in dictation, you will not be required in most settings to provide these units where they are not dictated. In the laboratory section of the report, for example, it is common practice for physicians to dictate just the name of a particular test and its numeric value, though virtually all of those values have a corresponding unit of measure that can be verified in a reputable laboratory resource. There are some facilities that do require their transcriptionists to include the units of measure with each laboratory value, whether dictated or not; however, this scenario is rare and is not common practice.

A dictator will rarely, if ever, dictate the unit of measure in its abbreviated form. A physician will not say that the patient was given "50 M G of Tylenol." Rather, he will dictate that the patient was given "50 milligrams of Tylenol," and the MT will be expected to abbreviate those units appropriately.

12.1 Metric Units

One of the complex aspects of this particular chapter is the contradiction that can be found in some areas between what is identified in the International System of Units or what is identified as part of the metric system and what is commonly encountered in transcription. It will be important to understand that the SI system is an evolved metric system that is now being widely adopted worldwide. There is still some inconsistency, however, in whether a value is reported in older metric units or the new SI units, though most units are similar.

12.1.1 International System of Units (SI)

The International System of Units (Système International d'Unités, abbreviated SI) is the system of metric measurements adopted in 1960 at the Eleventh General Conference on Weights and Measures of the International Organization for Standards. Since the 1977 recommendation of the 30th World Health Assembly that SI units be used in medicine, some medical journals use the SI to a limited degree, some use it only in conjunction with conventional units, and some have not yet adopted it. The adoption of SI in the documentation of patient care is likewise sporadic, but it is sufficiently widespread, in whole or in part, to warrant the attention of medical transcriptionists. It should be noted that, although some units from the apothecary system remain in use, all elements of the apothecary system have been dropped from the compendium of the United States Pharmacopeia (USP) system. Additionally, the accelerated movement toward international adoption of the electronic patient record is likely to strengthen the adoption of the SI in order to facilitate communication across borders.

12.1.2 Basic Units and Properties

The SI is founded in seven (7) SI base units representing an invariable physical measure.

base unit	SI symbol	basic property
meter	m	length
kilogram	kg	mass
second	s	time
ampere	A	electric current
kelvin	K	thermodynamic temperature
candela	cd	luminous intensity
mole	mol	amount of substance

Two supplementary units of the SI are:

radian	rad	plane angle
steradian	sr	solid angle

12.1.3 Derived Units

Other quantities, called *derived quantities*, are defined in terms of the seven base quantities via a system of quantity equations. The *SI derived units* for these derived quantities are obtained from these equations and the seven SI base units.

area	square meter	m^2
volume	cubic meter	m^3
speed/velocity	meter per second	m/s
acceleration	meter per second squared	m/s^2
wave number	reciprocal meter	m^{-1}
mass density	kilogram per cubic meter	kg/m^3
specific volume	cubic meter per kilogram	m^3/kg
current density	ampere per square meter	A/m^2
electric field	volt per meter	V/m
magnetic field strength	ampere per meter	A/m
substance concentration	mole per cubic meter	mol/m^3
luminance	candela per square meter	cd/m^2
mass fraction	kilogram per kilogram	kg/kg=1
frequency	hertz	Hz
pressure	pascal	Pa
force	newton	N

Note: Hertz, pascal, and newton are eponyms but are not capitalized when they are spelled out, even when they stand alone unaccompanied by a numeric value, except in instances (not typically encountered in health care) where the individuals associated with the naming of those units are referenced.

12.1.4 Prefixes and Symbols

The 20 SI prefixes used to form decimal multiples and submultiples of SI units are:

factor	prefix	symbol
10^{24}	yotta-	Y
10^{21}	zetta-	Z
10^{18}	exa-	E
10^{15}	peta-	P
10^{12}	tera-	T
10^{9}	giga-	G
10^{6}	mega-	M
10^{3}	kilo-	k
10^{2}	hecto-	h
10	deca-	da
10^{-1}	deci-	d
10^{-2}	centi-	c
10^{-3}	milli-	m
10^{-6}	micro-	μ *(See Note below)*
10^{-9}	nano-	n
10^{-12}	pico-	p
10^{-15}	femto-	f
10^{-18}	atto-	a
10^{-21}	zepto-	z
10^{-24}	yocto-	y

Note: Despite the fact that the symbol for *micro* continues to be μ in the international community and outside of health care, this symbol now appears on the dangerous abbreviations list, as outlined in Chapter 9 of this text, when combined with other units that may potentially be misread as "milli" instead of "micro." Currently, The Joint Commission specifies only *micrograms* and *microunits* on its list of dangerous uses of the symbol and recommends:

EXAMPLE

mcg *not* μg
microunits *not* μU *or* mcU (since "units" must be spelled out)

All other uses of the *micro* symbol (μ) are considered acceptable, and the symbol should be used where electronic environments facilitate its insertion.

It is important to note that the kilogram is the only SI unit with a prefix as part of its name and symbol. Because multiple prefixes may *not* be used, in the case of the kilogram the prefix names outlined above are used with the unit name "gram" and the prefix symbols are used with the unit symbol "g."

EXAMPLE

10^{-6} kg = 1 mg (one milligram)
not:
10^{-6} kg = 1 μkg (one microkilogram)

12.1.5 Abbreviation

Abbreviate most units of measure that accompany numerals and include virgule constructions. Use the same abbreviation for singular and plural forms. Do not use periods with abbreviated units of measure.

EXAMPLE

1 g
20 g
40 mm/h

The following are abbreviations for the metric units of measure most commonly used in medical reports. Do not use periods.

cm	centimeter
dL	deciliter
g	gram
L	liter
mEq	milliequivalent
mg	milligram
mL	milliliter
mm	millimeter
mmHg	millimeter of mercury
mmol	millimole
msec, ms	millisecond

Use these abbreviations only when a numeric quantity precedes the unit of measure. Do not add an s to indicate plural form.

12.1.6 Capitalization
Do not capitalize most metric units of measure or their abbreviations. Learn the obvious exceptions, and consult appropriate references for guidance.

EXAMPLE

cm	centimeter
dB	decibel
Hz	hertz
L	liter
mmHg	millimeter of mercury

12.1.7 Punctuation

Unit symbols are *not* followed by a period unless they occur at the end of a sentence.

EXAMPLE

> The wound measured 3 cm.
> *or:*
> The wound was 3 cm in length.
> *not:*
> The wound was 3 cm. in length.

Do *not* use a hyphen to form a compound modifier between a numeric value and its metric unit. According to the National Institute for Science and Technology:

In the expression for the value of a quantity, the unit symbol is placed after the numerical value and a space is left between the numerical value and the unit symbol. Even when the value of a quantity is used in an adjectival sense, a space is left between the numerical value and the unit symbol. This rule recognizes that unit symbols are not like ordinary words or abbreviations but are mathematical entities, and that the value of a quantity should be expressed in a way that is as independent of language as possible.

EXAMPLE

> 3 cm wound
> *not:*
> 3-cm wound
>
> 2 x 2 cm lesion
> *not:*
> 2 x 2-cm lesion *or* 2-x-2-cm lesion

12.1.8 Plurals

Metric unit symbols are unaltered in the plural.

EXAMPLE

> 1 cm, 2 cm, 10 cm
> *not:*
> 1 cm, 2 cms, 10 cms

12.1.9 Exponential Expressions

When technology does not readily allow exponents to be expressed as super-scripts, abbreviations like *cu* and *sq* are acceptable. Do not place the exponent numerals on the line in these expressions as they are not easily read when expressed in this manner.

EXAMPLE

10^5 *or* 10 to the 5th
3 m^2 *or* 3 sq m (*not* m2)
9 m^3 *or* 9 cu m (*not* m3)

12.1.10 Multiplication of Numbers

The SI uses the multiplication sign to express multiplication of values. The lowercase *x* should be used to express:

EXAMPLE

2 x 8 cm^2 burn (area)
3.2 x 4.3 x 4.9 m^3 cube (volume)
2 x 2 table (matrixes)
x30,000 (magnification)
4.6 x 10^9/L (scientific notation)

12.1.11 Concentrations

Concentrations can be expressed using a virgule (/) in place of the word *per* when the following conditions have been met: (1) The construction involves at least one *metric* unit of measure, and (2) at least one element includes a specific numeric quantity.

EXAMPLE

The CD4+ cell count was 200/mcL.
Blood volume was 70 mL/kg of body weight.

Hemoglobin level was 14 g/dL.
but:
Hemoglobin levels are reported in grams per deciliter.

Do *not* use the virgule in place of *per* when a prepositional phrase intervenes between the two units of measure.

> She was given 4.5 mEq of potassium per liter.
> He was advised to take 81 mg of aspirin per day.

Do *not* use the virgule in place of *per* when neither element in the expression represents a unit of measure (when both elements are numeric) or when there are two numeric values accompanying different units of measure, particularly in drug concentration expressions. When the units differ or the units and/or elements are unknown, a virgule should not be used to imply direct relationship. *Exception*: If it can be confirmed that such an expression is part of the legally registered trademark for a medication, express the concentration with a virgule as indicated by the manufacturer.

> The patient was prescribed Advair 250 per 50 b.i.d.
> I called in a prescription for Hydro-Tussin HD 200 mg per 10 mL.
> *but:*
> I will start her on Nortrel 0.5/35 for pregnancy prevention and management of her PMS. (legally trademarked name)

12.2 Conventional (Nonmetric) Units

Transcriptionists in the US will also find that old Imperial units and apothecary units are still used in certain areas of our healthcare system. This, of course, will come as no surprise to any American MT student who has likely grown up with the reality that the United States has not fully adopted the metric system. Our healthcare documentation is a reflection of this reality. In any given patient record, you will find references that range from older apothecary units (*drops, drams*) to English units (*pounds, ounces, feet*) to metric units (*mg, cm, mL*). Fortunately, these occur consistently in their contexts, at least within the US healthcare system. Height and weight, for example, are always dictated in English units, while the weight of the organs in an autopsy or pathology report is usually reported and recorded in metric units. Fortunately, the transcriptionist is rarely ever left wondering which unit is being referred to and will likely not encounter a flip-flop in usage in these areas. The only exception to this, of course, will be for MTs who transcribe in countries where the metric system may be more widely utilized. A transcriptionist transcribing for Canadian facilities will encounter some differences in style there and will probably encounter metric measurements virtually everywhere in a report. If those same transcriptionists perform work for US healthcare providers, however, they may find themselves hearing different units being dictated in the same contexts.

12.2.1 Basic Units and Properties

Spell out common nonmetric units of measure (ounce, pound, inch, foot, yard, mile, etc.) to express weight, depth, distance, height, length, and width, except in tables. Do not use an apostrophe or quotation marks to indicate feet or inches, respectively (except in tables).

EXAMPLE

    4 pounds
    5 ounces
    14 inches
    5 feet

12.2.2 Abbreviation

Do not abbreviate most nonmetric units of measure, except in tables. Use the same abbreviation for both singular and plural forms; do not add *s*.

EXAMPLE

    5 feet 3 inches
    not:
    5' 3" *or* 5 ft. 3 in.

    2 pounds
    not:
    2 lbs *or* 2#

Do not use a comma or other punctuation between units of the same dimension.

EXAMPLE

    The infant weighed 5 pounds 3 ounces.
    He is 5 feet 4 inches tall.

12.2.3 Compound Modifiers

Use a hyphen to join a number and a *nonmetric* unit of measure when they are used as an adjective preceding a noun.

EXAMPLE

> 5-inch wound
> 8-pound 5-ounce baby girl

12.2.4 Concentration

When expressions of concentration involve *nonmetric* units of measure, spell out the word *per* and do not use the virgule, since the virgule implies an abbreviated expression and nonmetric units are not abbreviated in the record. *Exception:* Use a virgule when the expression combines a metric unit with a nonmetric unit.

EXAMPLE

> Heart rate was 120 beats per minute.
> She takes 5 mg of Valium per day.
> She weighs in 3 days per week.
> *but:*
> Her IV was set to run at 10 mcg/min while she was in the ER.

It is important to note that a *molar* solution contains 1 mol (1 g by molecular weight) of solute in 1 L of solution. The SI style for reporting molar solutions is *mol/L*. For solutions with millimolar concentrations, *mmol/L* is used. For solutions with micromolar concentrations, the convention is to use *µmol/L*.

EXAMPLE

> The gel was incubated after applying 10 mL of a solution of 4 mmol/L potassium chloride and 5 mL of a solution of 1 mol/L sodium chloride.

12.2.5 Units of Time

Do not abbreviate expressions of English units of time except in virgule constructions. Do not use periods with such abbreviations.

minute	min
second	s
week	wk
month	mo
hour	h
day	d
year	y

The patient is 5 days old.
He will return in 1 week for followup.
40 mm/h
q.4 h.

12.2.6 Temperature

Degrees: Express temperature degrees with numerals except for zero.

zero degrees
36 degrees
36 °C

Use minus (not the symbol) to indicate temperatures below zero.

minus 48 °C

If the temperature scale name (Celsius, Fahrenheit, Kelvin) or abbreviation (C, F, K) is not dictated, it is not necessary to insert it.

38 °C
or:
38 degrees Celsius
or:
38 degrees

Use the degree symbol (°) if available, immediately followed by the abbreviation for the temperature scale. If the degree symbol is not available, write out *degrees* (and the temperature scale name, if dictated). Per the SI convention, a space should exist between the numeric value and its unit of measure.

EXAMPLE

98 °F
or:
98 degrees Fahrenheit

Note: The inclusion of a space between the numeric value and the degree symbol when expressing temperature values represents a change from recommendations provided in the previous editions of this text. SI convention clearly outlines that the space is only dropped with the degree symbol in expressions of planar angles (*See 12.2.7—Angles below*). AHDI has chosen to adopt this SI standard over that outlined in the *AMA Manual of Style*, which we believe represents an error in application.

Celsius: Metric-system temperature scale, designed by and named for Celsius, a Swedish astronomer. Also known as centigrade scale, but Celsius is the preferred term. Normal human temperature on the Celsius scale is 36.7 degrees, often rounded to 37 degrees. In the Celsius system, zero degrees represents the freezing point of water; 100 degrees represents the boiling point at sea level. Abbreviation: C (no period).

EXAMPLE

37 °C
or:
37 degrees Celsius

Fahrenheit: Temperature scale designed by and named for Fahrenheit, a German-born physicist who also invented the mercury thermometer. Normal human temperature on the Fahrenheit scale is 98.6 degrees. Abbreviation: F (no period).

EXAMPLE

96.5 °F
or:
96.5 degrees Fahrenheit

Kelvin: Temperature scale based on Celsius but not identical. It is used to record extremely high and low temperatures in science. The starting point is zero, representing total absence of heat and equal to minus 273.15 degrees Celsius. To convert to Kelvin from Celsius, subtract 273.15 from the Celsius temperature.

12.2.7 Angles

In expressing planar or rotational angles in orthopedics, write out *degrees* or use the degree symbol (°). When using the symbol, per SI convention, do *not* space between the number and the symbol.

EXAMPLE

> The patient was able to straight leg raise to 40 degrees.
> *or:*
> The patient was able to straight leg raise to 40°.

Use the degree symbol (°) when expressing planar or rotational angles in imaging studies.

EXAMPLE

> Positioning the patient's head at a 90° angle allowed for efficient acquisition of data over a 180° arc.
> Coronary cineangiography was done to LAO 60° and RAO 30°.

Trend Note: Some electronic environments and proprietary transcription platforms do not allow for use of the degree symbol. In those instances, spell out *degrees*. Since the word *degrees* is a *nonmetric* unit, keep in mind that compound modifying expressions should be hyphenated when the word is spelled out.

EXAMPLE

> 90-degree angle
> 180-degree arc
> *but:*
> an angle of 90 degrees
> a view of 360 degrees

12.3 Quick Reference Guides

The following tables are included for quick reference to both SI and
Conventional units of measure.

12.3.1 Units by Type

Basic Property	Metric or SI Units	Nonmetric Units
length	meter (m)	fingerbreadth, inch, feet, yard, mile
mass	gram (g), kilogram (kg)	ounce, pound
time		second (s), minute (m)
electrical current electrical voltage electrical resistance	ampere (A) volts (V) ohms	
temperature	degrees Celsius (C) kelvin (K)	degrees Fahrenheit (F)
luminous intensity	candela (cd)	
amount of substance	mole (mol)	
area	square meter (m²)	square inch, square yard
volume	cubic meter (m³)	cubic inch, cubic yard
frequency	hertz (Hz)	
energy, work	joule (J)	
pressure	pascal (Pa)	pounds per square inch (psi)
force	newton (N)	
mass density	kilogram per cubic meter (kg/m³)	pounds per cubic foot
speed, velocity	meter per second (m/s)	feet per second
acceleration	meter per second squared (m/s²)	feet per second squared
electric field strength	volt per meter (V/m)	
radiation	milliCuries (mCi)	

12.3.2 Common Prefixes

Prefix	Fractional Unit
deci-	one-tenth
centi-	one-hundredth
milli-	one-thousandth
micro-	one-millionth
nano-	one-billionth
pico-	one-trillionth
deka-	10 units
hector-	100 units
kilo-	1000 units
mega-	one million units
giga-	one billion units
tera-	one trillion units

12.3.3 Metric Conversions

Nonmetric Symbol	Known Quantity	Multiply by	To Find	Metric Symbol
in.	inches	2.54	centimeters	cm
ft	feet	30	centimeters	cm
ft	feet	0.3	meters	m
yd	yards	0.9	meters	m
	miles	1.6	kilometers	km
sq in	square inches	6.5	square centimeters	cm²
sq ft	square feet	0.09	square meters	m²
sq yd	square yards	0.8	square meters	m²
	square miles	2.6	square kilometers	km²
oz	ounces	28	grams	g
lb	pounds	0.45	kilograms	kg
tsp	teaspoons	5	milliliters	mL
tbsp	tablespoons	15	milliliters	mL
fl oz	fluid ounces	30	milliliters	mL
c	cups	0.24	liters	L
pt	US pints	0.47	liters	L
qt	US quarts	0.95	liters	L
gal	US gallons	3.8	liters	L
cu ft	cubic feet	0.03	cubic meters	m³
cu yd	cubic yards	0.76	cubic meters	m³

References

Taylor, B.N. Guide for the Use of the International System of Units. May 2007. 11 Nov. 2007. < http://physics.nist.gov/Pubs/SP811/contents.html>

Section 4
Specialty Standards

CHAPTER

13

Pharmacology

Introduction

As far back as ancient times, healers and physicians have turned to pharmacology to treat symptoms and cure disease. No generation, however, has witnessed a greater evolution, application, and use of drugs than our current one. Although there is a growing trend in medicine to seek alternative remedies, most of these are still based on herbal pharmacology, and despite the emergence of these new remedies, traditional medicine is still by far the treatment of choice in the US healthcare system. The application of medicinal remedies in the management and treatment of disease is a core component of patient care and, thus, a critical presence in documentation.

13.1 Chemical Nomenclature

Pharmacology is based on fundamental chemistry, or the synergy created by interaction and bonding of basic chemical elements. Most of these elements are found either in the human body, in large quantities or trace amounts, or in the drugs formulated to cure and/or manage disease. How these elements bond with each other to form a compound as well as how they interact with each other both outside and within the human body can be critical to the predication of a drug's efficacy *and* the potential harm or benefit that drug may have on a patient. Likewise, the balance of the basic elements in the human body is critical to homeostasis, or physical well-being, so these chemical references form the basis of most laboratory testing and evaluation as well.

13.1.1 Elements and Symbols
Names of elements are not capitalized. The symbols for chemical elements always include an initial capital letter; if there is a second letter, it is always lowercase. Never use periods or other punctuation with chemical symbols.

The following is a list of some of the more commonly encountered elements from the periodic table, with their symbols.

barium	Ba	iron	Fe
calcium	Ca	lead	Pb
carbon	C	magnesium	Mg
cesium	Cs	mercury	Hg
chlorine	Cl	nitrogen	N
cobalt	Co	oxygen	O
copper	Cu	potassium	K
gadolinium	Gd	silver	Ag
gallium	Ga	sodium	Na
gold	Au	sulfur	S
hydrogen	H	technetium	Tc
iodine	I	zinc	Zn

Some elements are uniquely used with *lasers*:

EXAMPLE

aluminum
argon
chromium
erbium
garnet
helium
holmium
neodymium
rhodamine
ruby
thulium
yttrium

Often these elements are combined and abbreviated in laser references.

yttrium-aluminum-garnet (YAG) laser
thulium-holmium-chromium-yttrium-aluminum-garnet (THC:YAG) laser
neodymium-doped yttrium-aluminum-garnet (Nd:YAG) laser

13.1.2 Compounds

Lowercase the names of chemical compounds written in full. Never use hyphens in chemical elements or compounds, whether used as nouns or adjectives. These should only be capitalized when abbreviated. *Exception:* Some *isotopes* are joined to the chemical name with a hyphen; refer to an appropriate drug resource for verification (*See 13.3.7—Isotopes below*).

carbon dioxide
not:
Carbon Dioxide
but:
CO2

Note: Do not confuse the capital "O" in oxygen references to the number 0.

13.1.3 Chemical Names and Concentrations

Do not capitalize chemical names, except at the beginning of a sentence.

acetylsalicylic acid
oxygen

Use brackets to express chemical concentration. When concentrations are expressed as percentages, use the percent sign rather than the spelled-out form, and do not use brackets.

[HCO_3-] *or* [HCO3-]
15% HNO_3 *or* HNO3

13.1.4 Formulas

Use parentheses for innermost units, adding brackets, then braces, if necessary. (Note that this is different from regular text, which uses brackets for the innermost parenthetical insertion and parentheses for the outermost.) Italics may also be used for some portions; consult chemistry references. Two examples of chemical formulas follow.

EXAMPLE

chlorphenoxamine hydrochloride
2-[1-(4-chlorophenyl)-1-phenylethoxy]-N,N-dimethylethanamine hydrochloride

hydroxychloroquine sulfate
7-chloro-4-{4-[ethyl(2-hydroxyethyl)amino]-1-methylbutylamino}-quinoline sulfate

13.1.5 Biochemical Terminology

Write out biochemical terms in healthcare documents because their abbreviations may not be readily recognized by healthcare professionals. Use abbreviated forms only in tables and in communications among biochemical specialists.

The following are examples of biochemical groups, terms, and abbreviations (3-letter and/or 1-letter):

amino acids of proteins	
phenylalanine	Phe, F
proline	Pro, P
tryptophan	Trp, W

common ribonucleosides	
adenosine	Ado, A
cytidine	Cyd, C
uridine	Urd, U

bases and nucleosides	
cytosine	Cyt
purine	Pur
uracil	Ura

sugars and carbohydrates	
fructose	Fru
glucose	Rib

13.2 Pharmacology

Medical transcriptionists should be familiar with the types, classifications, descriptions, and applications of core drug groups. In addition, you will be expected to recognize many commonly prescribed drugs by specialty and use as well as the rules for *how* this information should be represented in writing. As always, the focus is on clarity of communication in the record.

13.2.1 Drug Approval

Drugs intended for clinical use in health care go through several phases of development before they are approved by the FDA for human use. Specific clinical studies, including testing in animals, are typically performed after the manufacturer has obtained *investigational new drug (IND)* approval from the FDA. Once approved, the manufacturer applies for a nonproprietary, or generic name, for the drug under investigation. Development of the drug must comply with the Declaration of Helsinki and undergo institutional review board approval as well as informed consent from patients in order to be used in studies. Development typically follows these phases of clinical study or trial:

- Phase 1: Studies conducted in healthy volunteers to assess safety, effects, metabolism, kinetics, and drug interactions.
- Phase 2: Studies conducted to establish therapeutic efficacy and determine dose range.
- Phase 3: Trials typically randomized, controlled studies that assess safety/ efficacy in a large sample of patients (2000-3000) for whom the drug is anticipated to be effective.

These 3 phases represent a time frame of typically 2 to 10 years, with an average of 5 to 6 years. FDA approval typically follows within 1 year of the end of the third phase of clinical trials.

Drugs marketed or prescribed in the United States *must* have FDA approval. The FDA also approves the labeling for the newly approved drugs in terms of indications/conditions for which the drug can be *marketed*. The FDA does not, however, approve the other unanticipated indications/conditions for which the drug may ultimately be *prescribed*, which are generally referred to as *off-label prescriptions*.

13.2.2 Drug Naming and Classification

Brand Name: The brand, or proprietary, name is the manufacturer's name for a drug; it is the same as the trademark name. It may suggest a use or indication, and it often incorporates the manufacturer's name. Capitalize brand names and trademark names.

EXAMPLE

Tagamet
Bayer

Use of idiosyncratic capitalization is optional.

EXAMPLE

pHisoHex
or:
Phisohex

Trade Name: The trade name is a broader term than trademark, identifying the manufacturer but not the product. Capitalize trade names.

EXAMPLE

Dr. Scholl's

Code Name: The code name is the temporary designation for an as-yet-unnamed drug; it is assigned by the manufacturer. It may include a code number or code designation (number-letter combination).

Chemical Name: The chemical name describes the chemical structure of a drug. The American Chemical Society, which is the internationally recognized source for such names, follows a set of guidelines established by chemists. Do not capitalize chemical names.

EXAMPLE

acetylsalicylic acid
hydrogen peroxide

Generic Name: The generic name is also known as the nonproprietary name, the established, official name for a drug. In the United States, it is created by the US Adopted Names Council (USAN). International nomenclature is coordinated by the World Health Organization. The nonproprietary name is regulated internationally to ensure consistent usage and no duplication with other drugs. Generic names are in the public domain; their use is unrestricted. Do not capitalize generic names. When the generic name and brand name of a medication sound alike, use the generic spelling unless it is certain that the brand name is being referenced.

EXAMPLE

D: aminophylline
T: aminophylline
not:
T: Aminophyllin

Note: For MTs who prepare clinical manuscripts for their physician clients/ employers, be aware that the AMA recommends use of the nonproprietary name for all drugs referenced in formal publication to ensure research credibility that is not clouded by the perceived bias of using and clinically referencing a proprietary drug in formal literature.

Transcriptionists should be well aware of both generic and brand names for common drugs so there is no confusion when both are used interchangeably, even in the same report. When a generic reference is dictated and later in the same dictation the brand is used (or vice versa), neither reference should be edited or changed.

EXAMPLE

D: The patient was told on her last visit to take Tylenol t.i.d. as needed for her intermittent headaches.....She will return in 2 months and is instructed to continue taking her acetaminophen as needed.
T: She will return in 2 months and is instructed to continue taking her acetaminophen as needed.
not:
T: She will return in 2 months and is instructed to continue taking her Tylenol as needed.

Drugs of Abuse Scheduling: Transcriptionists should also be familiar with references to the classification schedule for drugs of abuse. The Controlled Substances Act of 1970 established by the Drug Enforcement Administration (DEA) mandated regulation of the manufacturing and dispensing of drugs deemed dangerous and potentially addictive. This law divided drugs of potential abuse into the following 5 schedules:

Schedule I: Drugs deemed to have a high risk for abuse/dependence for which there is no current recognized clinical application/use.

EXAMPLE

PCP
heroin
LSD
MDMA
marijuana
methaqualone

Schedule II: Drugs deemed to have a high risk for abuse/dependence that also have current clinical application/use.

EXAMPLE

opium
morphine
coca
cocaine
methadone
methamphetamine

Schedule III: Drugs deemed to have some risk for abuse/dependence that also have a high degree of clinical application/use.

EXAMPLE

amphetamine
barbiturate
Valium
Xanax
anabolic steroids
codeine

Schedule IV: Drugs deemed to have a limited risk for abuse/dependence that also have a high degree of clinical application/use.

chloral hydrate
meprobamate
paraldehyde
phenobarbital

Schedule V: Drugs deemed to have a low risk for abuse/dependence that are used for clinical research or represent the above drugs used in limited amounts for specific applications.

Note: Drug abuse schedules have historically been expressed using roman numerals, but many resources cite these schedules using arabic numerals. Defer to facility preference when transcribing these references in the record.

Slang or street references to illicit drugs should be included in quotation marks.

The patient says he has been up all night "hitting the pipe."
He finally admitted he is a "speedball" user.

When slang or brief forms of the actual drug name are referenced, either put the slang term in quotation marks or use the formal drug name.

She denies any "coke" use in the last 3 months.
or
She denies any cocaine use in the last 3 months.

13.2.3 Forms and Routes

Part of the approval process with the FDA involves a clear identification of the form or forms the drug will be manufactured in as well as the anticipated routes of administration that are deemed to be the safest and most effective for the patient. Transcriptionists should be familiar with all potential forms and routes that will be dictated by the author as well as any abbreviated forms used to express these.

The following are the most common forms of pharmacologic administration:

- tablet
- capsule
- cream
- ointment
- lotion
- powder
- liquid (elixirs, syrups, tinctures, sprays, and foams)
- suspension and emulsion
- suppository
- transdermal
- pellet/bead

When any of these forms are abbreviated as part of the dosage instructions, it is not necessary to expand them.

EXAMPLE

Tylenol 2 tabs b.i.d. p.r.n.
She was told to increase her dose to 2 caps instead of one.

In addition to the form of administration, there are various routes by which medications may be administered, which are outlined below:

- oral
- sublingual
- rectal
- vaginal
- topical
- transdermal
- inhalation
- parenteral
- intradermal
- subcutaneous
- intramuscular
- intravenous
- intra-articular
- intracardiac
- endotracheal
- intrathecal
- intra-arterial
- umbilical

Some of these routes are commonly abbreviated by the author, and it is not necessary to expand them, but care should be taken to use the appropriate abbreviations for these terms.

> oral—p.o. *not* po *or* PO
> subcutaneous—subcu *not* subQ *or* subq
> intramuscular—IM *not* I.M., i.m., *or* im
> intravenous—IV *not* I.V., i.v., *or* iv
> endotracheal—ET *not* E.T., e.t., *or* et

Note: In most instances, it is acceptable to use these abbreviated routes even when they are not used in direct correlation to a dosage instruction. Also, some institutions have historically required their transcriptionists to include periods with *I.V.* to avoid its misinterpretation as a roman numeral. It is the position of AHDI, however, that this is unnecessary since there would rarely be a context in which this would be used where meaning would be ambiguous.

> The patient is able to tolerate p.o. quite well.
> EMT began IV hydration in the field.

13.2.4 Dosage Schedules

Dose refers to the amount to be administered at one time, or total amount administered. *Dosage* means regimen and is usually expressed as a quantity per unit of time.

> dose   5 mg
> dosage   5 mg q.i.d.

Use lowercase abbreviations with periods for Latin abbreviations that are related to doses and dosages. Do not use abbreviations found on the dangerous abbreviations list provided in Chapter 9 of this text. Avoid using all capitals because they emphasize the abbreviation rather than the drug name. Avoid lowercase abbreviations without periods because some may be misread as words. *Do not translate. (see examples next page)*

abbreviation	Latin phrase	English translation
a.c.	ante cibum	before food
b.i.d.	bis in die	twice a day
gtt.	guttae	drops (better to spell out drops)
n.p.o.	nil per os	nothing by mouth
n.r.	non repetatur	do not repeat
p.c.	post cibum	after food
p.o.	per os	by mouth
p.r.n.	pro re nata	as needed
q.4 h.	quaque 4 hora	every 4 hours
q.h.	quaque hora	every hour
q.i.d.	quater in die	4 times a day
t.i.d.	ter in die	3 times a day
u.d.	ut dictum	as directed

Note: We have inserted a space after the numeral 4 in q.4 h. on the advice of the ISMP so that the number is more easily and clearly read.

Invalid Latin abbreviations such as q.a.m. (every morning) and mixed Latin and English abbreviations such as q.4 hours (every 4 hours) have become commonplace. However, as with all abbreviations, avoid those that are obscure (like a.c.b. for before breakfast) or dangerous. For example, b.i.w. is both obscure and dangerous. It is intended to mean twice weekly, but it could be mistaken for twice daily, resulting in a dosage frequency seven times that intended.

It is acceptable to express a range in dosage times in abbreviated format.

EXAMPLE

q.2–3 h.
q.4–6 h.

Note: AHDI continues to discourage dropping periods in lowercase abbreviations that might be misread as words (for example, bid and tid). If you must drop the periods, use all capitals, but keep in mind that the overuse of capitals, particularly in relation to drug doses and dosages, would draw more attention to the capitalized abbreviations than to the drug names themselves.

13.2.5 System of Measurement

Most pharmaceutical measurements for weight and volume are in the metric system. Although some units from the apothecary and avoirdupois systems remain in use, it should be noted that all elements of the apothecary system have been dropped from the compendium of the United States Pharmacopeia system (USP).

apothecary system	
weight	**liquid measure**
1 grain (gr)	1 minim
1 scruple (20 gr)	1 fluidram (60 minims)
1 dram (60 gr)	1 fluidounce (8 fluidrams)
1 ounce (480 gr)	1 pint (16 fluidounces)
1 pound (5760 gr)	1 gallon (4 quarts or 8 pints)

Note: Either fluidounce or fluid ounce is an acceptable spelling.

avoirdupois system
1 grain
1 ounce (437.5 grains)
1 pound (16 ounces or 7000 grains)

13.2.6 Punctuation

Do not use commas to separate drug names from doses and instructions. In a series of drugs for each of which the dose and/or instructions are given, use commas to separate each complete entry. *Exception:* Use semicolons or periods when entries in the series have internal commas. Medications may also be listed vertically. *(see examples next page)*

The patient was discharged on Coumadin 10 mg daily.

The patient was discharged on Carafate 1 g q.i.d., 40 minutes after meals and at bedtime; bethanechol 25 mg p.o. q.i.d.; and Reglan 5 mg at bedtime on a trial basis.

He was sent home on Biaxin 500 mg b.i.d., Atrovent inhaler 2 puffs q.i.d., and Altace 5 mg daily.

CURRENT MEDICATIONS
1. Lescol 2 mg at bedtime.
2. DiaBeta 5 mg 1 q.a.m.
3. Aspirin 325 mg 1 daily.
4. Xanax 0.25 mg t.i.d. p.r.n.

Some drug names, particularly those for topical preparations, include a percentage of active drug contained in the preparation. Use the percent symbol (%) and indicate these percentages after the drug name.

D: The patient was treated with metronidazole lotion point seven five.
T: The patient was treated with metronidazole lotion, 0.75%.

13.3 Drug Nomenclatures

Some of the nomenclatures outlined in this section are rather obscure and rarely encountered. Depending on the setting, an MT may spend an entire career without transcribing some of these terms. However, those MTs employed or contracted by a physician or practice that is involved in research, case studies, and clinical trials will likely be asked to transcribe records and prepare manuscripts in which these terms are referenced. More detailed scientific data and references to chemical formulas and processes that you would not typically find in patient record will be frequently referenced by practitioners involved in research. In the instance of that research being documented for formal publication in a medical journal, understanding the appropriate style for transcribing that data will be very valuable to the MT in that setting and an asset to the physician(s) in that practice.

13.3.1 Hormones

Many drugs are identical to or are derived from naturally occurring biological products, like hormones. When they are given as drugs, however, they are typically assigned a different name than their endogenous counterparts. In formal publication, the AMA recommends inclusion of the native name in parentheses when the therapeutic name for a drug may be less familiar.

Hypothalmic hormones: Identified by the suffix *–relin*, hypothalmic hormones *stimulate* the release of pituitary hormones. Hypothalmic hormones that *inhibit* release are identified by the suffix *–relix*.

Native Substance	Diagnostic/Therapeutic Agent
thyrotropin-releasing hormone (TRH)	protirelin
luteinizing hormone-releasing hormone (LHRH) or gonadotropin-releasing hormone (GnRH)	buserelin acetate, gonadorelin acetate (or hydrochloride), histrelin, lutrelin acetate nafarelin acetate
growth hormone-releasing factor (GHRF)	somatorelin
growth hormone release-inhibiting factor (GHRIF, somatostatin)	detirelix acetate

EXAMPLE

> *In formal publication:*
> D: After venipuncture, protirelin was injected.
> T: After venipuncture, protirelin (synthetic thyrotropin-releasing hormone) was injected.

Growth hormone: Be familiar with the common therapeutic names for growth hormone. The *som–* prefix is used for growth hormone derivatives.

Native Substance	Diagnostic/Therapeutic Agent
growth hormone	somatrem, somidobove, sometribove, somagrebove, somalapor, somenopor, sometripor, somfasepor

Thyroid hormones: References to the primary hormones (thyroxine and triiodothyronine) are commonly encountered in the record, and the abbreviation can be used when dictated.

Description	Therapeutic Agent
levorotatory thyroxine (T4)	levothyroxine sodium
triiodothyronine (T3)	liothyronine sodium
dextrorotatory triiodothyronine	dextrothyroxine sodium
liothyronine and levothyroxine sodium	liotrix sodium

13.3.2 Insulin

Insulin may be administered intravenously, subcutaneously, or intramuscularly. There are now forms of insulin that may also be inhaled. Insulin types derived from human DNA are referred to as human insulin; the synthetic types are generally modified types of porcine insulin. Below are some examples of insulin types, including both proprietary and nonproprietary names:

human insulin injection	Humulin
insulin lispro injection	Humalog
insulin aspart injection	NovoLog
insulin glargine injection	Lantus
prompt insulin zinc suspension	Semilente
insulin zinc suspension	Lente
extended human insulin zinc suspension	Ultralente
insulin isophane suspension	NPH

Note: NPH is one of the few exceptions to the rule for spelling out drug names. It can be transcribed in abbreviated form.

The above insulin injections and suspensions can be combined. When expressed in their nonproprietary forms, the concentrations should be expressed as percentages. When their proprietary names are referenced, the concentrations are expressed in virgule (/) construction.

70% human isophane suspension with 30% human insulin injection	Humulin 70/30
50% insulin isophane suspension with 50% human insulin injection	Humulin 50/50

13.3.3 Interferons

Interferons are a class of glycoproteins that exert antineoplastic, antiviral, and immuno-modulating effects. Use nonproprietary names as discussed below. For trade names and additional guidance, consult the USAN dictionary or other appropriate reference.

For general classes of compounds or single compounds, follow the lowercase interferon by the spelled-out Greek letter; use the Greek symbol in abbreviations. *Note:* alfa is the correct spelling in these terms, not alpha.

EXAMPLE

interferon alfa	IFN-α
interferon beta	IFN-β
interferon gamma	IFN-γ

For individual, pure, identifiable compounds with nonproprietary names, add a hyphen, an arabic numeral, and a lowercase letter.

EXAMPLE

interferon alfa-2a
interferon alfa-2b
interferon gamma-1a
interferon gamma-1b

For names of mixtures of interferons from natural sources, add a hyphen, a lowercase *n*, and an arabic numeral.

EXAMPLE

interferon alfa-n1
interferon alfa-n2

13.3.4 Interleukins

Interleukins are a class of proteins that are secreted mostly by macrophages and T lymphocytes; they induce growth and differentiation of lymphocytes and hematopoietic stem cells. There are 12 interleukin derivatives. With the exception of interleukin 3, interleukin derivatives end in *–kin*, so they can readily be identified by this suffix.

-nakin	interleukin 1 derivatives
-onakin	interleukin 1a derivatives
-benakin	interleukin 1b derivatives
-leukin	interleukin 2 derivatives
-trakin	interleukin 4 derivatives
-penkin	interleukin 5 derivatives
-exakin	interleukin 6 derivatives
-eptakin	interleukin 7 derivatives
-octakin	interleukin 8 derivatives
-nonakin	interleukin 9 derivatives
-decakin	interleukin 10 derivatives
-elvekin	interleukin 11 derivatives
-dodekin	interleukin 12 derivatives

Note: Interleukin 3 can be identified by the suffix *–plestim* and falls under the category of colony-stimulating factors (see below).

13.3.5 Colony-Stimulating Factors

Colony-stimulating factors are naturally occurring glycoproteins that regulate the proliferation, differentiation, and maturation of hematopoietic growth factors. They belong to a class of soluble immune system proteins known as *cytokines*.

Granulocyte colony-stimulating factors (G-CSFs) can be identified by the suffix –grastim.

filgrastim
lenograstim
Pd-grastim

Granulocyte-macrophage colony-stimulating factors (GM-CSFs) can be identified by the suffix –gramostim.

ecogramostim
molgramostim
regramostim
sargramostim

Macrophage colony-stimulating factors (M-CSFs) can be identified by the suffix –mostim.

cilmostim
lanimostim
mirimostim

Interleukin 3 (IL-3) factors can be identified by the suffix –plestim.

muplestim
daniplestim

Combined forms, or conjugates, of 2 types of colony-stimulating factors can be identified by the suffix –distim.

leridistim
milodistim

Stem-cell stimulating factors (SCSFs) can be identified by the suffix *–cestim*.

ancestim

13.3.6 Erythropoietins

The common stem for *erythropoietin* blood factors is *–poietin*. The words *alfa, beta,* and *gamma* are added to designate preparations with variable composition and carbohydrate activity.

epoetin alfa
epoetin beta
epoetin gamma

13.3.7 Isotopes

Isotopes are atoms of the same element that have different atomic masses. They are used in reference to radioactive drugs. When the element name, not the symbol, is used, place the isotope number on the line after the name in the same font and type size; do not superscript or subscript. Space between the element name and the isotope number. Do not hyphenate either the noun or the adjectival form.

iodine 128
technetium 99m

When the element symbol is used, place the isotope number as a superscript immediately before the symbol. In environments where superscripting is prohibited, use the following format: element symbol, space (not hyphen), isotope number (on the line). It is also acceptable to spell out the element name followed by the isotope number.

^{128}I *or* I 128 *or* iodine 128
^{99m}Tc *or* Tc 99m *or* technetium 99m

Section 4: Specialty Standards

For trademarked isotopes, follow the style of the manufacturer. In trademarks, the isotope is usually joined to the rest of the name by a hyphen; it may or may not be preceded by the element symbol.

> Glofil-125
> Hippuran I 131

13.3.8 Protocols and Multi-Drug Regimens

Commonly encountered in oncology and immunology, multi-drug regimens are often indicated by protocol designations or protocol acronyms. Abbreviations for multiple-drug regimens are acceptable if widely used and readily recognized, particularly within the specialty setting.

> MOPP (methotrexate, vincristine sulfate, prednisone, and procarbazine)

Some chemotherapy protocols combine abbreviations designating the type of cancer with treatment and drug abbreviations.

> BRAJCEF (BR = breast cancer, AJ = adjuvant therapy, C = cyclophosphamide, E = epirubicin, F = fluorouracil)
>
> LUAVPG (LU = lung, AV = advanced, P = platinum, G = gemcitabine)

13.3.9 Vitamins

The letters commonly used to refer to vitamins generally refer to the substances that occur naturally in food or in the human body. With the exception of vitamins A, E, and B complex, synthetic vitamins administered therapeutically are given designation or drug names that help to differentiate them from their naturally occurring counterparts. Lowercase *vitamin*, capitalize the letter designation, and use arabic numerals (in subscript form if available). Do not use a hyphen or space between the letter and numeral.

> vitamin B12 *or* vitamin B_{12}
> B12 vitamin *or* B_{12} vitamin

vitamin	drug name
vitamin B1	thiamine hydrochloride
vitamin B2	riboflavin
vitamin B6	pyridoxine hydrochloride
vitamin B12	cyanocobalamin
vitamin C	ascorbic acid
vitamin D	cholocalciferol
vitamin D2	ergocalciferol
vitamin D3	cholecalciferol
vitamin K1	phytonadione
vitamin K3	menadione

13.3.10 Herbals and Supplements

Herbals and dietary supplements are not assigned an international proprietary name (INN) by the USAN and are not regulated as drugs in the United States. According to the Dietary Supplement Health and Education Act of 1994, Congress has defined a dietary supplement to be "a product taken by mouth that contains a 'dietary ingredient' intended to supplement the diet." The law further identifies those ingredients as vitamins, minerals, herbs, and other botanicals, amino acids, and substances.

Herbal medicines are typically named and referred to in literature either by their common names or their genus and species names, but no consistent international nomenclature exists for naming any of these substances.

Do *not* capitalize medicinal herb names used in alternative medicine. Do capitalize the proper nouns that accompany them.

EXAMPLE

mugwort
saffron
ginseng

St. John's wort
St. James weed

Do not confuse the medicinal herb names with their genus/species names. When these are used, capitalize the genus, but not the species, name. *(See 7.3.6—Organisms).*

EXAMPLE

> Crocus sativus (saffron)
> Zingiber officinale (ginger)
> Hypericum perforatum (St. John's wort)

CHAPTER

14

Cardiology

Introduction

Heart disease continues to be the major cause of disability and death in the United States, and recent focus on heart disease in women has brought even greater attention to the factors of lifestyle, genetics, diet, infection, and immunity in the diagnosis and treatment of cardiovascular disease. Given the fact that advancements in the treatment of cardiovascular disease are constantly emerging onto the clinical scene, medical transcriptionists need to have a particularly thorough understanding of this specialty in an acute care setting.

14.1 Anatomy, Physiology, and Pathology

Cardiology patients present to and are admitted to the hospital for a wide variety of complex conditions, including hypertension, stroke, heart failure, cardiac arrhythmias, valvular disease, congenital heart disease, and pulmonary emboli (to name a few). The documentation of these conditions will frequently include references to the anatomical structure of the heart, its sounds (both normal and abnormal), and peripheral vascular indications.

14.1.1 Heart Sounds

There are 4 sounds and 4 components assessed on auscultation of the heart. Abbreviate heart sounds and components as follows, placing numerals on the line or using subscripts.

first heart sound	S1 *or* S$_1$
second heart sound	S2 *or* S$_2$
third heart sound	S3 *or* S$_3$
fourth heart sound	S4 *or* S$_4$
aortic valve component	A2 *or* A$_2$
mitral valve component	M1 *or* M$_1$
pulmonic valve component	P2 *or* P$_2$
tricuspid valve component	T1 *or* T$_1$

Heart sounds should be written out in full when used in general reference or at the beginning of a sentence.

EXAMPLE

> Third heart sounds are usually indicative of congestive heart failure.
> *but:*
> The S3 is often indicative of congestive heart failure.

14.1.2 Murmurs

Murmurs are graded from soft to loud and are written in arabic numerals. Systolic murmurs are graded on a scale of 1 to 6, and diastolic murmurs are graded on a scale of 1 to 4.

grade 1	barely audible, must strain to hear
grade 2	quiet, but clearly audible
grade 3	moderately loud
grade 4	loud
grade 5	very loud; audible with stethoscope partly off the chest
grade 6	so loud that it can be heard with stethoscope just above chest wall

Place a virgule between the murmur grade and the scale used (2/6 = a grade 2 murmur on a scale of 6). It is not unusual for dictators to use "out of" or "over" to express these grades.

grade 1/6 systolic murmur

Express partial units as indicated.

D: grade 4 and a half over 6 murmur
T: grade 4.5 over 6 murmur
or:
T: grade 4.5/6 murmur

D: grade 4 to 5 over 6 murmur
T: grade 4 to 5 over 6 murmur
or:
grade 4/6 to 5/6 murmur
not:
grade 4-5/6 murmur

D: to-and-fro SDM
T: to-and-fro systolic-diastolic murmur

Bruits: A bruit is an abnormal heart sound or murmur heard on auscultation. The plural form is bruits but because of the French origin of the word, often the final s is not pronounced and the singular and plural forms sound the same: "broo-ee."

Spell out the following abbreviations even when they are dictated in phono-cardiographic tracings.

ASM	atrial systolic murmur
CM	continuous murmur
DM	diastolic murmur
DSM	delayed systolic murmur
ESM	ejection systolic murmur
IDM	immediate diastolic murmur
LSM	late systolic murmur
PSM	pansystolic murmur
SDM	systolic-diastolic murmur
SEM	systolic ejection murmur
SM	systolic murmur
AEC	aortic ejection click
AOC	aortic opening click
C	click
E	ejection sound
EC	ejection click
NEC	nonejection click
PEC	pulmonary ejection click
OS	opening snap
SC	systolic click
SS	summation sound
W	whoop

14.1.3 Jugular Venous Pulse

Contours of the jugular venous pulse are expressed with words and single letters. In formal publication, the single letters should be expressed in italics; in healthcare documentation, in regular type.

a wave, a wave
x descent, x descent
z point, z point
c wave, c wave
x' descent, x prime descent
v wave, v wave
y descent, y descent
y trough, y trough
b wave, b wave

prominent *a* wave
increased *v* wave

14.1.4 Cardiac Muscle

Terms related to cardiac muscle are typically abbreviated and do not require expansion, although in formal publication, it is appropriate to expand on first mention and abbreviate thereafter. Do not abbreviate unless dictated that way, however.

A band	actin-myosin overlap
H band	Hensen
M line	mesophragma
T tubules	tubulus transversus
Z line	Zuckung
TnC	troponin C
TnI	troponin I
TnT	troponin T
cTnC	troponin C, cardiac form
cTnI	troponin I, cardiac form
cTnT	troponin T, cardiac form

14.2 Diagnostic Testing and Procedures

The management of cardiovascular disease involves a wide array of highly specialized radiologic and diagnostic procedures. Electrocardiography, vector cardiography, electrophysiologic studies, ultrasound, nuclear cardiology, radiology, catheterization, and pulmonary function testing are among the complex studies that an MT will encounter when transcribing in either the acute care setting or in private practice. Since these conditions are common and so often chronic, the MT will encounter references to them and their related studies in almost every medical specialty.

14.2.1 Laboratory Tests

Abbreviate most laboratory tests used to diagnose and manage cardiovascular disease. In formal publication, cellular or molecular terms (such as lipoproteins) should be expanded on first reference, especially if they are new, unusual, or not commonly encountered.

EXAMPLE

CK-MB
tPA
acyl CoA
HDL
HDL_1
HDL_2
HDL-C
HDL-R
HMG Coa
IDL
IDL-C
IDL-R
LDL
LDL-C
LDL-R
LPL
LPL_{188}
LP-X
LRP_1
LRP_2
VHDL
VLDL-C
VLDL-R

Expand *–apo* to *apolipoprotein* at first mention when combined with terms such as:

apo AI
apo AII
apo AIV
apo(a)
apo D
apo E

14.2.2 EKG and Tracing

ECG and EKG are acceptable abbreviations for *electrocardiogram, electrocardiography, electrocardiographic.* Transcribe as dictated.

Leads: Electronic connections for recording by means of electrocardiograph. Where subscripts are called for but are not available, standard-size numerals and letters on the line may be used.

Standard bipolar leads: Use roman numerals.

lead I
lead II
lead III

Augmented limb leads: Use a lowercase *a* followed by a capital V, then a capital R (right), L (left), or F (foot).

aVR
aVL
aVF

Precordial leads: Use a capital V followed by an arabic numeral. Enter the numeral in the same point size on the line with the V, with no space between, or use subscripting.

V1, V2, V3, V4, V5, V6, V7, V8, V9
or:
$V_1, V_2, V_3, V_4, V_5, V_6, V_7, V_8, V_9$

Right precordial leads: Use a capital V followed by an arabic numeral and capital R. Enter the numeral and R in the same point size on the line with the V, with no space between, or use subscripting.

V3R
V4R
or:
V$_3$R
V$_4$R, etc.

Ensiform cartilage lead: Use a capital V followed by a capital E in the same point size on the line with the V, with no space between, or subscript the E.

VE or V$_E$

Third interspace leads: Use an arabic numeral followed by capital V and an arabic numeral. Enter the numeral following the V as a subscript or in the same point size on the line, with no space between.

3V1, 3V2, 3V3, etc.
or:
3V$_1$, 3V$_2$, 3V$_3$, etc.

Esophageal leads: Use a capital E followed by an arabic numeral either subscripted or on the line in the same point size, with no space between.

E15, E24, E50, etc.
or:
E$_{15}$, E$_{24}$, E$_{50}$, etc.

Sequential leads: Repeat the V. Do not use a hyphen or dash.

> leads V1 through V5
> *or:*
> V_1 through V_5
> *not:*
> V1 through 5 *or* V_1 through $_5$
> *not:*
> V1-V5 *or* V_1-V_5
> *not:*
> V1-5 *or* V_{1-5}

Tracing: In general, for electrocardiographic deflections, use all capitals, but larger and smaller Q, R, and S waves may be differentiated by capital and lowercase letters, respectively. Do not place a hyphen after the single letter except when the term is used as an adjective.

> Q wave, q wave
> QS wave, qs wave
> R wave, r wave
> S wave, s wave
> R' wave, r' wave
> S' wave, s' wave
>
> *Note:* R' and S' are dictated as "R prime" and "S prime."
>
> J junction
> J point
> P wave
> QT interval, prolongation, etc.
> QTc, QTC, *or* corrected QT interval
> PR interval, segment, etc.
> QRS axis, complex, configuration, etc.
> ST segment
> T wave
> Ta wave
> U wave

Use a hyphen with tracing terms when they are used as adjectives preceding and modifying a noun.

> T-wave abnormality
> ST-segment depression
> non-Q-wave myocardial infarction

For QRS axis, use a plus or a minus sign followed by arabic numerals and a degree sign to express the number of degrees, or write out degrees.

> QRS +60°
> *or:*
> QRS +60 degrees

Note: There is no such thing as an ST wave or an ST-T wave, but it is common practice for providers to dictate the ST segment and the T wave together. Care should be taken to transcribe these references in a way that does not imply an ST wave or ST-T wave.

> D: STT wave abnormality
> T: ST and T-wave abnormality
> *or:*
> T: ST-T-wave abnormality
>
> *not:*
> T: STT-wave abnormality
> *or:*
> T: ST-T wave abnormality

14.2.3 Echocardiography

Expand abbreviated references to echocardiographic methods on first mention or when used in diagnostic and operative titles.

EXAMPLE

2DE	2-dimensional echocardiogram/echocardiography
3DE	3-dimensional echocardiogram/echocardiography
4DE	4-dimensional echocardiogram/echocardiography
CW Doppler	continuous-wave Doppler echocardiogram/echocardiography
IVUS	intravascular ultrasonography
TEE	transesophageal echocardiogram/echocardiography

When only the dimension is abbreviated, expansion is not necessary.

EXAMPLE

D: two D echo
T: 2D echocardiogram

The following indices are commonly encountered on echocardiographic evaluation and should be spelled out in diagnostic and procedural titles as well as on first reference in formal publication:

EXAMPLE

AVA	aortic valve area
EF	ejection fraction
EPSS	E point septal separation
FAC	fractional area change
FS	fractional shortening
IVS, IVST	interventricular septal thickness
LVID	left ventricular internal dimension
MVA	mitral valve area
PHT	pressure half time
PW, PWT	posterior wall thickness
RVID	right ventricular internal dimension
SAM	systolic anterior motion of the mitral valve
d *or* ed	end diastole
s *or* es	end systole

14.2.4 Pacemaker Codes

Cardiac pacemakers are expressed as 3- to 5-letter codes representing functionality and operation. Each of these letters corresponds to the operation of the pacemaker at each of five positions described below:

Chambers Paced: O (none), A (atrium), V (ventricle), D (dual), *or* S (single)
Chambers Sensed: O (none), A (atrium), V (ventricle), D (dual), *or* S (single)
Response to Sensing: O (none), T (triggered), I (inhibited), D (dual)
Rate Modulation: O (none), R (rate modulation)
Multisite Pacing: O (none), A (atrium), V (ventricle), D (dual)

Note: "None" is expressed with the letter O, not the numeral 0.

Thus, pacemakers are described using a 3-letter or 5-letter combined code based on the above indicators.

EXAMPLE

> DDIR pacing (dual-chamber, dual-sensed, inhibited response, rate modulating)
> VVI pacemaker (paced ventricle, sensed ventricle, inhibited response)
> DDDR pacing (dual-chamber, dual-sensed, dual-response)

14.2.5 Cardioversion/Defibrillation

A similar code as that assigned to pacemakers exists for implantable cardioverter/defibrillators.

Shock Chamber: O (none), A (atrium), V (ventricle), D (dual)
Antitachycardia Pacing Chamber: O (none), A (atrium), V (ventricle), D (dual)
Tachycardia Detection: E (electrocardiogram), H (hemodynamic)
Antibradycardia Pacing Chamber: O (none), A (atrium), V (ventricle), D (dual)

Thus, cardioverter/defibrillators are described using a 3-letter or 4-letter combined code based on the above indicators.

DDH defibrillator (dual-shock, dual-chamber, hemodynamic)
VOEO defibrillator (ventricular shock chamber, no antitachycardia pacing chamber, electrocardiogram tachycardia detection, no antibradycardia pacing chamber)

14.3 Classification Systems

Classification systems and terms are frequently used to identify and define conditions, and each system has a specific method for classifying and expressing those values. Some are expressed with arabic numbers and some are expressed with roman numerals. Some are so organized that specific expressions may require a blend of numbers and letters, both uppercase and lowercase, some with hyphens and some without. Each classification system is unique, and transcriptionists should consult a reputable resource or dictionary when questioning the expression of any classification system.

14.3.1 Angina

Unstable angina: The *Braunwald* system is used to classify unstable angina and is reported as class I through III. Express these classes using roman numerals. Express subclassification using capital letters and roman numerals.

EXAMPLE

Braunwald class I
Braunwald class IIIB

Exertional angina: The *Canadian Cardiovascular Society (CCS)* system is used to classify exertional angina as class I through IV. Express these classes using roman numerals.

EXAMPLE

CCS class I
CCS class II

14.3.2 Myocardial Infarction

Two classification systems exist to quantify cardiac function and status following a myocardial infarction.

Cardiac function: The *Forrester* classification system is used to describe cardiac function after myocardial infarction. Use roman numerals to express classes I through IV.

EXAMPLE

> Forrester class I
> Forrester class II

Cardiac status: The *Killip* classification system is used to describe cardiac status after myocardial infarction. Use roman numerals to express classes I through IV.

EXAMPLE

> Killip class I
> Killip class II heart failure

14.3.3 Heart Failure

The *NYHA* classification system is a widely adopted classification of cardiac failure that was developed by the New York Heart Association. Use roman numerals to express classes I through IV.

I	asymptomatic
II	comfortable at rest, symptomatic with normal activity
III	comfortable at rest, symptomatic with less than normal activity
IV	severe cardiac failure, symptomatic at rest

EXAMPLE

> The patient has been diagnosed with cardiac failure, class III.
> I have been following this patient for NYHA class II failure.

14.3.4 Atrial Fibrillation

The American College of Cardiology and the American Heart Association (ACC/AHA) have classified atrial fibrillation as *paroxysmal, persistent,* and *permanent.* These terms are defined below:

- *Paroxysmal:* Recurrent, intermittent atrial fibrillation that previously terminated without specific therapy. Paroxysmal atrial fibrillation is self-limited.
- *Persistent:* Recurrent, sustained atrial fibrillation that was previously terminated by therapeutic intervention. Persistent atrial fibrillation may be the first presentation, a culmination of recurrent episodes of paroxysmal atrial fibrillation or long-standing atrial fibrillation (greater than one year). Persistent atrial fibrillation is not self-limited, but may be converted to sinus rhythm by medical or electrical intervention.
- *Permanent:* Continuous atrial fibrillation which cannot be converted to normal sinus rhythm by pharmacologic or electrical techniques.

14.3.5 Coronary Artery Angiography (TIMI)

Assessment of thrombolysis in myocardial infarction (TIMI) through coronary artery angiography is expressed using a grading system for coronary perfusion. This is performed to evaluate reperfusion achieved by thrombolytic therapy. Express grades 0 through 3, from lowest flow (or severest blockage) to highest flow, using lowercase *grade* and arabic numerals.

EXAMPLE

The patient had TIMI grade 3 flow at 90 minutes following thrombolytic therapy.

CHAPTER

15

Genetics

Introduction

The identification and study of genetic abnormalities and defects has become an area of increased clinical focus over recent years. The applications of genetic research are far-reaching, and significant research into the cause and cure of most major diseases and illnesses today is being directed at genomics, which is focused on manipulating human genes to identify and/or eliminate traits in our DNA. Most genes function by encoding synthesis of proteins and enzymes at the cellular level. The absence or defection of a gene can result in an array of different effects and defects. Being able to detect and/or manipulate those defects will greatly alter the course of preventative medicine in the future.

15.1 Human Gene Nomenclature

Gene nomenclature has been established by the *Human Gene Nomenclature Committee (HGNA)*, one of 7 committees that are part of the *Human Genome Organisation (HUGO)*, which is responsible for gene mapping and name validation. At current estimate, there are approximately 30,000 genes of which more than 20,000 are currently represented by valid names and active symbols.

15.1.1 DNA, RNA, and Amino Acids
Deoxyribonucleic acid (DNA) includes the bases thymine (T), cytosine (C), adenine (A), and guanine (G). DNA contains the genetic code and is found in the chromosomes of humans and animals. DNA expressions and their abbreviations include:

EXAMPLE

complementary DNA	cDNA
double-stranded DNA	dsDNA
single-stranded DNA	ssDNA

Ribonucleic acid (RNA) includes the bases cytosine, adenine, guanine, and uracil (U). RNA is functionally associated with DNA. RNA expressions and their abbreviations include:

EXAMPLE

heterogeneous RNA	hnRNA
messenger RNA	mRNA
ribosomal RNA	rRNA
small nuclear RNA	snRNA
transfer RNA	tRNA

Amino acids: Write out in text. In tables, use 3-letter or 1-letter abbreviations.

EXAMPLE

phenylalanine	Phe	F
proline	Pro	P
tryptophan	Trp	W

For general reference, a complete list of standard amino acids is provided below:

alanine, cysteineaspartic acid, glutamic acid, phenylalanine, glycine, histidine, isoleucine, lysine, leucine, methionine, asparagine, proline, glutamine, arginine, serine, threonine, selenocysteine, valine, tryptophan, and tyrosine

15.1.2 Genes and Gene Symbols

Genes are the molecular units of heredity. They are assigned an approved gene name, a gene description, and an approved gene symbol.

EXAMPLE

Gene Name: the alpha-fetoprotein gene
Description: α-fetoprotein gene
Symbol: AFP

Gene names are usually named for the molecular product of the gene, the function of the gene, or the condition associated with the gene (if known). The gene description typically may include Greek letters, which can be referenced in formal publication but should be avoided in healthcare documentation. When the gene is referred to in dictation, the gene name should be used, not the description.

D: testing for the beta two microglobulin gene
T: testing for the beta-2-microglobulin gene
not:
T: testing for the β2-microglobulin gene

When gene symbols and names are officially designated, variable naming conventions are used to identify their related genes. Often this is accomplished by a sequential numbering system based off the *stem*, or root symbol, for the gene family.

Gene Name: tumor necrosis factor
Root Symbol: TNF
Genes: TNF, TNFA1P1, TNFAIP2, TNFAIP3, TNFRSF1A, etc.

Human gene symbols usually consist of 3 to 7 characters that represent an abbreviated form of the gene name or other attribute of the gene. They should be expressed with uppercase letters. They may contain, but never start with, arabic numerals. They do not contain Greek letters, roman numerals, superscripts, subscripts, or punctuation. When there is potential for misinterpretation, the gene symbol should be italicized to differentiate it from a similarly named entity or product of the gene. This may be necessary in formal publication but is not always possible in healthcare documentation, where italicized characters are avoided. For transcriptionists who work specifically in the area of genetics and genetic research, it may be appropriate to adopt this practice. In general, however, gene name symbols do not have to be italicized.

BRCA-1, BRCA-2
CFTR
SYN1
but:
ABO (in formal publication to differentiate gene from the ABO blood group system)
EPO (in formal publication to differentiate gene from erythropoietin—Epo)

Gene symbols do not immediately follow the term in the gene name that they appear to abbreviate; rather, they should follow the term *gene* in the expression.

Huntington disease gene, HD
not:
Huntington disease (HD) gene

The cystic fibrosis transmembrane conductance regulator gene, CFTR, is implicated in cystic fibrosis.
not:
The cystic fibrosis transmembrane conductance regulator (CFTR) gene is implicated in cystic fibrosis.

15.1.3 Alleles

Alleles identify alternative forms of a gene and describe, or are characterized by, variant sequences, or *mutations*, of a gene. Because they are a variant form of a particular gene, they are expressed as a combined form of the gene name or symbol and a suffix that identifies the allele itself. Allele symbols consist of the gene symbol plus an asterisk followed by the allele designation.

HBB*6B
APOE*E4

15.1.4 Genotype and Phenotype

A *genotype* is made up of a set of alleles for a single individual. Human beings have 2 of each nonsex chromosome and thus have 2 alleles for each autosomal gene. The simplest genotype would be described with 1 gene and the names of 2 alleles. More complex genotypes consist of 2 or more allele symbol *pairs*. In formal publication, allele groupings are expressed by placement of alleles above and below a horizontal line:

$$\frac{ADA*1}{ADA*2}$$

If referenced in healthcare documentation, however, this expression is not readily reproduced. These should then be expressed on the same line and separated by a virgule:

> ADA*1/ADA*2

A *single space* separates alleles on the same chromosome from alleles on another chromosome.

> AMY1*A PGM1*2/AMY1*B PGM1*1

Semicolons are used to separate pairs of alleles at unlinked loci.

> ADA*1/ADA*2; ADH1*1/ADH1*1; AMY1*A/AMY1*B

Commas are used to express that alleles on either side of the virgule are on the same chromosome pair but not on which chromosome of the pair specifically.

> PGM*1/PGM1*2, AMY1*A/AMY1*B

Note: The above complexity of allele expression will likely only be relevant and necessary information for transcriptionists working specifically in genetics. In those settings, clear direction from the dictator will be necessary in making sure these variable forms are expressed correctly, particularly in formal publication.

The *phenotype* represents the collection of traits in an individual as a result of his/her genotype. The phenotype is often an abbreviated expression of the more detailed genotype. No italics are used to express phenotypes and spaces are used rather than asterisks. Seek a reputable genetics reference or resource to verify expression of all genotypes and phenotypes.

Genotype	Phenotype
ADA*1/ADA*1	ADA 1
ABO*A1/ABO*O	ABO A1

15.1.5 Oncogenes and Tumor Suppressor Genes

Oncogene refers to a gene that normally plays a role in healthy growth or activity but when mutated can actively foster the growth of cancer. They were originally identified in viruses and thus can be referred to as *retroviral genes* or *retroviral oncogenes*. Express as three-letter lowercase terms derived from names of associated viruses. Italics are used in formal publications, but regular type is used in medical transcription.

EXAMPLE

> abl
>
> mos
>
> sis
>
> src

The prefix *v-* (virus) or *c-* (cellular or chromosomal counterpart) indicates the location of the oncogene. The c-prefixed oncogenes are also known as proto-oncogenes and may be alternatively expressed in all capitals, without the prefix. Italics are used in formal publications, but regular type is preferred in medical transcription. Note: The prefix is never italicized.

Tumor suppressor genes normally restrict cellular growth, but when they are missing or are being inactivated by mutation, they allow cells to grow at an uncontrolled rate. They are expressed with capital letters and arabic numerals like other human genes.

EXAMPLE

> CDKN1A
>
> DCC
>
> NF1

15.2 Chromosomes

Genetic testing can be performed to establish the identity of an individual or the relationship between individuals as in forensic medicine or paternity testing. It can be used to detect hereditary disorders in newborns, both prior to and after birth. The application of genetic testing to the specialty of oncology is increasingly more prevalent. Screening for oncogenes that indicate a predetermined risk for certain cancers is now a standard practice for many oncologists.

There are 46 chromosomes in human cells, occurring in pairs and numbered from largest to smallest from 1 through 22. The sex chromosomes are designated by X and Y, with both X and Y in males and two X's in females. The non-sex chromosomes, or numbered chromosomes, are also called autosomes.

15.2.1 Group Designations
A chromosome can be referred to by number or by group.

chromosome	group
1-3	A
4, 5	B
6-12, X	C
13-15	D
16-18	E
19, 20	F
21, 22, Y	G

EXAMPLE

chromosome 16
a chromosome in group E
a group-E chromosome
an E group chromosome

Certain terms are used to generally describe conditions related to chromosomal abnormalities:

EXAMPLE

trisomy: an extra chromosome in any one of the autosomes or either sex chromosome
trisomy D: an extra chromosome in a group-D chromosome, either the 13th, 14th, or 15th chromosome
trisomy 21: an extra 21st chromosome (Down syndrome)

A plus or minus in front of the chromosome number means there is either an extra chromosome or an absent chromosome within that pair.

> trisomy 21 = female karyotype: 47,XX +21

The plus or minus following the chromosome number means that part of the chromosome is either extra or missing.

> cri du chat syndrome = male karyotype: 46,X6 5p-

15.2.2 Arms and Bands

Arms: Each chromosome has a short arm and a long arm. The short arm is designated by a p, the long arm by a q, immediately following the chromosome number (no space between). Each arm is divided into regions (from 1 to 4); place the region number immediately following the arm designation. Regions are divided into bands, again joined without a space. If a subdivision is identified, it follows a decimal point placed immediately after the band number.

20p	20th chromosome, short arm
20p1	20th chromosome, short arm, region 1
20p11	20th chromosome, short arm, region 1, band 1
20p11.23	20th chromosome, short arm, region 1, band 1, subdivision 23

A translocation occurs when a segment normally found in a certain arm of a chromosome appears in a different location; it may be written as a small t with the from and to sites in parentheses, e.g., $t(14q21q)$, meaning from long arm of 14 to long arm of 21. A more complex designation such as $t(2;6)(q34;p12)$ means from region 3 band 4 of the long arm of chromosome 2 to region 1 band 2 of the short arm of chromosome 6. The chromosome numbers appear in a separate set of parentheses from the arm, region, and band information.

A ring chromosome is one that has pieces missing from the end of each arm, and the two arms have joined at the ends.

Bands: Use capital letters to refer to chromosome bands, which are elicited by special staining methods.

band	stain
C bands *or* C-banding	constitutive heterochromatin
G bands *or* G-banding	Giemsa
N bands *or* N-banding	nucleolar organizing region
Q bands *or* Q-banding	quinacrine
R bands *or* R-banding	reverse-Giemsa

15.2.3 Karyotypes

A *karyotype* is the chromosome complement of an individual, tissue, or cell line. It describes an individual's chromosome complement: the number of chromosomes plus the sex chromosomes present in that individual. Place a comma (without spacing) between the chromosome number and the sex chromosome. Use a virgule to indicate more than one karyotype in an individual.

EXAMPLE

normal human karyotypes:	46,XX (female)
	46,XY (male)
some abnormal karyotypes:	47,XXY
	45,X0
	48,XXX
	45,X/46,XX

15.3 Nonhuman Gene Nomenclature

Gene terminology related to laboratory mice/rats, bacteria, and viruses is often seen in clinical research and formal publication because of the common use of those species in the study of disease in humans as well as the primary identification of certain genes associated with them. While again not likely to be encountered by the average healthcare documentation specialist, reference to this terminology will play a key role in the preparation of formal manuscripts for those MTs employed in the genetics domain.

15.3.1 Vertebrates

Mouse and rat gene symbols are expressed similarly to human gene symbols in that they are short (3 to 5 characters) and are descriptive. However, what differentiates their expression from human genes is that they are expressed in *lowercase* (except for the expression of Greek letters). They also should be italicized in formal publication.

EXAMPLE

Human Gene Symbol	Description	Mouse/Rat Symbol
AFP	alpha-fetoprotein	*Afp*
B2M	beta-2 microglobulin	*B2m*

15.3.2 Bacteria
Bacterial gene terms are typically expressed as italicized, lowercased, 3-letter abbreviations. The phenotypes are expressed with initial capital letters.

EXAMPLE

Gene Symbol	Phenotype
araA	*AraA*
asr	*Asr*
soda	*SodA*

15.3.3 Viruses
HIV and other retroviruses consist of 3 main *structural* genes and a number of *regulatory* genes. These are expressed as lowercased, italicized abbreviations.

EXAMPLE

Structural:
env
gag
pol

Regulatory:
nef
rev
tat
vif
vpr
vpu
vpx

CHAPTER

16

Hematology/Oncology

16.1 Hematology

Hematology is the branch of medicine that is concerned with the study of the blood—its formed elements, blood typing, hemostasis, etc.—and the identification and treatment of blood diseases and disorders.

16.1.1 Blood Groups/Types

Blood groups are determined by erythrocyte antigens that are identified as having common immunologic properties. There are over 600 recognized red blood cell antigens organized by the International Society of Blood Transfusion (ISBT) into groups which belong to approximately 29 systems. The most common blood group nomenclature is the *ABO system,* which is a simple alphabetic naming system for blood groups. This is almost exclusively the blood system encountered in healthcare documentation, though some of the other blood nomenclatures may be referenced in formal publication.

Use single or dual letters, sometimes with a subscript letter or number. If subscripts are not available, place the numeral immediately following and on the line with the letter.

EXAMPLE

group A
group A_1 *or* group A1
group A_{1B} *or* group A1B

Other systems: Other common blood group systems include Auberger, Diego, Duffy, Kell, Kidd, Lewis, Lutheran, Rh (not Rhesus), Sutter, and Xg. Consult laboratory references for guidance in expressing terms related to these and other blood groups.

Blood Types: Write out *negative* or *positive* rather than – or +, because the minus or plus sign is easily overlooked.

Her blood type is B negative.
She has a B-negative blood type.
not:
She has a B- blood type.

16.1.2 Erythrocytes

Diseases and conditions arising from red blood cell disorders comprise a significant portion of any hematology/oncology practice. Peripheral blood smears and red cell evaluation will typically involve identification of the quantity and morphology of red cells to diagnose erythrocyte disorders. Transcriptionists should be familiar with the terms used to describe red cell morphology:

spherocytes
anisocytosis
target cells
Howell-Jolly bodies
acanthocytes
megalocytes
stippling
crystals
stomatocytes
drepanocytes
Rouleaux

As part of a complete blood count (CBC), red cell quantification and function is evaluated. Abbreviations for red cell testing should be transcribed as dictated and do not require expansion.

> RBC, rbc (acceptable for either *red blood cell(s)* or *red blood count*)
> hemoglobin
> hematocrit
> MCV
> MCH
> MCHC
> RDW

Hemoglobin and hematocrit: These values are often dictated "H and H" or "H over H." For clarity, translate the abbreviations into their respective terms.

EXAMPLE

> D: H and H 11.8 and 35.3.
> T: Hemoglobin 11.8 and hematocrit 35.3.

When red cell counts are dictated as a percentage, transcribe as dictated. Do not add a percent sign (%) unless it is dictated.

EXAMPLE

> D: MCHC 34 percent
> T: MCHC 34%

16.1.3 Leukocytes

White blood cells are one of several types of formed elements in the blood and their primary role/function is in immune response to infection and foreign bodies. Each of the 5 leukocytes is present in a healthy human body in the following percentages:

EXAMPLE

> neutrophils 65%
> lymphocytes 25%
> monocytes 6%
> eosinophils 4%
> basophils 1%

Knowing these baseline percentages is important in identifying a variation in these percentages and recognizing that such variations are often diagnostically significant. As part of a complete blood count (CBC), white cell quantification is evaluated. Abbreviations and brief forms related to white cell testing should be transcribed as dictated.

WBC, wbc (acceptable for either *white blood cell(s)* or *white blood count*)
PMNs, polys
neutrophils
basophils, basos
lymphocytes, lymphs
monocytes, monos
eosinophils, eos
basophils, basos
bands, stabs
segmented neutrophils, segs

Differential blood count: Part of a white blood cell count that includes polymorphonuclear neutrophils (PMNs, polys, segmented neutrophils [segs]), band neutrophils (bands, stabs), lymphocytes (lymphs), eosinophils (eos), basophils (basos), and monocytes (monos). Differential counts may be given as whole numbers or as percents; total should equal 100 in either case.

White blood count of 4800, with 58% segs, 7% bands, 24% lymphs, 8% monos, 1% eos, and 2% basos.
or:
White blood count of 4800, with 58 segs, 7 bands, 24 lymphs, 8 monos, 1 eo, and 2 basos.

16.1.4 Lymphocytes

T lymphocytes (T cells) and *B lymphocytes (B cells)* are the most common lymphocytes. T means thymus-derived, B means bursa-derived. In general, do not use the extended forms. Do not hyphenate except when used as an adjective preceding a noun.

T cells
T-cell count

Pre– and pan–: Use a hyphen to join *pre–* or *pan–* to the following letter or word.

pre-T cell
pan-B lymphocyte
pan-thymocyte

Subsets of T lymphocytes: Use a virgule (not a hyphen) to express helper/inducer and cytotoxic/suppressor subsets of T lymphocytes. Helper/inducer T lymphocytes are also known as helper cells or helper T lymphocytes. Cytotoxic/suppressor T lymphocytes are also called suppressor cells. Use a hyphen (not a virgule or colon) in the phrase helper-suppressor ratio.

helper-suppressor ratio
not:
helper/suppressor ratio
not:
helper:suppressor ratio

Surface antigens: Join arabic numerals (on the line) to the letter to express surface antigens of T lymphocytes.

T3
T8
T11

16.1.5 Platelets and Hemostasis

Hemostasis refers to the process of platelet plug formation (*primary hemostasis*) and coagulation or clotting (*secondary hemostasis*).

Transcribe *primary hemostasis* terms as dictated and refer to a reputable resource or dictionary to verify accurate expression of these when dictated in their abbreviated forms, as the use of mixed capital letters, lowercase letters, hyphenation, and arabic numerals can vary from one hemostatic term to the next. Some examples are provided below (*see next page*).

EXAMPLE

beta-thromboglobulin	BTG
diacylglycerol	DAG
glycoprotein VI	GpVI
inositol triphosphate	IP_3
platelet activating factor	PAF

Secondary hemostasis primarily involves reference to terms related to clotting factors and variant factors. When transcribing *clotting factors,* lowercase *factor* and use roman numerals.

EXAMPLE

factor I	fibrinogen
factor II	prothrombin
factor III	thromboplastin
factor IV	calcium ions
factor V	proaccelerin
factor VI	(none currently designated)
factor VII	proconvertin
factor VIII	antihemophilic factor
factor IX	Christmas factor
factor X	Stuart factor/Prower factor
factor XI	plasma thromboplastin antecedent
factor XII	Hageman factor/glass factor
factor XIII	fibrin-stabilizing factor

Clotting factor variants: Abnormal or variant forms for clotting factors related to locations should be transcribed as dictated, with careful attention paid to the proper noun eponyms associated with many of these factor variants.

EXAMPLE

factor V Cambridge
factor V Leiden
factor X San Antonio
fibrinogen Paris
prothrombin Barcelona
prothrombin Himi I

Hemophilias: Transcriptionists should be familiar with the correlation between hemophilia classifications and associated clotting factor deficiencies.

hemophilia A	factor VII deficiency
hemophilia B	factor IX deficiency
hemophilia C	factor XI deficiency

von Willebrand (factor VIII): This glycoprotein is involved in coagulation and is deficient in von Willebrand disease. Express as dictated using the newer and preferred abbreviations and terminology below:

factor VIII
factor VIII:Ag
VII:c
vWF
vWF Ag
RCoF

In addition, von Willebrand *disease* is classified by variant using *type* and roman numerals.

type I
type IIA
type IIB
type III
Normandy 1 (use arabic numeral)

Complement factors are involved in antigen-antibody reactions and inflammation. Immediately follow a capital C, B, P, or D with an arabic numeral on the line.

C1
C7

Add a lowercase letter (usually *a* or *b*) for fragments of complement components.

C5a
Bb

Platelet factors: Use arabic numerals for platelet factors (abbreviation: *PF*).

platelet factor 3
PF 3 (Note: Space between PF and the numeral.)

Activated form: Add a lowercase *a* to designate a factor's activated form.

factor Xa

16.1.6 Histocompatibility

Human leukocyte antigens (HLA) are genetic markers on white blood cells. Just as red cell antigens determine blood type, HLA antigens determine tissue type. Express with capital-lowercase combinations and hyphens. Check appropriate references for guidance.

HLA-DR5   associated with Hashimoto thyroiditis
B8, Dw3   associated with Graves disease

Major histocompatibility complex, class I antigens:

HLA-D
HLA-DR

Major histocompatibility complex, class II antigens:

> HLA-B27
> HLA-DRw10

Examples of antigenic specificities of major HLA loci:

> HLA-A
> HLA-B
> HLA-C
> HLA-D

16.1.7 Smears and Stains

Peripheral blood smears are performed to evaluate the morphology of blood elements, primarily erythrocytes, to determine the presence of blood disorders and hematologic disease or pathology. Stains are widely used in the laboratory to differentiate and identify cellular elements of both blood and tissue. References to stains used in peripheral blood smears and other histologic evaluation should be transcribed as dictated, keeping in mind that a number of them are eponyms and need to follow the rules for eponyms (*See 8.2.7— Eponyms*). Common histology stains are provided below.

> Hematoxylin (general staining)
> eosin (general staining)
> Toluidine blue (general staining)
> Masson trichrome stain (connective tissue staining)
> Mallory trichrome stain (connective tissue staining)
> Weigert stain (elastic fiber staining)
> silver stain (nerve fiber staining)
> Wright stain (blood cell staining)
> Orcein stain (elastic fiber staining)

Peripheral blood smears and bone marrow aspirate microscopic evaluations are generally performed using *Wright* stain. The hematologist will often designate how many slides were evaluated.

EXAMPLE

> D: Evaluation of bone marrow aspirate was performed using 2 Wright's slides.
> T: Evaluation of bone marrow aspirate was performed using 2 Wright slides.

References to *myeloid* and *erythroid* series should be transcribed as dictated, being careful to express ratios accurately.

EXAMPLE

> D: Myeloid to erythroid ratio was 1 to 1.
> T: Myeloid-to-erythroid ratio was 1:1.
> *not:*
> T: Myeloid:erythroid ratio was 1:1.
>
> D: M to E was 1:1.
> T: Myeloid-to-erythroid ratio was 1:1.

16.1.8 Flow Cytometry

Flow cytometry is performed on cells in liquid suspension (i.e., blood, bone marrow, body fluids, or tissue cell suspensions) that have been incubated with fluorescently tagged antibodies directed against specific cell surface proteins. A number of different antibody panels are used, depending on the clinical question to be answered. It is ordered in hematology most frequently to identify the antibodies bound to certain cell types that are diagnostically significant for myeloproliferative disorders, such as acute leukemias, lymphomas, and lymphoproliferative disorders.

An *acute leukemia panel* is designed to determine whether leukemic blasts are of myeloid or lymphoid origin, and to further classify the cells as B or T cell, monocytic, megakaryocytic, etc. The panel includes the following antibodies:

myeloid	CD13, CD33
B cell	CD10, CD19, and kappa and lambda light chains
T cell	CD2, CD5, CD7
megakaryocyte	CD61
stem cell	CD34
immature lymphoid	TdT

A *lymphoma panel* is performed using 3-color flow cytometry. The panel includes the following antibodies:

| B cell | CD19, CD20, and kappa and lambda light chains |
| T cell | CD2, CD5 |

If a *large granular lymphocyte (LGL)* disorder is suspected, an *LGL panel* is performed, which includes the following antibodies:

| T cell | CD3, CD4, CD8 |
| NK | CD16, CD56, CD57 |

There are many other antibodies that can be tested for by flow cytometry, but they are all expressed like those above with capital letters and arabic numerals.

Flow cytometry showed a B-cell CLL, positive CD20, positive CD38, and positive ZAP-70. These cells were CD5-positive, CD19-positive, CD23-positive, and CD38-positive, and they had predominant lambda light chains. This is a picture consistent with chronic lymphocytic leukemia.

16.2 Oncology

Oncology is the branch of medicine that is concerned with the identification, treatment, and management of tumors and related cancers. It often involves the diagnostic staging and grading of malignancy, genetic testing, and variable treatments with both chemotherapy and radiotherapy.

16.2.1 Cancer Staging and Grading

Express cancer stages with *stage* and roman numerals. For subdivisions of cancer stages, add capital letters on the line and arabic suffixes, without internal spaces or hyphens.

EXAMPLE

> stage 0 (indicates carcinoma in situ)
> stage I, stage IA
> stage II, stage II3
> stage III
> stage IV, stage IVB

Express histologic grades using *grade* and arabic numerals.

EXAMPLE

> grade 1
> grade 2
> grade 3
> grade 4

TNM staging system for malignant tumors: System for staging malignant tumors, developed by the American Joint Committee on Cancer and the Union Internationale Contre le Cancer.

T	tumor size or involvement
TX	primary tumor cannot be assessed
T0	no evidence of primary tumor
Tis	carcinoma in situ
N	regional lymph node involvement
NX	regional lymph nodes cannot be assessed
N0	no regional lymph node metastasis
M	extent of metastasis
MX	extent of metastasis cannot be determined
M0	no metastasis
M1	distant metastasis

To express degree of positive finding in any of these areas, use arabic numerals. When they are combined to represent a complete staging expression, use arabic numerals *without* spacing between each delineation.

Note: This represents a change in recommendation from that outlined in the 2nd edition of this text.

T2N0M0 (stage I equivalent for many types of cancer)

The combinations that define individual stages differ from one cancer type and anatomic location to another. In other words, the TNM expression for stage II disease is different for each type of cancer.

stage IIA lung cancer = T1N1M0
stage IIA pancreatic cancer = T3N0M0

Staging indicators are used along with TNM criteria to define cancers and assess stages. These are expressed with capital letters and arabic numerals.

grade	GX, G1, G2, G3, G4
host performance	H0, H1, H2, H3, H4
lymphatic invasion	LX, L0, L1, L2
residual tumor	RX, R0, R1, R2
scleral invasion	SX, S0, S1, S2
venous invasion	VX, V0, V1, V2

Prefixes: Lowercase prefixes on the line with TNM and other symbols to indicate criteria used to describe and stage the tumor, e.g., cTNM, aT2.

letter	determining criteria
a	autopsy staging
c	clinical classification
p	pathological classification
r	retreatment classification
y, yp	classification during or following treatment with multiple modalities

Chapter 16: Hematology/Oncology

Suffixes: The T, N, M, and other symbols used for staging may be followed by suffixes in addition to the common X, O, and numerals. These further delineate qualities such as size, invasiveness, and extent of metastasis:

Ta	M1a	N1a	pN1a	pN0
Tis	M2a	N2a	pN1mi	pN0(i)
T1b		N2b	pN0(sn)	pN0(i+)
T1c		N2c	pN3c	pN0(mol)
T1a1				pN0(mol+)
T2a				
T2(m)				
T2(5)				
T3a				

16.2.2 Classification Systems

There is a classification system assigned to virtually every type of cancer that qualifies the location and extent of disease. Those provided below represent the most common cancer staging/grading systems, but it is by no means exhaustive. Consult a reputable resource or dictionary to verify appropriate expression of any classification system that may be new or unfamiliar.

Astler-Coller: Staging system for colon cancer from the least involvement at stage A and B1 through the most extensive involvement at stage D.

> The patient's Astler-Coller B2 lesion extends through the entire thickness of the colon wall, with no involvement of nearby nodes.

Broders index: Classification of aggressiveness of tumor malignancy developed in the 1920s by AC Broders. Reported as grade 1 (most differentiation and best prognosis) through grade 4 (least differentiation and poorest prognosis). Lowercase grade; use arabic numerals.

> Broders grade 3

Cervical cytology: Three different systems are currently in use for cervical cytology: the Papanicolaou test (Pap smear), the CIN classification system, and the Bethesda System.

The Bethesda System is the standardized nomenclature system for reporting cervical cytology and Papanicolaou test results. Abbreviate only if dictated.

EXAMPLE

> atypical squamous cells of undetermined significance (ASCUS)
> endocervical/transformation zone (EC/TZ)
> atypical squamous cells (ASCs)
> loop electrosurgical excision procedure (LEEP)

CIN is an acronym for cervical intraepithelial neoplasia and is expressed with arabic numerals from grade 1 (least severe) to grade 3 (most severe). Place a hyphen between CIN and the numeral.

EXAMPLE

> CIN-1, CIN-2, CIN-3
> *or:*
> CIN grade 1, CIN grade 2, CIN grade 3

The Papanicolaou test uses roman numerals to classify cervical cytology samples from class I (within normal limits) through class V (carcinoma).

EXAMPLE

> Pap I
> Pap II

A cervical cytology sample that is within normal limits in the Bethesda system corresponds with a Pap class I or II; Bethesda's atypical squamous cell of undetermined significance (ASCUS) corresponds with Pap class III; Bethesda's low-grade squamous intraepithelial lesion (LGSIL) corresponds with Pap class III and CIN grade 1; and Bethesda's high-grade squamous intraepithelial lesion (HGSIL) corresponds with Pap classes III and IV and CIN grades 2 and 3. In the Bethesda system, the next higher level is labeled simply "carcinoma," corresponding with Pap class V and with "carcinoma" in the CIN system.

Clark level: Describes the invasion level of primary malignant melanoma of the skin from the epidermis. Use roman numerals I (least deep) to IV (deepest). Lowercase *level.*

Clark level I	into underlying papillary dermis
Clark level II	to junction of papillary and reticular dermis
Clark level III	into reticular dermis
Clark level IV	into the subcutaneous fat

Dukes classification: Named for British pathologist Cuthbert E. Dukes (1890-1977). It classifies the extent of operable adenocarcinoma of the colon or rectum. Do not use an apostrophe before or after the *s.* Follow Dukes with a capital letter.

Dukes A	confined to mucosa
Dukes B	extending into the muscularis mucosae
Dukes C	extending through the bowel wall, with metastasis to lymph nodes

When the Dukes classification is further defined by numbers, use arabic numerals on the same line with the letter, with no space between.

EXAMPLE

| Dukes C2 |

FAB classification: French-American-British morphologic classification system for acute nonlymphoid leukemia. Express with capital M followed by arabic numeral (1 through 6); do not space between the M and the numeral.

M1	myeloblastic, no differentiation
M2	myeloblastic, differentiation
M3	promyelocytic
M4	myelomonocytic
M5	monocytic
M6	erythroleukemia

FAB staging of carcinoma utilizes TNM classification of malignant tumors
(*See TNM staging below*).

> FAB T1N1M0

FAB staging can be further delineated using the *Rai classification* and *Binet staging* systems.

Rai classification is expressed using lowercase *stage* and roman numerals 0 to IV:

stage 0	Patients at low risk, have lymphocytosis, and a high lymphocyte count defined as more than 15,000 lymphocytes per cubic millimeter (> 15,000/mm3).
stage I	Patients at intermediate risk and have lymphocytosis plus enlarged lymph nodes.
stage II	Patients at intermediate risk but have lymphocytosis plus an enlarged liver or enlarged spleen, with or without lymphadenopathy.
stage III	Patients at high risk, have lymphocytosis plus anemia, and a low red blood cell count (hemoglobin < 11 g/dL), with or without lymphadenopathy, hepatomegaly, or splenomegaly.
stage IV	Patients at high risk but have lymphocytosis plus thrombocytopenia (< 100–103 /dL).

Binet staging further classifies FAB stages and is expressed using lowercase *stage* and capital letters A through C.

> Binet stage A (fewer than 3 areas of enlarged lymphoid tissue)
> Binet stage B (greater than 3 areas of enlarged lymphoid tissue)
> Binet stage C (anemia plus thrombocytopenia)

FIGO staging: Federation Internationale de Gynécologie et Obstétrique system for staging gynecologic malignancy, particularly carcinomas of the ovary. Expressed as stage I (least severe) to stage IV (most severe), with subdivisions within each stage (a, b, c). Lowercase *stage*, and use roman numerals. Use lowercase letters to indicate subdivisions within a stage.

EXAMPLE

DIAGNOSIS
Ovarian carcinoma, FIGO stage IIc.

Gleason tumor grade: Also known as *Gleason score.* The system scores or grades the prognosis for adenocarcinoma of the prostate, with a scale of 1 through 5 for each dominant and secondary pattern; these are then totaled for the score. The higher the score, the poorer the prognosis. Lowercase *grade* or *score*, and use arabic numerals.

EXAMPLE

DIAGNOSIS
Adenocarcinoma of prostate, Gleason score 8.

Gleason score 3 + 2 = 5.
Gleason 3 + 3 with a total score of 6.

Jewett classification of bladder carcinoma: Use capitals as follows:

EXAMPLE

0	in situ (Note: this is the letter O, not a zero)
A	involving submucosa
B	involving muscle
C	involving surrounding tissue
D	involving distant sites

DIAGNOSIS
Bladder carcinoma, Jewett class B.

Karnofsky rating scale, Karnofsky status: Scale for rating performance status of patients with malignant neoplasms. Use arabic numerals: 10, 20, 30, 40, 50, 60, 70, 80, 90, 100. (Normal is 100, moribund is 10.)

Multiple Endocrine Neoplasm: Express using capitalized letters followed by a space and arabic numerals (1 through 3). Capitalize subclassification letters following the arabic numeral.

EXAMPLE

MEN 1
MEN 2
MEN 2A
MEN 2B
MEN 3

16.2.3 Chemotherapy Protocols

Commonly encountered in oncology and immunology, multi-drug regimens are often indicated by protocol designations or protocol acronyms. Abbreviations for multiple-drug regimens are acceptable if widely used and readily recognized, particularly within the specialty setting.

EXAMPLE

MOPP (methotrexate, vincristine sulfate, prednisone, and procarbazine)

Some chemotherapy protocols combine abbreviations designating the type of cancer with treatment and drug abbreviations.

EXAMPLE

BRAJCEF (BR = breast cancer, AJ = adjuvant therapy, C = cyclophosphamide, E = epirubicin, F = fluorouracil)

LUAVPG (LU = lung, AV = advanced, P = platinum, G = gemcitabine)

Chemotherapy treatment often necessitates supplemental treatment for anemias and low red/white cell counts that result from excessive cellular destruction secondary to chemotoxicity. Transcriptionists should be familiar with the medications such as those below. Refer to a reputable resource or dictionary to confirm spelling and expression.

EXAMPLE

Procrit
Neulasta
Aranesp
Epogen

16.2.4 Radiation Therapy

Radiotherapy (radiation therapy) refers to the use of ionizing radiation to eradicate cancerous cells. It can be used alone or in conjunction with chemotherapy. When the latter is true, this is typically referred to as *concomitant radiotherapy*.

The amount of radiation used in radiation therapy is measured in *Gray (Gy)* or *centigray (cGy)* and varies depending on the type and stage of cancer being treated. The typical dose for curative cases of solid epithelial tumor ranges from 60 to 80 Gy; for lymphoma tumors, 20 to 40 Gy. Total doses are typically fractionated over a period of days to allow cells time to recover and respond.

EXAMPLE

> The patient will be treated with radiotherapy in the adjuvant setting and will receive 2 Gy fractional treatments for a total of 60 Gy.

Radiation therapy is delivered externally through a number of conventional methods:

EXAMPLE

> external beam radiotherapy (EBRT *or* XBRT)
> 2-dimensional external beam radiotherapy (2DXRT)
> 3-dimensional conformal radiotherapy (3DCRT)
> intensity-modulated radiation therapy (IMRT)

Radiotherapy can also be delivered internally by means of infusion, ingestion, or radioactive seed implantation. This is typically accomplished through treatment with isotopes. *Isotopes* are atoms of the same element that have different atomic masses. They are used in reference to radioactive drugs. When the element name, not the symbol, is used, place the isotope number on the line after the name in the same font and type size; do not superscript or subscript. Space between the element name and the isotope number. Do not hyphenate either the noun or the adjectival form.

EXAMPLE

> iodine 128
> technetium 99m

When the element symbol is used, place the isotope number as a superscript immediately before the symbol. In environments where superscripting is prohibited, use the following format: element symbol, space (not hyphen), isotope number (on the line). It is also acceptable to spell out the element name followed by the isotope number.

^{128}I or I 128 or iodine 128
^{99m}Tc or Tc 99m or technetium 99m

For trademarked isotopes, follow the style of the manufacturer. In trademarks, the isotope is usually joined to the rest of the name by a hyphen; it may or may not be preceded by the element symbol.

Glofil-125
Hippuran I 131

CHAPTER

17

Dermatology/Allergy/
Immunology

Introduction

Dermatology as a specialty is focused on the identification, treatment, and management of diseases and disorders involving the skin and connective tissues. These can range from congenital defects to neoplasms to viral or bacterial infections to allergies and disorders of the immune system. Because of the close link between allergic and immunologic response to manifestations of the skin and connective tissues, these specialties are often closely associated with each other, and testing for many dermatologic conditions involves evaluation of immunologic components.

17.1 Dermatology/Allergy

Dermatologists perform many specialized diagnostic procedures including microscopic examination of skin biopsy specimens, cytological smears, patch tests, photo tests, potassium hydroxide (KOH) preparations, fungus cultures, and other microbiologic examination of skin scrapings and secretions. Treatment methods used by dermatologists include externally applied, injected, and internal medications, selected x-ray and ultraviolet light therapy, and a range of dermatologic surgical procedures. This is a highly specialized clinical area not typically encountered, with the exception of the identification and treatment of malignancies, in the acute care setting. Transcriptionists in the outpatient setting should be familiar with the concepts outlined below.

17.1.1 Terminology
Most of the terms encountered in dermatology involve both descriptive terms of visible abnormalities and clinical terms, often derived from Latin, that correlate to conditions, syndromes, and diseases. Transcriptionists should be familiar with the pluralization of Latin terms

(*See 8.1.11—Foreign Terms*), particularly when dictators are not always careful to dictate these correctly.

singular	plural
lentigo	lentigines
naris	nares
nasal ala (one "wing")	nasal alae (both "wings")
comedo	comedones

The plural forms of Latin terms that consist of a noun-adjective combination are often difficult to determine. (In Latin, the adjective must agree in number, gender, and case with the noun it modifies.) In the following list we show such terms in their singular and plural forms; they are all in the nominative case.

singular	plural
verruca vulgaris	verrucae vulgares
condyloma acuminatum	condylomata acuminata
nevus araneus	nevi aranei

Sometimes the genitive case (used in Latin to show possession) is misread as a plural, causing confusion. The following terms consist, for the most part, of a noun in the nominative case plus a noun in the genitive case.

Latin term	English translation
pruritus vulvae	itching of the vulva
muscularis mucosa	muscular (layer) of mucosa
incontinentia pigmenti	bronzing of the skin

Be familiar with Latin terms for conditions that do not take plural forms. Consult a reputable dictionary or resource to confirm appropriate expression.

molluscum contagiosum
lupus erythematosus
erythema nodosum

Many dermatologic terms arise from other foreign language, such as French. Express these using appropriate accent and diacritical marks. In electronic environments where these symbols cannot be facilitated, omit them.

café au lait *or* cafe au lait
tache cérébral *or* tache cerebral
tache bleuâtre *or* tache bleuatre
but:
peau d'orange

Be careful not to confuse dermatologic terms and conditions ending in the suffix *–form* with those ending in *–forme*. Consult a reputable dictionary or resource to confirm appropriate expression.

filiform
herpetiform
zosteriform
scarlatiniform
morbilliform
but:
erythema multiforme
glioblastoma multiforme

Pay particular attention to Latin terms that can be both singular and plural to ensure the appropriate expression is used in clinical context, even when dictated in error.

D: The patient had multiple actinic keratosis of the upper trunk.
T: The patient had multiple actinic keratoses of the upper trunk.

D: The patient had multiple areas of actinic keratoses of the upper trunk.
T: The patient had multiple areas of actinic keratosis of the upper trunk.

Apply the rules for possessive eponyms to those eponymic terms common to dermatology/allergy documentation.

Nikolsky sign
Koebner phenomenon
Osler nodes
Janeway spots
Beau lines
Rumpel-Leede test

17.1.2 Testing and Procedures

Refer to an appropriate resource or reputable dictionary to confirm expression and reporting of any tests or procedures not outlined below.

Allergy Testing: Multiple tests can be undertaken to assess for allergic sensitivity and response.

prick testing (pinpoint introduction of allergen into the skin)
scratch testing (abrading the skin to introduce allergen)
challenge testing (introduction of allergen by oral, inhaled, or other routes)
patch testing (allergens applied to a patch placed on the skin)
RAST (radioallergosorbent) testing (blood test)

Mohs: A highly specialized surgical technique in which all remaining visible parts of a tumor are excised and skin is removed layer by layer and examined under a microscope while the patient is undergoing surgery. Skin continues to be removed until cancer is no longer detected.

Mohs
not:
Moh's
not:
Mohs'

17.1.3 Classification Systems

ABCDEs: Acronym used to describe key characteristics of melanoma detection. Should be expressed as an abbreviation if dictated.

EXAMPLE

Asymmetry (A)
Border irregularity (B)
Color variation (C)
Diameter (D)
Evolving (E)

Breslow thickness: Term used to describe the correlation between tumor depth/invasion and the 5-year survival rate after surgical removal of the tumor, first identified by Alexander Breslow, MD, in 1975.

EXAMPLE

less than 0.76 mm
0.76-1.50 mm
1.51-2.50 mm
2.51-4.0 mm
4.1-8.0 mm
more than 8.0

Burns: Classified as 1st, 2nd, 3rd, and 4th degree, according to burn depth. AHDI recommends dropping the hyphen in the adjectival form. Expressing ordinals as numerals is preferred to writing them out.

EXAMPLE

1st degree burn *or* 1st degree burn
3rd degree burn *or* 3rd degree burn

Rule of Nines: Formula based on multiples of 9 for determining percentage of burned body surface. This formula does not apply to children because a child's head is disproportionately large.

head	9%
each arm	9%
each leg	18%
anterior trunk	18%
posterior trunk	18%
perineum	1%

Decubitus ulcers: Classified using roman numerals from stage I (nonblanchable erythema of intact skin) through stage IV (full-thickness skin loss with extensive tissue destruction).

Note: The phrase *decubitus ulcers* should be used when the erroneous plural *decubiti* is dictated.

D: The patient has 2 stage II decubiti and 1 stage III decubitus ulcer.
T: The patient has 2 stage II decubitus ulcers and 1 stage III decubitus ulcer.
or:
T: The patient has 2 stage II and one stage III decubitus ulcers.

Clark level: Describes invasion level of primary malignant melanoma of the skin from the epidermis. Use roman numerals I (least deep) to IV (deepest). Lowercase *level.*

Clark level I	into underlying papillary dermis
Clark level II	to junction of papillary and reticular dermis
Clark level III	into reticular dermis
Clark level IV	into the subcutaneous fat

Note: Breslow depth and Clark level of epidermal involvement are often dictated together.

The lesion was classified as Breslow depth 0.74 mm, Clark level II-III.

17.2 Immunology

The primary focus of immunology is the function and management of the immune system. It has correlations to almost every clinical specialty because of the number of diseases, syndromes, and conditions that have immunologic implications and origins. For the working transcriptionist, the connection to immunologic terminology will fall primarily in the domain of laboratory tests and values ordered to assess/manage immunologic health and function.

17.2.1 CD Cell Markers

CDs, or *clusters of differentiation*, refer to the classification system for identifying cellular surface antigens, of which there are more than 200. CD terms should be expressed with capital *CD*, arabic numerals, and lowercase subclassification letters.

CD1a
CD3d
CD4
CD10
CD41

17.2.2 Cytokines/Chemokines

Cytokines are glycoproteins produced after stimulation or activation of immune cells. In close proximity and in small concentrations, they can facilitate immune and inflammatory reactions, repair processes, and cell growth and differentiation. Cytokines are grouped into families and subfamilies.
(see examples next page)

chemokine families
interleukin 1/toll-like receptors
platelet-derived growth factor family (PDGF)
receptor tyrosine kinases
transforming growth factor beta (TGF-beta *or* TGF-ß)
tumor necrosis factor (TNF)
type 1 hematopoietins
type II interferons

Chemokines are a cytokine family that consists of 40 cytokines with critical functions in the immune system. Chemokines are classified into 4 subfamilies based on cysteine (C) residues and amino-acid (X) residues.

CXC
CC
XC
CX3C

Chemokine subfamilies are formed by combining the chemokine family classification with a subfamily code to form the *systematic name*.

CXC	CXCL1
	CXCL4
	CXCL5
	CXCL6
	CXCL8
	CXCL14
CC	CCL1
	CCL3
	CCL5
	CCL7
	CCL21
XC	XCL1
	XCL2
CX3C	CX3CL1

17.2.3 HLA/Histocompatibility

Human leukocyte antigens (HLA) are genetic markers on white blood cells. Just as red cell antigens determine blood type, HLA antigens determine tissue type. Express with capital-lowercase combinations and hyphens. Check appropriate references for guidance.

EXAMPLE

HLA-DR5	associated with Hashimoto thyroiditis
B8, Dw3	associated with Graves disease

Major histocompatibility complex, class I antigens:

EXAMPLE

HLA-D
HLA-DR

Major histocompatibility complex, class II antigens:

EXAMPLE

HLA-B27
HLA-DRw10

Examples of antigenic specificities of major HLA loci:

EXAMPLE

HLA-A
HLA-B
HLA-C
HLA-D

17.2.4 Immunoglobulins

Immunoglobulins are the glycoproteins that constitute antibodies. These are identified by the abbreviation *Ig* followed by a class designation. *IgG* refers to the class of immunoglobulins most abundant in serum. The 5 classes of immunoglobulins, from most to least abundant, are:

EXAMPLE

IgG
IgA
IgM
IgD
IgE

Ig Prefixes: Expand these terms on first mention in formal publication.

EXAMPLE

mIgM	monomeric IgM
mIgM	membrane-bound IgM
pIg	polymeric immunoglobulin
pIgA	polymerized IgA
pIgR	receptor for polymeric immunoglobulin
sIg	surface immunoglobulin
sIgM	surface IgM
sIgA	surface IgA

Note: Be careful not to confuse immunoglobulin references with other similar abbreviations.

EXAMPLE

IGF-1 (insulin growth factor)
not:
IgF-1

17.2.5 Interferons

Interferons are a class of glycoproteins that exert antineoplastic, antiviral, and immuno-modulating effects. Use nonproprietary names as discussed below. For trade names and additional guidance, consult the USAN dictionary or other appropriate reference.

For general classes of compounds or single compounds, follow the lowercase interferon by the spelled-out Greek letter; use the Greek symbol in abbreviations. *Note:* alfa is the correct spelling in these terms, not alpha.

EXAMPLE

interferon alfa	IFN-α
interferon beta	IFN-β
interferon gamma	IFN-γ

For individual, pure, identifiable compounds with nonproprietary names, add a hyphen, an arabic numeral, and a lowercase letter.

EXAMPLE

interferon alfa-2a
interferon alfa-2b
interferon gamma-1a
interferon gamma-1b

For names of mixtures of interferons from natural sources, add a hyphen, a lowercase *n*, and an arabic numeral.

EXAMPLE

interferon alfa-n1
interferon alfa-n2

17.2.6 Interleukins

Interleukins are a class of proteins that are secreted mostly by macrophages and T lymphocytes; they induce growth and differentiation of lymphocytes and hematopoietic stem cells. There are 12 interleukin derivatives. With the exception of interleukin 3, interleukin derivatives end in *–kin*, so they can readily be identified by this suffix.

-nakin	interleukin 1 derivatives
-onakin	interleukin 1a derivatives
-benakin	interleukin 1b derivatives
-leukin	interleukin 2 derivatives

(continued next page)

-trakin	interleukin 4 derivatives
-penkin	interleukin 5 derivatives
-exakin	interleukin 6 derivatives
-eptakin	interleukin 7 derivatives
-octakin	interleukin 8 derivatives
-nonakin	interleukin 9 derivatives
-decakin	interleukin 10 derivatives
-elvekin	interleukin 11 derivatives
-dodekin	interleukin 12 derivatives

Note: Interleukin 3 can be identified by the suffix *–plestim* and falls under the category of colony-stimulating factors (see below).

17.2.7 Colony-Stimulating Factors

Colony-stimulating factors are naturally occurring glycoproteins that regulate the proliferation, differentiation, and maturation of hematopoietic growth factors. They belong to a class of soluble immune system proteins known as *cytokines.*

Granulocyte colony-stimulating factors (G-CSFs) can be identified by the suffix *–grastim.*

EXAMPLE

> filgrastim
> lenograstim
> Pd-grastim

Granulocyte-macrophage colony-stimulating factors (GM-CSFs) can be identified by the suffix *–gramostim.*

EXAMPLE

> ecogramostim
> molgramostim
> regramostim
> sargramostim

Macrophage colony-stimulating factors (M-CSFs) can be identified by the suffix *–mostim.*

> cilmostim
> lanimostim
> mirimostim

Interleukin 3 (IL-3) factors can be identified by the suffix *–plestim.*

> muplestim
> daniplestim

Combined forms, or conjugates, of 2 types of colony-stimulating factors can be identified by the suffix *–distim.*

> leridistim
> milodistim

Stem-cell stimulating factors (SCSFs) can be identified by the suffix *–cestim.*

> ancestim

17.2.8 Lymphocytes

Lymphocytes are the cells that carry out antigen-specific immune responses. T *lymphocytes (T cells)* and *B lymphocytes (B cells)* are the most common lymphocytes. In general, do not use the extended forms. Do not hyphenate except when used as an adjective preceding a noun. A third group of lymphocytes is called *natural killer cells (NK cells).*

> T cells
> T-cell count
> NK cells

Pre– and pan–: Use a hyphen to join *pre–* or *pan–* to the following letter or word.

> pre-T cell
> pan-B lymphocyte
> pan-thymocyte

B lymphocytes: The prefixes *pre–* and *pro–* are used to delineate cell development.

> pro-B cell
> pre-B cell

Subsets are named with capital letters and arabic numerals.

> CD5+ B cells
> B1 B cells

T lymphocytes: The main types of T lymphocytes should be expanded at first mention in formal publication and then expressed with subscripted delineation.

> helper T cells: T_H cells
> cytotoxic T cells: T_C cells

Use a virgule (not a hyphen) to express helper/inducer and cytotoxic/suppressor subsets descriptions of T lymphocytes. Helper/inducer T lymphocytes are also known as helper cells or helper T lymphocytes. Cytotoxic/suppressor T lymphocytes are also called suppressor cells. Use a hyphen (not a virgule or colon) in the phrase helper-suppressor ratio.

> helper-suppressor ratio
> *not:*
> helper/suppressor ratio
> *not:*
> helper:suppressor ratio

Surface antigens: Join arabic numerals (on the line) to the letter to express surface antigens of T lymphocytes.

> T3
> T8
> T11

Most helper T cells express the cell marker *CD4* and most cytotoxic T cells express the cell marker *CD8*. Presence or absence of a marker on a T cell is expressed with a plus (+) or minus (–) sign, superscripted in formal publication.

> CD4+, CD4$^+$
> CD4-, CD4$^-$
> CD4+CD8-, CD4$^+$CD8$^-$

The terms *negative* and *positive* are spelled out and used to describe combinations of CD4 and CD8 marker findings.

> CD4+CD8-, CD4-CD8+   "single-positive lymphocytes"
> CD4-CD8-   "double-negative lymphocytes"
> CD4+CD8+   "double-positive lymphocytes"

CHAPTER

18

Orthopedics/Neurology

Introduction

Few specialties provide as diverse and rich a language than those found in the field of orthopedics and neurology. Where else will you encounter such unusual phrases and acronyms as *FOOSH (fell on outstretched hand), catch and clunk test, boutonnière deformity, breakdancer's thumb, Stookey reflex, microknurling,* and *matricectomy*? With myriad tests associated with reflex, sensation, mobility, gait, and neurological function, the eponyms alone can keep an MT running to the reference books. In addition, no other specialty can boast such a surprising repertoire of unique surgical instruments and materials (*rasps, rongeurs, curettes, saws, cement, plates, pins, screws, wires, reamers, perforators, retractors,* etc.). Orthopedic surgery could very well be described as "applied anatomical carpentry," as the methods and techniques used to reinforce and correct the deformities and conditions of the skeleton are very similar to those applied to any other *structure*.

18.1 Orthopedics

Orthopedics is a specialty that concerns itself primarily with the diagnosis and treatment of diseases and disorders (hereditary, developmental, traumatic, inflammatory, and degenerative) of the musculoskeletal system. In recent years, it has become a specialty so diverse and highly specialized that many orthopedic surgeons have chosen to focus on a particular area of the body (i.e., upper extremity, back, knees, maxillofacial, etc.). Each anatomical area has its own terms, tests, and style applications.

18.1.1 Anatomic Terms

Do not capitalize the names of anatomic features (except the eponyms associated with them).

EXAMPLE

> os frontale
> zygomatic bone
> ligament of Treitz

Posture-based terms:

EXAMPLE

anterior	nearer the front
posterior	nearer the rear
superior	nearer the top
inferior	nearer the bottom

Region-based terms:

EXAMPLE

cranial, cephalic	nearer the head
caudal	nearer the tail or lower end
dorsal	nearer the back
ventral	nearer the belly side or anterior surface

Directional and positional terms: Form directional adverbs by replacing the adjectival suffix (*–al*, *–or*, *–ic*) with the suffix *–ad*, meaning *–ward*. Use these forms in the same type of constructions in which *–ward* forms are used.

EXAMPLE

> caudad
> cephalad
> craniad
> laterad
> orad
> superiad
> ventrad

Do not substitute the –*ad* form when the adjective itself or the –*ly* adverb has been used correctly.

> It extends caudally from...
> the anterior incision

Use a combining vowel to join directional and positional adjectives.

> mediolateral

Latin and English names: It is common practice to mix the English and Latin names of anatomic parts, e.g., using English for the noun and Latin for the adjectives. These may be transcribed as dictated or edited to either their English or Latin forms.

> latissimus dorsi muscle
> peroneus profundus nerve
> palpebrales arteries

18.1.2 Angles

In expressing angles in orthopedic testing, write out *degrees* or use the degree sign (°).

> The patient was able to straight leg raise to 40 degrees.
> *or:*
> The patient was able to straight leg raise to 40°.

18.1.3 Terminology

Crepitance, crepitation, crepitus: These terms are all synonymous. The adjectival form is *crepitant* (*crepitants* is not a word). Although *crepitance* is not found in dictionaries, its frequent usage has made it acceptable, though MTs should defer to facility preference, especially in a non-verbatim environment, for editing *crepitance* to *crepitates*.

Fingerbreadth: Commonly used unit of measure associated with physical measurement (by hand) of distance on physical examination. Plural form is *fingerbreadths*, not *fingersbreadth*.

Fluctuation, fluctuance: These terms are synonymous. *Fluctuants* is not a word. The adjectival form is *fluctuant*.

Hyphenated forms: Refer to a reputable dictionary or resource to confirm combined anatomical terms as single-word vs. hyphenated compounds.

EXAMPLE

> anterolateral
> dorsiflexion
> fracture-dislocation

Planes: Term used to describe an imaginary flat surface and frequently dictated to provide anatomic orientation. The planes of the body and its structures include those listed below. Check appropriate references (anatomy books and medical dictionaries) for additional planes.

EXAMPLE

frontal	A vertical plane dividing the body or structure into anterior and posterior portions. Also known as coronal plane.
sagittal	Lengthwise vertical plane dividing the body or structure into right and left portions; midsagittal plane divides the body into right and left halves. Also known as median plane.
transverse	Plane running across the body parallel to the ground, dividing the body or structure into upper and lower portions. Also known as horizontal or axial plane.

Possessive eponyms: Follow the rules for possessive eponyms by dropping the 's, even when dictated, but be careful to confirm whether an eponym ends in s.

EXAMPLE

> D: The patient had positive Tinel's and Phalen's signs.
> T: The patient had positive Tinel and Phalen signs.
> *not:*
> T: The patient had positive Tinels and Phalens signs.
>
> *but:*
>
> D: The patient had a positive Homans sign.
> T: The patient had a positive Homans sign.
> *not:*
> T: The patient had a positive Homan sign.
> *not:*
> T: The patient had a positive Homan's sign.

Reflexes: Assessment is graded on a scale of 0 to 4. Express as an arabic numeral followed (or preceded) by a plus sign (except 0, which stands alone). Lowercase the word *grade*.

grade	meaning
0	absent
+1 or 1+	decreased
+2 or 2+	normal
+3 or 3+	hyperactive
+4 or 4+	clonus

When reflexes are expressed as a range using *over*, repeat the denominator for clarity of expression.

D: grade 2 to 3 plus over 4
T: grade 2+/4 to 3+/4
not:
T: grade 2-3+/4
not:
T: grade 2+-3+/4

Do not use plus signs without the numeral, i.e., do not use +, ++, +++, ++++.

Knee reflexes were grade 3+/4.
not:
Knee reflexes were grade +++/4.

Sign, test, score: Do not capitalize these words even when they are associated with eponyms. Do capitalize the eponyms that precede them.

drawer sign
fabere test
Bancroft sign
Cozen test

18.1.4 Surgical Instruments

Wires, pins, and screws: These materials, typically used in orthopedics, are generally measured in portions of an inch, though frequently metric equivalents are used instead. In the case of pins and screws, typically the size expressed represents the *thread diameter*, which is not the same as the *head diameter*. Transcribe as dictated. When a number alone is given to identify this surgical hardware, it cannot be assumed that the number represents a measurement and could instead represent a numbering system of identification for that particular product. Again, transcribe as dictated; do not add a unit of measure or express as a decimal/fraction when this information is unknown.

> D: a three thirty two Steinmann pin
> T: a 3/32-inch Steinmann pin
>
> D: a four point five cortex screw
> T: a 4.5 cortex screw
> *or:*
> T: a 4.5 mm cortex screw
>
> D: a number sixteen pin
> T: a #16 pin
> *not:*
> T: a 16 mm pin
> *not:*
> T: a 16 inch pin

When more than one dimension is used to identify a screw or pin (i.e., thread diameter and thread length), express these dimensions fractionally, being careful to express thread diameters as decimals when indicated.

EXAMPLE

> D: a six five sixteen cancellous bone screw
> T: a 6.5/16 cancellous bone screw
> *or:*
> T: a 6.5/16 mm cancellous bone screw

Note: In the example above, it should be assumed that since the author dictated "six five" and not "sixty-five," the expression is intended to represent the phrase "six point five," the most common expression of thread diameters.

Kirschner wires, or K-wires, are measured in portions of an inch but are written using decimals and expressed in thousands. Be careful to include the zero *after* the decimal point, as physicians do not typically dictate it.

EXAMPLE

> D: a four five K wire and a six two K wire
> T: a 0.045 K-wire and a 0.062 K-wire

18.1.5 Classification Systems

Catterall hip score: Rating system for Legg-Perthes disease (pediatric avascular necrosis of the femoral head). Use roman numerals I (no findings) through IV (involvement of entire femoral head).

Crowe classification: System for classifying developmental dysplasia of the hip.

grade I	less than 50% subluxation
grade II	50% to 75% subluxation
grade III	75% to 100% subluxation

Garden: System for classifying subcapital fractures of the femoral neck. Lowercase *stage* and use arabic numerals: stage 1 (incomplete) through stage 3 (most complete).

LeFort: Classification system for facial fractures. Use roman numeral I, II, or III. Do not space between *Le* and *Fort*.

EXAMPLE

LeFort I

Mayo: Classification system for olecranon fractures. Use roman numerals and capital letters.

type	description
I	undisplaced
IA	noncomminuted
IB	comminuted
II	displaced, stable
IIA	noncomminuted
IIB	comminuted
III	displaced, unstable
IIIA	noncomminuted
IIIB	comminuted

Neer staging: System for classifying shoulder impingement.

stage	description
I	inflammation and edema of the rotator cuff
II	degenerative fibrosis
III	partial or full-thickness tear

Neer-Horowitz: Classification for proximal humeral physeal fractures in children. Use roman numerals I (less than 5 mm displacement) through IV (displaced more than two-thirds the width of the shaft).

EXAMPLE

Neer-Horowitz II

Outerbridge scale: Assesses damage in chondromalacia patellae. Lowercase *grade*. Use arabic numerals 1 (minimal) through 4 (excessive).

EXAMPLE

DIAGNOSIS
Chondromalacia patellae, grade 3.

Salter: Classification system for epiphyseal fractures. Use roman numerals I (least severe) through VI (most severe).

EXAMPLE

Salter III fracture

Schatzker: Classification system for tibial plateau fractures in terms of injury and therapeutic requirements. Lowercase *type* and use roman numerals: type I (least complicated) through type VI (most complicated).

Salter-Harris: Classification system for fractures involving the physis in children. Use roman numerals I (fracture across the physis only) through V (crush injury to physis).

EXAMPLE

Salter-Harris fracture type II.

stress fractures: Lowercase *grade* and use roman numerals I (local symptoms, negative radiographs, positive bone scan) through IV (local symptoms, actual bone fracture identified on radiographs, positive bone scan). Note: A grade 0 indicates an asymptomatic patient with negative radiographs and negative bone scan.

18.2 Neurology

As a specialty, neurology is concerned with the identification, treatment, and management of diseases and disorders of the nervous system, including the brain and spine. It should not be confused with psychiatry, which focuses on mental and social function.

18.2.1 Cranial Nerves

Use arabic or roman numerals for cranial nerve designations. Be consistent. (Defer to client/facility preference.)

EXAMPLE

cranial nerve 12	cranial nerve XII
cranial nerves 2-12	cranial nerves II-XII

Ordinals should be expressed using arabic numerals.

EXAMPLE

12th cranial nerve

The cranial nerves, including their English and Latin names, are as follows:

number	English name	Latin name
1 *or* I	olfactory	olfactorius
2 *or* II	optic	opticus
3 *or* III	oculomotor	oculomotorius
4 *or* IV	trochlear	trochlearis
5 *or* V	trigeminal	trigeminus
6 *or* VI	abducens	abducens

(continued next page)

7 or VII	facial	facialis
8 or VIII	vestibulocochlear	vestibulocochlearis
9 or IX	glossopharyngeal	glossopharyngeus
10 or X	vagus	vagus
11 or XI	accessory	accessorius
12 or XII	hypoglossal	hypoglossus

Use the English names when designating cranial nerves.

EXAMPLE

The oculomotor, trochlear, and abducens nerves are responsible for ocular movement.

18.2.2 Vertebrae, Spinal Nerves, and Spinal Levels

Sharing a common nomenclature, these entities are derived from spinal anatomic regions:

region	vertebrae	spinal nerves
cervical	C1 through C7	C1 through C8
thoracic	T1 through T12	T1 through T12
lumbar	L1 through L5	L1 through L5
sacrum	S1 through S5	S1 through S5
coccyx	4 fused	coccygeal nerve

Portions of a vertebra may be referred to as follows, i.e., without the term *vertebra*:

EXAMPLE

C3 spinous process
L4 lamina
transverse process of T10

Use a hyphen to express the space between two vertebrae (the intervertebral space). It is not necessary to repeat the same letter before the second vertebra, but it may be transcribed if dictated.

> C1-2 *or* C1-C2
> L5-S1

It is preferable to repeat the letter before each numbered vertebra in a list.

> The lesion involves C4, C5, and C6.
> *not:*
> The lesion involves C4, 5, and 6.
> *not:*
> The lesion involves C4, 5, 6.

When expressing a range between two *nonadjacent* vertebrae where the word *through*, not *to*, is used, spell out and do not hyphenate. To hyphenate, especially in reference to fusions, would imply an erroneous construction.

> D: We performed a fusion of T10 through T12.
> T: We performed a fusion of T10 through T12.
> *not:*
> T: We performed a fusion of T10-T12.

Note: In the example above, to express this as *T10-T12* would imply that T10 was fused to T12 rather than a procedure that involved fusion of T10 to T11 and T11 to T12.

Do not use a single hyphen to express a range when more than two vertebrae are specifically dictated within the range.

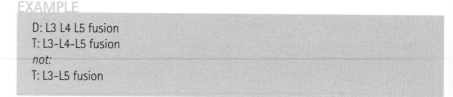

> D: L3 L4 L5 fusion
> T: L3-L4-L5 fusion
> *not:*
> T: L3-L5 fusion

Disk/disc: Most medical lexicographic resources as well as *The AMA Manual of Style* 10th edition indicate the use of *disk* for all anatomical terms other than ophthalmologic use. However, *Terminologia Anatomica* retains the use of *disc* in reference to spinal terminology. Transcriptionists should be aware that the preferred trend is for use of *disk*; however, many orthopedists still prefer the guidelines outlined in *Terminologia Anatomica* and may direct an MT to use *disc* in transcription of spinal terminology. This same rule applies to terms like *orthopedic* vs. *orthopaedic*; the Old English spellings are still referenced in *Terminologia Anatomica*, and therefore some orthopedists still defer to that usage. The preferred trend, however, is to use the modern spellings.

References to disks should be expressed with hyphens in similar fashion to the corresponding intervertebral spaces.

EXAMPLE

C7-T1 disk
L5-S1 disk

18.2.3 Diagnostic Testing and Procedures

Electroencephalographic Terms: Test performed to measure electrical activity in the brain. EEG is the abbreviation for electroencephalogram, electroencephalography, and electroencephalograph.

Use capital letters to refer to anatomic areas. Use lowercase letters to refer to relative electrode positions. Use odd numbers to refer to electrodes placed on the left. Use even numbers to refer to those on the right. The letter *z* refers to midline (zero) electrodes.

EXAMPLE

A1, A2	earlobe electrodes
Cz, C3, C4	central electrodes
F7, F8	anterior temporal electrodes
Fpz, Fp1, Fp2	frontal pole; prefrontal electrodes
Fz, F3, F4	frontal electrodes
Oz, O1, O2	occipital electrodes
Pg1, Pg2	nasopharyngeal electrodes
Pz, P3, P4	parietal electrodes
T3, T4	midtemporal electrodes
T5, T6	posterior temporal electrodes

Trend note: Previous style guides, including the second edition of this text, recommended subscripting the arabic numerals and lowercase letters in the expressions above. The preferred trend is now to express those on the same line without subscripting.

Express *frequency* in cycles per second (c/s or cps) or hertz (Hz).

EXAMPLE

16 c/s *or* 16 cps *or* 16 Hz

Some terms commonly used in EEG reports:

EXAMPLE

10-20 International System for electrode placement
alert, drowsy, and sleeping states
alpha range
alpha rhythm
alpha waves
amplitude
artifact
background rhythm
beta rhythms
bisynchronous
central sleep spindles
cycles per second (c/s, cps)
delta brush
delta spikes
delta waves
frontal sharp transient
hyperventilation
lambda rhythm
lateralizing focus
mu pattern
occipital driving
paroxysmal, paroxysms
photic stimulation
rhythmic activity
sharp elements
sharp waves
sleep spindles
slow transients

(continued next page)

slow waves
spike and dome complex
spike and wave pattern
spikes
spindles
Standard International lead placements
symmetrical activity
synchronous
theta activity
theta frequency
21-channel recording
vertex waves
voltage
wave bursts

Evoked potential testing: Measurement of stimulated electrical signals.

BAEPs	brainstem auditory evoked potentials
SSEPs	somatosensory evoked potentials
VEPs	visual evoked potentials
PVEPs	pattern visual evoked potentials
FVEPs	flash visual evoked potentials

Similar to electrode terminology for EEGs, evoked potential testing uses additional and/or modified electrodes:

BAEP electrodes:	
Ac	contralateral earlobe
Ai	ipsilateral earlobe
EAM	external auditory meatus
EAMc	contralateral EAM
EAMi	ipsilateral EAM
M1 M2	mastoid process
Mc	contralateral M
Mi	ipsilateral M

SSEP electrodes:	
AC	anterior cervical
C1 prime	near EEG C1
C2 prime	near EEG C2
C3 prime	near EEG C3
C4 prime	near EEG C4
C2S, C5S	C2, C5 spinous processes
Cc	contralateral C3 prime or C4 prime
Ci	ipsilateral C3 prime or C4 prime
CP	midway between C3 or C4 and P3 or P4
CPc	contralateral CP
CPi	ipsilateral CP
Cz prime	near 10-20 Cz
EP	Erb point
EP1, EP2	left and right EP
Epi	ipsilateral EP
Fpz prime	near EEG Fpz
IC	iliac crest
L2S, L3S	L2, L3 spinous processes
LN	lateral neck
LNi	ipsilateral LN
PFd, PFp	popliteal fossa (distal, proximal)
REF	reference
T6S, T10S, T12S	T6, T10, T12 spinous processes

VEP electrodes:	
I	inion
LO	left occipital
LT	left posterior temporal
MF	midfrontal
MO	midoccipital
MP	midparietal
RO	right occipital
RT	right posterior temporal
V	vertex

Waveforms for evoked potential testing are classified as *P* for positive or *N* for negative plus an arabic numeral indicating the number of milliseconds between stimulus and response in normal adults.

EXAMPLE

VEP: N75, N100, N155, P75, P100, P135
SSEP: N9, N11, N13, N15, N18, N20, N34, N35, P9, P11, P13, P15, P27, P37

SSEPs were recorded from the brachial plexus, cervical spine at C2 (N13), and contralateral parietal area (N19) with a frontal reference.

Nerve conduction studies: Test performed to measure the electrical conduction of the motor and sensory nerves and to determine nerve conduction velocity (NCV) for diagnosing conduction delay and nerve entrapment disorders.

Motor nerve conduction studies record muscle response when electrical stimulation is applied to a peripheral nerve supplying that muscle. The time it takes for the electrical impulse to travel from the stimulation to the recording site, called *latency*, is measured and expressed in milliseconds (ms). The response, or *amplitude*, is measured in millivolts (mV).

Sensory nerve conduction studies are performed by electrical stimulation of a peripheral nerve and recorded from a sensory portion of the nerve, such as on a finger. Like the motor studies, sensory latencies are also measured in ms, but sensory amplitudes are measured in microvolts (mcV).

F-wave study uses stimulation of a motor nerve and recording of action potentials from a muscle supplied by the nerve.

H-reflex study uses stimulation of a nerve and recording of the reflex electrical discharge from a muscle in the limb.

Small-pain-fibers nerve conduction studies (spf-NCS) use an electrical stimulus with a neuroselective frequency to determine the minimum voltage causing conduction.

18.2.4 Classification Systems

Glasgow coma scale: Describes level of consciousness of patients with head injuries by testing the patient's ability to respond to verbal, motor, and sensory stimulation. Each parameter is scored on a scale of 1 through 5, and then totals are added together to indicate level of consciousness.

score	level of consciousness
14 or 15	normal
7 or less	coma
3 or less	brain death

Harvard criteria for brain death: In addition to body temperature equal to or higher than 32°C and the absence of central nervous system depressants, all of the following criteria must be met in order to establish brain death.

1	unreceptivity and unresponsiveness
2	no movement or breathing
3	no reflexes
4	flat electroencephalogram (confirmatory)

Hunt and Hess neurological classification: Classifies prognosis of patients with hemorrhage. Write out and lowercase *grade*; do not abbreviate. Use arabic numerals 1 through 4.

EXAMPLE

grade 3

Kurtzke disability score: Two-part scoring system to evaluate patients with multiple sclerosis. Part one evaluates functional systems (pyramidal, cerebellar, brainstem, sensory, bowel and bladder, visual, mental, and other). Part two is a disability status scale from 0 to 10. Use arabic numerals.

Rancho Los Amigos cognitive function scale: Neurologic assessment tool. Levels I through VIII are written with roman numerals.

I	no response
II	generalized response to stimulation
III	localized response to stimuli
IV	confused and agitated behavior
V	confused with inappropriate behavior (nonagitated)
VI	confused but appropriate behavior
VII	automatic and appropriate behavior
VIII	purposeful and appropriate behavior

CHAPTER

19

Obstetrics/Gynecology/ Pediatrics

Introduction

Certainly few specialties are more enjoyable to allied healthcare workers than obstetrics and gynecology. The areas of labor and delivery and neonatal intensive care are much sought after by many in the clinical setting. It's one of the few areas of the hospital where the majority of patients are happy to be there. Being a participant in the birth of a baby can be a rewarding branch of applied medicine. Medical transcriptionists likewise tend to enjoy the exposure to this specialty in the acute care setting, where a typical day for most hospital MTs will include a healthy mix of routine deliveries and C-sections. MTs are afforded a glimpse into the beginning of life for the next generation, and transcribing the birth of a healthy baby to parents plagued by years of infertility will always be a welcome joy.

Obstetrics, neonatology, and pediatrics find their intersection, of course, in the postnatal setting and are closely connected during that time. After discharge from the hospital, the neonate begins its own care history in the domain of pediatrics.

19.1 Obstetrics and Gynecology

The obstetric domain is focused on the entire process of conception, gestation, labor, and delivery, and houses its own unique terms, tests, procedures, and evaluation systems. In the gynecologic setting, an MT will encounter terminology, tests, and diagnoses related to vaginal, cervical, and uterine health as well as those that pertain to the ovulatory cycle, hormone regulation, and fertility. It is important to remember that this also includes the evolving reproductive health of women as they approach and transition through menopause.

19.1.1 Gynecologic Evaluation

A number of pertinent findings are recorded on routine pelvic examination, with some unusual and often confusing terminology associated with that evaluation.

Adnexa: Appendages or adjunct parts. The uterine adnexa consist of the ovaries, tubes, and ligaments. Adnexa is always plural, even when referring to only one side.

EXAMPLE

> The adnexa are normal.
> Left adnexa are normal.

BUS: Abbreviation referring to the *Bartholin glands, urethra, and Skene glands.* It does not refer to, as is often assumed, the *Bartholin, urethral, and Skene glands,* as there is no such entity as a "urethral gland," and should never be expanded that way or erroneously expressed as *BUS glands.* These 3 anatomic entities are visible or palpable features of the vaginal vestibule and in the abbreviation are listed as they occur from posterior to anterior. They represent an evaluation of 3 separate entities, so the abbreviation should take a plural verb.

EXAMPLE

> BUS normal
> *or:*
> BUS are normal

Pap smear: The brief form for *Papanicolaou,* which may be used if dictated. If the full word is dictated, transcribe in full. Be careful not to confuse *Pap* with *PAP,* which refers to *positive airway pressure* and relates to mechanical ventilation.

19.1.2 Obstetrical Course

Obstetrical history: GPA is the abbreviation for *gravida, para, abortus.* Accompanied by arabic numerals, *G, P,* and *A* (or *Ab*) describe the patient's obstetric history. Use arabic numerals. Roman numerals are not appropriate.

G	gravida (number of pregnancies)	
P	para (number of births of viable offspring)	
A *or* Ab	abortus (abortions)	
nulligravida	gravida 0	no pregnancies
primigravida	gravida 1, G1	1 pregnancy
secundigravida	gravida 2, G2	2 pregnancies
nullipara	para 0	no deliveries of viable offspring

Separate GPA sections by commas. Either the abbreviated or the spelled-out form may be used, whichever is dictated.

EXAMPLE

Obstetric history: G4, P3, A1.
or:
Obstetric history: gravida 4, para 3, abortus 1.

The *TPAL* system is used to describe obstetric history of a patient.

EXAMPLE

T   term infants
P   premature infants
A   abortions
L   living children

Separate TPAL numbers by hyphens.

EXAMPLE

Obstetric history: 4-2-2-4.

TPAL numbers need not be spelled out unless dictated that way, for example:

EXAMPLE

Obstetric history: 4 term infants, 2 premature infants, 2 abortions, 4 living children.

Sometimes, GPA terminology is combined with TPAL terminology, sometimes in abbreviated format, and should be transcribed as dictated.

D: The patient is gravida three, three, zero, zero, three.
T: The patient is gravida 3, 3-0-0-3.
or:
T: The patient is gravida 3, para 3-0-0-3

D: The patient is G three, P three, zero, zero, three.
T: The patient is G3, P3-0-0-3

D: The patient is gravida three, zero, zero, three.
T: The patient is gravida 3-0-0-3

Abort, abortion: Transcribe this term as dictated (editing only as necessary for grammar and clarity). Although the *AMA Manual of Style* prefers the term *terminate* to *abort*, AHDI does not recommend making this editorial change if *abort* is dictated.

D: abort
T: abort (not terminate)

Gestational age: This refers to the age of the embryo/fetus, calculated from the first day of the mother's last normal menstrual period. It is not the same thing as *conceptual age*, which begins counting fetal age from the time of conception. Gestational age is correlated to fetal weight and classified as follows:

Large for gestational age	Fetal weight measured above 90th percentile at 40 weeks' gestation (birth weight in excess of 8 pounds 13 ounces).
Macrosomia	Fetal weight measured above the defined limit at any point during gestation.
Normal for gestational age	Fetal weight measured within defined limit of "normal birth weight" (between 5 pounds 8 ounces and 8 pounds 12 ounces).
Small for gestational age	Fetal weight measured below 10th percentile at gestational age.

Fundal height: Measurement of gestational growth taken from the top of the pubic bone to the top of the uterus. After the 12th week of pregnancy, the number of centimeters should equal the number of weeks of pregnancy. If the measurement is larger, it may indicate a large-for-dates fetus or multiple fetuses. Express fundal height with arabic numerals and in centimeters.

> The patient is at 26 weeks' gestational age, and fundal height today measures 29 cm. We will therefore get an ultrasound to confirm dates and size on her next visit.

19.1.3 Labor and Delivery

Labor stages: There are 3 distinct stages of labor, expressed with lowercase *stage* and arabic numerals.

stage 1	(early labor)	Onset of contractions; dilatation of cervix from 0-3 cm
	(active labor)	Stronger, more consistent contractions; dilatation of cervix from 3-7 cm
	(transition)	Dilatation of cervix from 7-10 cm
stage 2	Pushing and delivery of baby	
stage 3	Delivery of placenta	

Evaluation of cervix: Once labor begins, the cervix begins to *dilate* and *efface*. Dilation is measured and expressed in centimeters (0-10 cm). A cervix at zero centimeters is more frequently described as *closed*. The cervix will also begin to soften and thin out, or *efface*. Effacement of the cervix is measured and expressed as a percentage, from 0% to 100%.

> When we checked the patient again at 10:30 a.m., the cervix was 5 cm and 80% effaced.

Many providers will abbreviate these references, which should be expanded by the transcriptionist.

> D: When we checked the patient again at 10:30 a.m., the cervix was 5 and 80.
> T: When we checked the patient again at 10:30 a.m., the cervix was 5 cm and 80%.

Measurement of station: In addition to the evaluation of the cervix, the examiner will determine the position of the descending fetal part (usually the head) in the birth canal. Station is expressed as -5 to +5, representing the number of centimeters below or above an imaginary plane through the ischial spines (station 0 is at the plane). It is often combined with the cervical findings during serial evaluation throughout labor. Again, when abbreviated, the transcriptionist should expand the reference for clarity.

> D: On examination, she was eight eighty minus one.
> T: On examination, she was 8 cm, 80%, and -1.
> *or:*
> T: On examination, she was 8 cm, 80%, and at -1 station.
> *not:*
> T: On examination, she was 880 minus 1. (or any other variation)

Cesarean section: Expressed as *cesarean section*, lowercase. Not *Cesarean, caesarean,* or *Caesarean.* Brief form is C-section, but do not use it unless it is dictated, and even then, do not use it in the operative title section of operative reports or discharge summaries.

19.1.4 Classification Systems

Cervical cytology: Three different systems are currently in use for cervical cytology: the Papanicolaou test (Pap smear), the CIN classification system, and the Bethesda System.

The Bethesda System is the standardized nomenclature system for reporting cervical cytology and Papanicolaou test results. Abbreviate only if dictated.

atypical squamous cells of undetermined significance (ASCUS)
endocervical/transformation zone (EC/TZ)
atypical squamous cells (ASCs)
loop electrosurgical excision procedure (LEEP)

CIN is an acronym for *cervical intraepithelial neoplasia* and is expressed with arabic numerals from grade 1 (least severe) to grade 3 (most severe). Place a hyphen between CIN and the numeral.

CIN-1, CIN-2, CIN-3
or:
CIN grade 1, CIN grade 2, CIN grade 3

The Papanicolaou test uses roman numerals to classify cervical cytology samples from class I (within normal limits) through class V (carcinoma).

Pap I
Pap II

A cervical cytology sample that is within normal limits in the Bethesda System corresponds with a Pap class I or II; Bethesda's atypical squamous cell of undetermined significance (ASCUS) corresponds with Pap class III; Bethesda's low-grade squamous intraepithelial lesion (LGSIL) corresponds with Pap class III and CIN grade 1; and Bethesda's high-grade squamous intraepithelial lesion (HGSIL) corresponds with Pap classes III and IV and CIN grades 2 and 3. In the Bethesda system, the next higher level is labeled simply "carcinoma," corresponding with Pap class V and with "carcinoma" in the CIN system.

FIGO staging: Federation Internationale de Gynécologie et Obstétrique system for staging gynecologic malignancy, particularly carcinomas of the ovary. Expressed as stage I (least severe) to stage IV (most severe), with subdivisions within each stage (a, b, c). Lowercase *stage*, and use roman numerals. Use lowercase letters to indicate subdivisions within a stage.

DIAGNOSIS
Ovarian carcinoma, FIGO stage IIc.

POP-Q classification: This system for pelvic organ prolapse quantification involves the assessment of 9 points of measurement.

Aa
Ba
C
D
Ap
Bp
PB
GH
TVL

These values represent quantitative measurements and should be expressed with arabic numerals (Aa 1, Ba +6, C +5, GH 6, PB 4, TVL 10, Ap -2, Bp 0, D 0). Once these quantitative measurements have been assessed, the patient is given a POP-Q stage of one to four, expressed in Roman numerals (like all stages) as I through IV.

EXAMPLE

The patient is POP-Q stage II.

19.2 Pediatrics

Most of the pediatric domain is focused on assessment of developmental milestones, treatment and management of normal childhood illnesses and inoculations, and identification of congenital abnormalities or genetic defects. Much depends on the provision of an accurate history on the part of the parent(s) or guardian(s). Much of the anatomical, physiological, and disease process terminology encountered in other specialties are rarely encountered in pediatrics.

19.2.1 Neonatology and Genetics

APGAR questionnaire: Acronym from initial letters of <u>a</u>daptability, <u>p</u>artnership, <u>g</u>rowth, <u>a</u>ffection, <u>r</u>esolve, referring to a family assessment instrument. Use all capitals. Do not confuse with Apgar score.

Apgar score: Assessment of newborn's condition in which pulse, breathing, color, tone, and reflex irritability are each rated 0, 1, or 2, at 1 minute and 5 minutes after birth. Some facilities assess at 1, 5, and 10 minutes after birth. Each set of ratings is totaled, and both totals are reported. It was named after Virginia Apgar, MD. Do not confuse with *APGAR questionnaire* (see above) for family assessment. Use initial capital only. Express ratings with arabic numerals. Write out the numbers related to minutes to avoid ambiguity between scores and minutes. Also, *Apgar score* is preferred to the coined term *Apgars* and should be expanded where facility guidelines allow for its expansion.

EXAMPLE

D: Apgars were seven ten.
T: Apgar scores were 7 and 10 at 1 and 5 minutes.
or:
T: Apgar scores were 7 at 1 minute and 10 at 5 minutes.
not:
T: Apgars were 7/10.
not:
T: Apgars were 7 and 10.

Genetic testing: There are 46 chromosomes in human cells, occurring in pairs and numbered 1 through 22, plus the sex chromosomes, an X and a Y in males and two X's in females. The non-sex chromosomes are also called autosomes. Refer to chromosomes by number or by group.

EXAMPLE

chromosome	group
1-3	A
4, 5	B
6-12, X	C
13-15	D
16-18	E
19, 20	F
21, 22, Y	G

chromosome 16
a chromosome in group E
a group-E chromosome

trisomy: an extra chromosome in any one of the autosomes or either sex chromosome

trisomy D: an extra chromosome in a group-D chromosome, either the 13th, 14th, or 15th chromosome

trisomy 21: an extra 21st chromosome (Down syndrome)

A plus or minus in front of the chromosome number means there is either an extra chromosome or an absent chromosome within that pair.

trisomy 21 = female karyotype: 47,XX +21

The plus or minus following the chromosome number means that part of the chromosome is either extra or missing.

cri du chat syndrome = male karyotype: 46,XY 5p-

Each chromosome has a short arm and a long arm. The short arm is designated by a p, the long arm by a q, immediately following the chromosome number (no space between). Each arm is divided into regions (from 1 to 4); place the region number immediately following the arm designation. Regions are divided into bands, again joined without a space. If a subdivision is identified, it follows a decimal point placed immediately after the band number.

20p	20th chromosome, short arm
20p1	20th chromosome, short arm, region 1
20p11	20th chromosome, short arm, region 1, band 1
20p11.23	20th chromosome, short arm, region 1, band 1, subdivision 23

A translocation occurs when a segment normally found in a certain arm of a chromosome appears in a different location; it may be written as a small t with the from and to sites in parentheses, e.g., $t(14q21q)$, meaning from long arm of 14 to long arm of 21. A more complex designation such as $t(2;6)(q34;p12)$ means from region 3 band 4 of the long arm of chromosome 2 to region 1 band 2 of the short arm of chromosome 6. The chromosome numbers appear in a separate set of parentheses from the arm, region, and band information.

A ring chromosome is one that has pieces missing from the end of each arm, and the two arms have joined at the ends.

Use capital letters to refer to chromosome bands, which are elicited by special staining methods.

EXAMPLE

band	stain
C bands *or* C-banding	constitutive heterochromatin
G bands *or* G-banding	Giemsa
N bands *or* N-banding	nucleolar organizing region
Q bands *or* Q-banding	quinacrine
R bands *or* R-banding	reverse-Giemsa

Karyotypes describe an individual's chromosome complement: the number of chromosomes plus the sex chromosomes present in that individual. Place a comma (without spacing) between the chromosome number and the sex chromosome. Use a virgule to indicate more than one karyotype in an individual.

EXAMPLE

normal human karyotypes:	46,XX (female)
	46,XY (male)
some abnormal karyotypes:	47,XXY
	45,X0
	48,XXX
	45,X/46,XX

19.2.2 Pediatric Immunizations

Transcriptionists in the pediatric setting should be familiar with recommended immunization schedules for children and adolescents as determined by the Department of Health and Human Services (HHS) and the Centers for Disease Control (CDC).

Capitalize vaccine/immunization references in the record. Do *not* capitalize their disease name counterparts. It is acceptable to abbreviate most vaccines/ immunizations in the record, but only if they are specifically dictated that way. Otherwise, spell them out. Do not abbreviate them in the diagnosis area. If abbreviated, be sure to verify the correct expression of the vaccine, as mixed capital letters and lowercase letters are common in vaccine abbreviations. (*see examples next page*)

disease entity name	vaccine name	abbreviation
hepatitis B	Hepatitis B	HepB
rotavirus	Rotavirus	Rota
diphtheria/tetanus/pertussis	Diphtheria, Tetanus, Pertussis	DTaP
Haemophilus influenzae	Haemophilus influenzae, type b	Hib
pneumococcus	Pneumococcal	PCV
poliovirus	Inactivated Poliovirus	IPV
influenza	Influenza	Influenza
measles, mumps, rubella	Measles, Mumps, Rubella	MMR
varicella	Varicella	Varicella
hepatitis A	Hepatitis A	HepA
meningococcus	Meningococcal	MPSV4
tetanus/diphtheria/pertussis	Tetanus, Diphtheria, Pertussis	Tdap
human papillomavirus	Human Papillomavirus	HPV

The following immunizations are recommended between the ages of 0-6 years, with ideal range of recommended age in parentheses:

HepB (1-2 months, 6-18 months)
Rota (2-6 months)
DTap (15-18 months)
Hib (12-15 months)
PCV (12-15 months)
IPV (6-18 months)
Influenza (yearly beginning at 6 months)
MMR (12-15 months)
Varicella (12-18 months or 4-6 years)
HepA (2 doses; 12-24 months)
MPSV4 (2-6 years)

The following immunizations are recommended between the ages of 7-18 years:

Tdap (booster dose; 11-12 years)
HPV (3 doses; 11-12 years)
MPSV4

19.2.3 Classification Systems

Ballard scale: A scoring system for assessing the gestational age of infants based on neuromuscular and physical maturity. Scores are converted to gestational age (in weeks). Express in arabic numerals.

score	age (weeks)
5	26
10	28
15	30
20	32
25	34
30	36
35	38
40	40
45	42
50	44

Tanner staging: System used to classify sexual maturity during puberty, or *thelarche*, in both males and females by evaluating pubic hair development in both sexes, genitalia development in males, and breast development in females. Express classifications using lowercase *stage* and arabic numerals.

Pubic hair (both male and female)	
Tanner stage 1	no pubic hair at all (prepubertal state)
Tanner stage 2	small amount of long, downy hair with slight pigmentation at the base of the penis and scrotum (males) or on the labia majora (females)
Tanner stage 3	hair more coarse; begins to extend laterally
Tanner stage 4	adult-like hair quality, extending across pubis but not medial thighs
Tanner stage 5	hair extends to medial surface of the thighs

(continued next page)

Genitals (male)	
Tanner stage 1	testicular volume less than 1.5 cc; penis size 3 cm or less (prepubertal state)
Tanner stage 2	testicular volume between 1.6 and 6 cc; scrotal thinning and enlargement; no change in penis size
Tanner stage 3	testicular volume between 6 and 12 cc; scrotum enlarges further; penis lengthens to about 6 cm
Tanner stage 4	testicular volume between 12 and 20 cc; scrotum enlarges further and darkens; penis increases in length to 10 cm
Tanner stage 5	testicular volume greater than 20 cc; adult scrotum and penis of 15 cm in length

Breasts (female)	
Tanner stage 1	no glandular tissue; areola follows the skin contours of the chest (prepubertal)
Tanner stage 2	breast bud forms; small area of surrounding glandular tissue; areolar widening begins
Tanner stage 3	breasts become slightly elevated; extend beyond the borders of the areola; more areolar widening but in contour with surrounding tissue
Tanner stage 4	increased breast size and elevation; areola/papilla secondary mounds form; projection from contour of the surrounding breast
Tanner stage 5	breast reaches final adult size; areola returns to contour of surrounding breast, with a projecting central papilla

Pediatric HIV classification: System developed by the Centers for Disease Control (CDC) for categorizing clinical manifestations of HIV disease among children. First developed in 1982, this classification system was revised by the CDC in 1994. In the new system, HIV-infected children are classified into mutually exclusive categories according to three parameters: *infection status, clinical status,* and *immunologic status.* Children infected with HIV or perinatally exposed to HIV may be classified into one of the following four clinical categories based on signs, symptoms, or diagnoses related to HIV infection:

Category N	not symptomatic
Category A	mildly symptomatic
Category B	moderately symptomatic
Category C	severely symptomatic

CHAPTER

20

Ophthalmology

Introduction

Ophthalmology is a highly specialized branch of medicine that deals with diagnosis, treatment, and management of diseases and conditions related to the visual pathways, including the eye, brain, and ancillary areas (lacrimal system and eyelids). The vast majority of transcriptionists will likely encounter little ophthalmology in general transcription unless specifically employed or contracted by an ophthalmology practice *or* exposed to ophthalmologic surgical procedures in the acute care setting. The language associated with the specialty is unique and often highly technical, and any MT working in ophthalmology should have reputable dictionaries and resources related to the specialty on hand to assist in accurate documentation in this arena.

20.1 Evaluation and Diagnostic Terms

Adnexa, adnexa oculi: As in obstetrics and gynecology, the term *adnexa* is always plural, and so is its expanded reference *adnexa oculi.* The term refers to the eyelids, lacrimal apparatus, and other eye appendages. Since all are examined together, the reference is always plural and should accompany a plural verb.

EXAMPLE

> D: On examination, the adnexa oculi is unremarkable.
> T: On examination, the adnexa oculi are unremarkable.

Disc vs. disk: Use *disc* for all references to the optic disc in ophthalmology.

Cup-disc ratio, cup-to-disc ratio: Refers to the ratio of the diameter of the optic cup to the diameter of the optic disc.

> cup-disc ratio of 0.5

Disc diameters: Abbreviated *DD*, disc diameters are used to measure relative distances from findings on the ocular fundus to the optic disc itself.

> The lesion was identified 2 DD superior to the fovea.

Disc areas: Abbreviated *DA*, disc areas are used to indicate relative size of findings on the ocular fundus in comparison to the size of the optic disc itself.

> The lesion measured 2 DA.
> Some minor ischemia was noted and determined to be less than 5 disc areas of retinal nonperfusion.

Greatest linear dimension: Reference measuring the greatest dimension between 2 points on the boundary of an ocular lesion.

> Lesion size was less than 5 disc areas, and greatest linear dimension was less than 3200 mcm.

Injection: This term is often used to indicate hyperemia or dilatation of the vessels in relation to evaluation of the eye. However, to avoid ambiguity or clarity of meaning, the AMA recommends changing *injection* to *hyperemia* or *vasodilation*. Defer to facility preference for making this editorial change in routine transcription but pay particular attention to this change in any manuscript prepared for formal publication.

> D: conjunctival injection
> T: conjunctival hyperemia

OD, OS, OU: These abbreviations which reference the eyes should be expanded when used in general reference. It is appropriate, and preferred, to abbreviate them when associated with visual testing and measured values.

OD	oculus dexter	right eye
OS	oculus sinister	left eye
OU	oculus uterque	each eye

Visual acuity was 20/20 OD and 20/40 OS.
but:
D: She complained of sensitivity to light OS.
T: She complained of sensitivity to light in the left eye.

Optic pressure: This is measured in millimeters of mercury (mmHg). Defer to facility/client preference for including this abbreviation even when it is not dictated.

20.2 Testing and Equipment

Visual acuity: Do not confuse *vision* with *visual acuity*, which refers to clearness of vision. *Distance acuity* is reported using the Snellen eye chart and measured in *Snellen fractions* (20/20, 20/15, etc.). The first number refers to the testing distance from chart to patient; the second number refers to the smallest row of letters that can be read by the patient.

EXAMPLE

20/20: able to read at 20 feet what a normal eye should be able to read at 20 feet
20/40: able to read at 20 feet what a normal eye should be able to read at 40 feet

The *Bailey-Lovie* acuity chart measures visual acuity using a base 10 logarithm of the minimum angle of resolution, or *logMAR*. A logMAR of 0.0 is equivalent to a Snellen 20/20.

Near visual acuity (or *reading vision*) is measured using Snellen equivalents or the Jaeger system (J values).

EXAMPLE

The patient has J7 near visual acuity.

Visual field: This refers to the total area in which objects can be seen in the peripheral vision when the eye is fixed on a single central point. This is measured by means of degrees from a central point (0° to 90°). Where able to do so, use the degree symbol; otherwise, spell out *degrees*.

EXAMPLE

> 85° temporally *or* 85 degrees temporally
> 55° nasally *or* 55 degrees nasally

Diopter: The power of an optical lens is measured in diopters. It is abbreviated *D* when used with corrective values, which should be expressed in arabic numbers. Measurement in negative diopters refers to nearsighted vision, while measurement of positive diopters refers to farsighted vision. The greater the degree of nearsighted or farsighted vision, the higher the lens prescription will be in diopters. For example, *-5.00 D* means the degree of nearsighted correction is 5.00 diopters of correction to obtain 20/20 vision.

EXAMPLE

> I explained to the patient that nearly 90% of all myopic patients have corrections of less than -6.00 D, which is in the mild-to-moderate range, and her correction is -10.00 D, which puts her in the category of severe myopia.

Lens diopters, refraction, axis measurements: Physicians will often combine these terms to describe the optic status of a patient. Express with a positive or negative sign (+ or −) and decimal values; space between each value, but do not separate with commas or other punctuation.

EXAMPLE

> D: She has a plus fourteen lens.
> T: She has a +14.00 lens.
>
> D: He has a plus twenty-five lens.
> T: He has a +0.25 lens.
>
> D: Refraction was plus one hundred, plus five hundred, axis ninety.
> T: Refraction was +1.00 +5.00 axis 90.
> *or:*
> T: Refraction was +1.00 +5.00 x 90.
>
> D: The patient had a plus two fifty add.
> T: The patient had a +2.50 add.

Electroretinogram: Abbreviated *ERG*, this study measures the mass retinal response, or electrical potentials, to a stimulus of light using a corneal electrode and neutral electrodes on the skin. Waves of an ERG should be expressed as follows:

a_1 *or* a1
a_2 *or* a2
b

For pattern electroretinogram (PERG), the waves are expressed as:

a_{pt} *or* apt
b_{pt} *or* bpt
c_{pt} *or* cpt

Goldmann perimetry: Visual field is often measured using the Goldmann system. This is expressed using a combination of roman numbers I through V to designate *spot size* followed by arabic numerals 1 through 4 and letters *a* through *e* to designate *luminance.* Each value should be joined by a hyphen.

1-4-3 isopter area
V-4-3 light

Lasers: Lasers are used extensively in ophthalmologic surgery and should be transcribed as dictated. Consult a reputable dictionary or resource for verification of expression.

argon laser
krypton laser
Nd:YAG laser
holmium:YAG laser

20.3 Classification Systems

Lens Opacities Classification System II (LOCS II) is used to classify age-related cataracts. It involves grading 4 features of the cataract by comparing the features seen against a standard set of transparencies. The classifications are expressed with lowercase *grade*, capital letters, and arabic numbers. This test is performed via slit-lamp examination.

Feature	Abbreviation	Grades
nuclear color	NC	NC0 through NCII
nuclear opalescence	N	N0 through NIV
cortical cataract	C	C0 Ctr (trace) CI through CV
posterior subcapsular	P	P0 through PIV

CHAPTER

21

Organisms and Pathogens

Introduction

Transcriptionists and editors in the acute care setting are likely to encounter many references to organisms and pathogens, both in the identification and treatment of disease and in diagnostic procedures performed in the microbiology area of the laboratory. Most of these are performed, of course, to confirm the presence or absence of an infectious process and to identify the specific organism at work. Many of the standards and directions outlined in this chapter relate specifically to the expression of organisms in formal publication, though an overall understanding of biological nomenclature and taxonomy is critical to any documentation specialist working in environments where these terms are used frequently.

21.1 Nomenclature

Biological nomenclature, or the *naming* of living things, refers to the assignment of names according to international rules. This involves a scientific name that represents a longer description—one that has been formally defined and is internationally adopted.

21.1.1 Scientific vs. Common Names

While scientific names are the *formal* names assigned to such organisms as fungi, bacteria, viruses, prokaryotes, etc., some of these entities also have widely used vernacular names, but because they do not always consistently correlate to the formally defined attribute or set of attributes associated with that scientific name, the *scientific name* should be used in formal publication, at least on first mention. Subsequently, vernacular names may be used. In formal publication, include the scientific name in parentheses after the vernacular name for clarity. *(see examples next page)*

> D: Of the 300 patients who participated in the study, 83 reported taking St. John's wort on a daily basis.
>
> T: Of the 300 patients who participated in the study, 83 reported taking St. John's wort *(Hypericum perforatum)* on a daily basis.

21.1.2 Taxonomy

Taxonomy refers to the classification, or organization, of scientifically named organisms to reflect their relationships to each other. Organisms are classified in taxonomic groups, called *taxa* (singular *taxon*) within different ranks.

EXAMPLE

Rank	Taxon
genus	*Homo*
species	*Homo sapiens*

Note: There has been some confusion, not clarified in the previous edition of this text, as to the difference between the genus and species names for organisms. The entire 2-word term, called the *binomial*, is the *species name*, not just the second term, or *specific name*. In the example above, it would not be correct to say that the genus is "*Homo*" and the species "*sapiens*." The genus is *Homo* and the species is *Homo sapiens*.

In formal publication, all scientific names should be italicized (higher ranking taxa are not typically italicized), but this is not recommended (or required) in transcription of health records. MTs who prepare formal manuscripts should be aware of which portions of the bacterial code require italics and which do not. In most clinical journals, taxa above the genus level are *not* italicized.

EXAMPLE

Rank	Taxon
kingdom	Procaryotae
division	Firmicutes
class	Firmibacteria
family	Bacillaceae
genus	*Staphylococcus*
species	*Staphylococcus aureus*

Be careful to differentiate between the formal terms for taxa and the common, or vernacular, terms. Either are acceptable in formal publication.

EXAMPLE

Formal Term	Vernacular
Vertebrata	vertebrates
Primates	primates
Hominidae	hominids
Fungi	fungi
Moniliaceae	moniliaceous molds
Procaryotae	prokaryotes
Mycobacteriaceae	mycobacteria
Chlamydiales	chlamydiae
Streptococcus pneumoniae	pneumococcus

21.1.3 Genus and Species Names

Use initial caps for all taxa, except for the second portion of the binomial species name.

EXAMPLE

Haemophilus influenzae
Escherichia coli
Staphylococcus aureus

It is acceptable to abbreviate the genus portion of a binomial species name, but only if dictated. In formal publication, spell out the genus portion on first mention and use the abbreviated genus portion thereafter. The use of a period after the genus name abbreviation is acceptable, but both AHDI and the AMA recommend dropping it.

EXAMPLE

H influenzae
E coli
S aureus

Do not begin a sentence with an abbreviated genus name; either expand or recast the sentence.

D: C difficile is the most likely culprit here.
T: Clostridium difficile is the most likely culprit here.
or:
T: The most likely culprit here is C difficile.

Do *not* capitalize genus names used in plural and adjectival forms, when they are used in the vernacular, or when they stand alone.

staphylococcus
group B streptococcus
staphylococci
staphylococcal infection
staph infection
strep throat

Do not abbreviate the genus name when the species name is included in full expression.

D: She has had 2 cases of Staph aureus in the last year.
T: She has had 2 cases of Staphylococcus aureus in the last year.

The suffixes *–osis* and *–iasis* indicate disease caused by a particular class of infectious agents or types of infection. Do *not* capitalize terms formed with these suffixes.

amebiasis
dermatophytosis

When organisms with genus names that begin with the same letter are mentioned in the same document or article, the full scientific name should be used on first mention to avoid genus ambiguity. Thereafter, the abbreviated genus portion is acceptable if dictated.

> D: Nosocomial infections caused by either S aureus or S faecalis are quite common.
> T: Nosocomial infections caused by either Staphylococcus aureus or Streptococcus faecalis are quite common. (abbreviate thereafter if dictated)

Do not use 2-letter abbreviations for the species name (even if dictated). If unable to confidently expand those based on previous expansion in the text, leave a blank and flag the report. When these 2-letter abbreviations are used as part of a longer disease-entity abbreviation, they are acceptable.

EHEC	enterohemorrhagic Escherichia coli
MRSA	methicillin-resistant Staphylococcus aureus

In formal publication, express changes in genus in parentheses with the qualifier *formerly*.

Helicobacter (formerly *Campylobacter*) *pylori*

Express changes in species by expressing the entire binomial in parentheses with the qualifier *formerly*.

Bacteroides ureolyticus (formerly *Bacteroides corrodens*)

21.1.4 Vernacular Names

In some cases, pathogens and infectious agents (and/or the diseases that result from them) are better known publicly by their vernacular names, and references to these (particularly on the part of the patient) may be encountered. In formal publication, these references may be included if the author is intentionally referencing the public identification, but the formal scientific name should also be included for credibility and clarity. In patient care documentation, these vernacular references should be retained *if* dictated, though it is preferable to include them in quotation marks.

EXAMPLE

> D: The patient has recently returned from a trip to China and is concerned that her symptoms may be indicative of bird flu.
>
> T: The patient has recently returned from a trip to China and is concerned that her symptoms may be indicative of "bird flu."

21.2 Bacteria

Rules for bacterial nomenclature can be found in the *International Code of Nomenclature of Bacteria.*

21.2.1 Changes in Taxonomy

It is not uncommon for changes to occur in both the naming of organisms as well as where they are taxonomically classified. Two significant and highly debated taxonomic changes have occurred, of which the transcriptionist should be aware.

EXAMPLE

| Chlamydia pneumoniae | *has become* | Chlamydophila pneumonia |
| Chlamydia psittaci | *has become* | Chlamydophila psittaci |

Transcriptionists should defer to client/provider preference but should be aware that the newer terminology is used by the Centers for Disease Control and Prevention and is being widely adopted in bacterial literature and lexicographic texts.

21.2.2 Gram Staining

Bacteria are frequently grouped according to their reactions to Gram stain. Follow the rules for capitalizing eponyms and lowercasing words derived from eponyms. Do not capitalize the general bacterial terms these eponyms modify.

gram-negative bacilli
gram-positive cocci
but:
The cultures were sent for Gram stain and C&S.

21.2.3 Laboratory Media

Do not capitalize the names of microorganisms when used in association with laboratory media.

bacteroides bile esculin agar
brucella agar

21.2.4 Salmonella and Serotypes

Salmonella is complex and its nomenclature continues to evolve. Previously assumed separate species have been determined to be strains. This means that the previously used binomial species expressions no longer apply to these strains, or *serotypes*.

Salmonella Typhi
not:
Salmonella typhi

In formal publication, serotypes of subspecies use should be expressed with the genus in italics, the abbreviation *ser* and the capitalized subspecies (not in italics). In the health record, avoid the use of italics.

Salmonella ser Typhi
Salmonella ser Enteritidis

21.2.5 Streptococci

Streptococci are uniquely grouped into Lancefield serologic groups, expressed with single capital letters.

> group A *Streptococcus pyogenes*
> group C streptococci
> group B beta-hemolytic streptococci

Proteins of *Streptococcus pyogenes*:

> M protein
> class I M protein
> class II M protein
> P substance
> R protein
> T substance

21.3 Viruses

Unlike bacteria, viruses are as frequently referred to (even in formal publication) by their common or vernacular terms unless the specific taxonomic group is required, in which case formal virus names are used.

> cytomegalovirus
> *or:*
> *Human herpesvirus 5*

21.3.1 Style Considerations

Virus terms that end in *–virales*, *–viridae*, or *–virinae* should be capitalized.

| betaherpesvirinae | *change to* | Betaherpesvirinae |
| parvoviridae | *change to* | Parvoviridae |

Words that end in *–virus* may or may not be formal terms and could represent genuses, species, or subspecific terms. In formal publication, it is preferred to provide the formal, taxonomic identity of a virus on first mention and use the informal term thereafter.

EXAMPLE

First mention: *Human herpesvirus 5* (cytomegalovirus)
Thereafter: cytomegalovirus

21.3.2 Capitalization and Italics

Formal virus names are expressed with initial capitals at each taxonomic rank. When a proper name accompanies those formal names, those proper names should likewise be capitalized.

EXAMPLE

Respirovirus
West Nile virus

Vernacular virus names are not expressed with capitals (unless a proper noun is part of the common name).

EXAMPLE

La Crosse virus

In formal publication, all formal viral names should be italicized (higher ranking taxa are not typically italicized), but this is not recommended (or required) in transcription of health records. MTs who prepare formal manuscripts should be aware of which portions of the bacterial code require italics and which do not. In most clinical journals, taxa above the genus level are *not* italicized.

EXAMPLE

Rank	Taxon
order	Mononegavirales
family	Paramyxoviridae
genus	*Respirovirus*
species	*Human parainfluenzavirus 1*

21.3.3 Formal and Vernacular Names

Formal names are used to delineate or intentionally express the taxonomic identification of a virus. Vernacular, or common, names are used to express physical entities when generally referenced. In formal publication, express the formal name on first reference and the vernacular name thereafter.

EXAMPLE

Human herpesvirus 4	Epstein-Barr virus
Human herpesvirus 3	varicella-zoster virus
Human immunodeficiency virus	HIV

21.3.4 Abbreviations

Formal viral species names should *not* be abbreviated. The vernacular, or common, names can be abbreviated according to acceptable international code.

EXAMPLE

hepatitis B virus (HBV)

21.3.5 Hepatitis Nomenclature

Use capital letters to designate type. Do not use a hyphen to connect the word *hepatitis* to the letter designating its type, but do use a hyphen to connect *non* to the letter.

EXAMPLE

hepatitis A
hepatitis C
non-A hepatitis
non-B hepatitis
non-A, non-B hepatitis
delta hepatitis

Related abbreviations:

HAV	hepatitis A virus
HBAg	hepatitis B antigen
HBsAg	hepatitis B surface antigen
HBIG	hepatitis B immunoglobulin
HBV	hepatitis B virus
anti-HAV	antibody to hepatitis A
anti-HBV	antibody to hepatitis B

Previous designations of viral hepatitis, such as infectious hepatitis, short-incubation-period hepatitis, long-incubation-period hepatitis, and serum hepatitis are no longer preferred but should be transcribed if dictated.

Child-Pugh score: This classification system measures the degree of end-stage liver failure resulting from prolonged hepatitis and cirrhosis—also frequently referred to as the *Child-Turcotte-Pugh classification*. First the following 5 measures of liver disease are scored from 1-3, with 3 being the most severe:

bilirubin
serum albumin
INR
ascites
hepatic encephalopathy

Then the chronic liver disease is classified into Child-Pugh classification A through C by totaling the scores of each of the 5 areas above.

Points	Class	Life expectancy
5-6	A	15-20 years
7-9	B	candidate for transplant
10-15	C	1-3 months

Resources

Sneath et al. *International Code of Nomenclature of Bacteria*. American Society for Microbiology. Revised 1990. Accessed 18 December 2007. <http://www.ncbi.nlm.nih.gov/books/bv.fcgi?indexed=google&rid=icnb.TOC>

CHAPTER

22

Psychiatry

Introduction

Transcriptionists working in the setting of a psychiatric facility or as part of an acute care facility will likely encounter the most detailed and interpretive reports related to this specialty, though most transcriptionists will encounter some of the terminology and references to mental status exam and findings in virtually every specialty in health care, as the interview process with any patient in a care encounter involves some assessment on the part of the provider of the patient's mental status, appearance, etc. For those working within the psychiatric specialty, however, the terminology and testing is unique and the care for how psychiatric findings are permanently expressed in the record is also unique. In few other areas of health care is a patient more reticent to be evaluated and diagnosed and to have their disorders classified and formally recorded. Often it is the family and friends of the patient who provide the most insight and reliable history, and frequent reference to previous medical records and reporting is often necessary throughout the course of psychiatric evaluation and care planning.

A transcriptionist working in the psychiatric setting will encounter the use of *direct quotation* probably more than any other specialty. There will be many instances where a patient will use colorful, descriptive, and often bizarre terms to describe their feelings, lifestyle, family members, etc. This material should always be transcribed *as dictated*, regardless of its grammatical or even clinical accuracy, and it should always be included in quotation marks. Transcriptionists should likewise be prepared to hear the provider reference new and unusual terms (i.e., *starter marriage, hanging game, torture survivor*) or rare and surprising phobias (i.e., *fear of air*). These should not be transcribed in quotation marks but should be expressed exactly as dictated.

Finally, it should be noted here that for obvious reasons, this is a clinical specialty where confidentiality is paramount. Patient cases should never be discussed with anyone and great care should be taken to protect the privacy of the record. This will often include strict facility policies governing how and when carbon copies are handled, and transcriptionists in this setting should adhere to facility guidelines in this regard.

22.1 Terminology

22.1.1 DSM and Psychiatric Diagnoses

The American Psychiatric Association has published 5 editions of its manual for classifying mental disorders. All 5 editions have been titled *Diagnostic and Statistical Manual of Mental Disorders (DSM)*, and each edition references its edition in abbreviated form with roman numerals.

> *DSM-I*
> *DSM-II*
> *DSM-III*
> *DSM-III-R (revised)*
> *DSM-IV*

Transcriptionists should be familiar with these abbreviations, as practitioners will often refer to the way a disorder may have been described or classified in a previous edition to differentiate it from the current edition.

Since the third edition, psychiatric diagnoses have been classified and expressed based on a system of assessment on several axes:

Axis I	Clinical/psychiatric disorders other than personality disorders and mental retardation.
Axis II	Personality disorders and mental retardation.
Axis III	General medical conditions.
Axis IV	Psychosocial and environmental problems.
Axis V	Global Assessment of Functioning.

When dictated, these should be expressed as above, with the axis reference capitalized and expressed in roman numerals, followed by a tab or indent and the findings for each axis.

Axis I	Major depressive disorder, single episode, without psychotic features. Alcohol abuse.
Axis II	Dependent personality disorder.
Axis III	None.
Axis IV	Threat of job loss.
Axis V	GAF 45 on admission; improved to 75 at time of discharge.

In settings where the ICD-9/ICD-10 code is also included as part of this diagnostic summary, a 3-column organization is typically used.

Axis I	296.3	Major depressive disorder, single episode, severe, without psychotic features.
	305.0	Alcohol abuse.
Axis II	301.6	Dependent personality disorder.
Axis III	None.	
Axis IV		Threat of job loss.
Axis V	GAF =3	(current)

22.1.2 Psychiatric Disorder Terms

According to the *AMA Manual of Style*, 10th edition, practitioners are strongly discouraged from using the terms *catatonic, manic, psychotic,* and *schizophrenic* to "describe normal variations of individual or group behavior, for which suitable descriptions are available." In other words, these terms should be used only when describing a formal diagnosis or disorder and not in describing the patient or normal variations of behavior. Other terms, such as *contradictory* for *schizophrenic; strange, disorganized,* or *senseless* for *psychotic; overactive* for *manic;* and *motionless* for *catatonic* should be used. The AMA further asserts that it is "dehumanizing" to refer to a patient as "a schizophrenic" and recommends the use of "patient with schizophrenia" or "the schizophrenic patient" instead. Transcriptionists in the psychiatric setting should be familiar with these recommendations and engage in dialogue with their provider employers/clients to set policy for handling these references in the record, but this is the decision of the practitioner and the MT should defer to that preference.

22.1.3 Mental Status Examination

Whether in a psychiatric setting or in general physical examination, the formal mental status exam involves evaluation of a set of observable and/or testable findings and responses. These findings and conclusions follow a fairly standard format:

Appearance
Sensorium
Activity/Behavior
Mood/Affect
Thought Content
Cognitive Function
Orientation
Memory
Judgment
Insight

Some or all of these areas may be tested/observed and recorded depending on patient history as well as the reason for examination.

Mini-Mental State Examination (MMSE): Providers will often refer to the "mini mental status exam," which is technically a reference to the *Mini-Mental State Examination*, a tool that can be used to systematically and thoroughly assess mental status. It is an 11-question measurement that tests five areas of cognitive function: orientation, registration, attention and calculation, recall, and language. The maximum score is 30. A score of 23 or lower is indicative of cognitive impairment. The formal name of the test should be transcribed even when the general term "mini mental" or "mini mental status" is dictated.

EXAMPLE

D: The patient had a mini mental status score of 27.
T: The patient had a Mini-Mental State Examination score of 27.

22.2 Classification Systems

22.2.1 Global Assessment of Functioning (GAF)
The GAF scale is used by mental health professionals to assess an individual's overall psychological functioning. This is typically reported in a psychiatric diagnosis as axis V. Use arabic numerals 0 (inadequate information) through 100 (superior functioning in a wide range of activities).

EXAMPLE

| Axis V | GAF = 60; flat affect. |

22.2.2 Global Assessment of Relational Functioning (GARF)
This scale is used by mental health professionals to measure an overall functioning of a family or other ongoing relationship. Use arabic numerals from 0 (inadequate information) to 100 (relational unit functioning satisfactorily from self-report of participants and from perspectives of observers).

22.2.3 Social and Occupational Functioning Assessment Scale (SOFAS)
This is an instrument used by mental health professionals to assess an individual's social and occupational functioning only. Use arabic numerals from 0 (inadequate information) through 100 (superior functioning in a wide range of activities).

22.3 Outline of Psychiatric/Psychological Testing

The following outline provides an overview of common tests utilized in assessing certain disorders and abilities in the psychiatric/cognitive function domain:

Major Depression
Hamilton-D (age > 18 years)
Beck Depression Inventory (age > 18 years)
Zung Depression Rating Scale
Geriatric Depression Scale

Anxiety Disorder
Hamilton Anxiety Scale

Competency
Protective placement

Psychosis
Rorschach
MMPI

Organicity
Bender
Plutchik
Luria-Nebraska

Post Traumatic Stress Disorder (PTSD)
Mississippi Scale for PTSD
MMPI
Sentence Completion Test
Millon

Personality profile
MMPI
Millon
NEOPI
Myers-Briggs

Dementia
Cognitive Capacity Screening Exam (CCSE)
Mattis Dementia Rating Scale (MDRS)
Dementia Rating Scale (DRS)
Mini-Mental State Examination
Plutchik Geriatric Rating Scale

Other Tests
Cal Verbal Learning Test
Selective Reminding Test
Controlled Oral Word Association
Multilingual Aphasia Exam
Apraxia Draw a Clock Test
Memory-Wexler Internal Memory Test
Executive Function-WI Card Sort Test

References

Moses, Scott MD. "*The Family Practice Notebook: Psychiatry*" 8 September 2007. 21 December 2007. <*http://www.fpnotebook.com/PSY84.htm*>

CHAPTER

23

Pulmonary/Respiratory

Introduction

Transcriptionists in the acute care setting will encounter frequent references to a patient's pulmonary status, both in emergent intervention and throughout a patient's hospital stay. Even patients who are admitted for other primary causes may require secondary respiratory support and treatment, particularly for underlying pulmonary disease or infection. Given the frequent correlation between infectious processes and pulmonary compromise, some pulmonologists will also specialize in the diagnosis and treatment of infectious diseases. Cardiovascular medicine likewise has its crossover into the domain of pulmonary function and management, and transcriptionists should be well familiar with this specialty and equipped with references and resource materials unique to respiratory therapy and care.

23.1 Terminology

A wide variety of terms related to respiration, blood gas measurements, ventilatory effort, etc., are encountered in this critical field, where a great deal of clinical intervention is emergent. Many of these are expressed with symbols or in abbreviated form, and care should be taken to ensure that the appropriate symbol or abbreviation is expressed.

23.1.1 Symbols

Primary symbols used in pulmonary and respiratory terminology are the first terms of an expression and are expressed as follows. It is important to note that the same letter may stand for one entity in respiratory mechanics and for another entity in gas exchange (e.g., *P* stands for *pressure* in respiratory mechanics but stands for *partial pressure* in gas exchange).
(see examples next page)

C concentration
F fractional concentration in dry gas
P *or* p pressure *or* partial pressure
Q volume of blood
V volume of gas
D diffusing (diffusion) capacity
R resistance *or* gas exchange ratio
S saturation
sG specific conductance

Secondary symbols for gas phase: These symbols immediately follow the primary symbol. Express as small capitals in formal publication. Use regular capitals in patient care documentation.

A *or* A alveolar
B *or* B barometric
E *or* E expired
ET *or* ET end-tidal
I *or* I inspired
L *or* L lung
T *or* T tidal

Secondary symbols for blood phase: These symbols immediately follow the secondary symbol for gas phase. Express as lowercase letters.

aw	airway
b	blood
a	arterial
c	capillary
f	ideal
p	pulse oximetry
v	venous

23.1.2 Abbreviations

Gas abbreviations: These are usually the last element of the term. Use regular capitals in patient care documentation. Use subscripts or place the numerals on the line.

EXAMPLE

CO_2 *or* CO2
O_2 *or* O2
N_2 *or* N2
CO *or* CO

Combine the above symbols for pulmonary and respiratory physiology terms.

EXAMPLE

PCO_2 (PCO2)	
or:	
pCO_2 (pCO2)	partial pressure of carbon dioxide
$PaCO_2$ (PaCO2)	partial pressure of arterial carbon dioxide
PO_2 (PO2)	
or:	
pO_2 (pO2)	partial pressure of oxygen
PaO_2 (PaO2)	partial pressure of arterial oxygen
V/Q	ventilation-perfusion ratio

Note: The above terms may be used without expansion, even at first mention in formal publication.

See 23.2.1—*Pulmonary Function Testing* for abbreviations related specifically to PFTs.
See 23.2.2—*Mechanical Ventilation* for abbreviations related specifically to airway management.

23.1.3 Nomenclature

Breaths per minute, respirations per minute: Spell out. Do not abbreviate.

EXAMPLE

Respirations: 18 breaths per minute.
not:
Respirations: 18 bpm.

21 respirations per minute
not:
21 rpm

Use virgules in references to respirations only in the following form:

EXAMPLE

Respirations: 21/min
not:
21 respirations/min

23.2 Diagnostics and Treatment

23.2.1 Pulmonary Function Testing

The following are some common abbreviations associated with PFTs, which should always be expanded at first mention in formal publication. Where technology does not enable the ready and easy use of subscripting, same-line numeric expression should be used.

Term	Expansion	Unit of Measure
CC	closing capacity	L
CV	closing volume	L
ERV	expiratory reserve volume	L
FEF	forced expiratory flow	L/min
$FEF_{25\%-75\%}$	FEF, midexpiratory phase	L/min *or* L/s
$FEF_{200-1200}$	FEF between 200 and 1200 of forced vital capacity	mL L/min *or* L/s

(continued next page)

FEV	forced expiratory volume	L
FEV$_1$	FEV in first second of expiration	L
FIVC	forced inspiratory vital capacity	L
FIO$_2$	fraction of inspired oxygen	mmHg
FVC	forced vital capacity	L
IRV	inspiratory reserve volume	L
IVC	inspiratory vital capacity	L
MVV	maximum voluntary ventilation	L/min
PEF, PEFR	peak expiratory flow rate	L/min
RV	residual volume	L
TLC	total lung capacity	L
VC	vital capacity	L

Other PFT Terminology		
DCO *or* DLCO	carbon monoxide diffusion capacity	
FEF$_{50}$	mid-expiratory flow rate (also called R$_{50}$)	
FIF	forced inspiratory flow	
FRC	functional residual capacity	
FVL	flow-volume loop	
SVC	slow vital capacity	
TV	tidal volume	

In addition to the above, there are several vital ratios that are measured and reported as part of pulmonary function testing. Follow the rules for expressing ratios (*See 11.3—Ratios*).

EXAMPLE

> D: FEV1 to FVC was 60 percent of predicted.
> T: FEV1-FVC was 60% of predicted.

23.2.2 Mechanical Ventilation

The following abbreviations are used in reference to mechanical ventilation and airway management. These should be expanded upon first mention in formal publication.

APRV	airway pressure release ventilation
BiPAP	bilevel positive airway pressure
CPAP	continuous positive airway pressure
ECMO	extracorporeal membrane oxygenation
ET	endotracheal tube
HFV	high-frequency ventilation
NIPPV	noninvasive positive pressure ventilation
NIV	noninvasive ventilation
PAV	proportional assist ventilation
PEEP	positive end-expiratory pressure

Note: Do not confuse *PAP (positive airway pressure)* for *Pap (Papanicolaou)*.

Venturi mask vs. Ventimask: Any mask that is designed based on the Venturi principle, (i.e., allowing for precise measurements of exact oxygen) may be referred to as a *Venturi mask* and likewise dictated interchangeably (and generically) as a *ventimask*. It is important to note, however, that *Ventimask* is a registered trade name. Since it may not be possible for the MT to ascertain whether the brand is being referenced as opposed to a general Venturi mask, it is best to either expand the reference to *Venturi mask* or use the capitalized brand *Ventimask*. Do not use *ventimask*.

Note: Transcriptionists should always be careful to check a reputable resource to determine manufacturer preference for capitalization and spelling of ventilator and CPAP names. For example, it is important to know that *pillows* is a style of CPAP mask and *not* a brand name.

Liters of oxygen: While the general rule for using numeric values with metric units dictates the use of a space between the numeric value and the unit of measure, it is common and *preferred* that the space be omitted when referencing liters of oxygen.

> She was put on O2 at a flow rate of 3L/min.
> The patient will be started on oxygen 2L via nasal cannula.

23.2.3 Polysomnography and Sleep Staging

The following physiologic parameters are simultaneously monitored during polysomnography, or sleep studies:

EEG	standard electrodes used
EOG (electro-oculogram)	tracings obtained from the left and right eyes
EMG (electromyogram)	submental and leg muscle EMGs
Respiratory function EKG	SaO2, expired CO2, and tidal volume

Sleep stages involve REM and non-REM sleep as well as five related and subsequent sleep stages, expressed with lowercase *stage* and arabic numerals:

> REM   rapid eye movement sleep
> NREM   non-rapid eye movement sleep
> sleep stage 1
> sleep stage 2
> sleep stage 3
> sleep stage 4

Note: Many sleep clinics also use the *Beck Inventory for Depression* assessment to determine likelihood of depression in patients with potential sleep disorders. It is used in conjunction with other pre-polysomnography assessment tools (*See 23.3.2—Epworth Sleepiness Scale*).

23.3 Classification Systems

23.3.1 Mallampati-Samsoon

This classification system is used by anesthesiologists and emergency medical personnel to assess the airway for ease or difficulty of intubation. The airway is examined and identified as class I through IV based on findings. Class I identifies a patient in whom intubation should be easy, and class IV identifies a patient in whom intubation would be almost impossible due to nearly complete obstruction of visible airway. Express with lowercase *class* and roman numerals.

class I	uvula, faucial pillars, and soft palate can all be visualized
class II	only faucial pillars and soft palate can be visualized
class III	only the soft palate can be visualized
class IV	only the hard palate can be visualized

23.3.2 Epworth Sleepiness Scale

This classification system uses a questionnaire to measure daytime sleepiness on a scale of 1 to 24 for the purposes of assessing potential sleep disorders, especially those related to apnea.

The patient uses the following scale to choose the most appropriate number for each situation:

0 = would *never* doze or sleep
1 = *slight* chance of dozing or sleeping
2 = *moderate* chance of dozing or sleeping
3 = *high* chance of dozing or sleeping

This scoring system is then used by the patient to score each of the following scenarios:

Sitting and reading
Watching TV
Being a passenger in a motor vehicle
Sitting inactive in a public place
Being a passenger in a motor vehicle for an hour or more
Lying down in the afternoon
Sitting and talking to someone
Sitting quietly after lunch (no alcohol)
Stopped for a few minutes in traffic while driving

The score for each scenario is then totaled, arriving at an overall Epworth score:

Less than 8	normal sleep function
8-10	mild sleepiness
11-15	moderate sleepiness
16-20	severe sleepiness
21-24	excessive sleepiness

EXAMPLE

The patient's Epworth Sleepiness Scale score is 16.

CHAPTER

24

Other Specialty Standards

Introduction

This chapter is designed to provide insight into standards of style related to miscellaneous clinical areas and specialties not previously covered in this text or specialties for which there were not sufficient style and standards issues to warrant a chapter of their own.

24.1 Radiology

X-ray: Refers both to the radiologic process and to radiation particles. Whether used as a noun, verb, or adjective, lowercase and hyphenate.

EXAMPLE

> His x-ray was not in the jacket. (noun)
> He was x-rayed yesterday. (verb)
> His x-ray films have been lost. (adjective)

Capitalize *x-ray* only when it is the first word in a sentence.

EXAMPLE

> X-rays taken on his last visit revealed some interstitial changes.

Avoid using the prefix *re-* with *x-ray*. Recast the sentence to avoid this usage.

EXAMPLE

> D: We are going to re-x-ray her on her next visit.
> T: We are going to x-ray her again on her next visit.

Plain vs. plane films: The correct term is *plain*, which refers to an x-ray that has been done without contrast as opposed to a CT scan or other study that may use contrast. When dictated, this is *not* a reference to a directional *plane* or surface.

EXAMPLE

> Plain film of the abdomen was negative.

b value: The *b factor* or *b value* measures the intensity, or strength, and timing of diffusion gradient in diffusion-weighted MRIs. These are expressed in seconds per square millimeter.

EXAMPLE

> Four gradient strengths resulted in b values of 0 and 1000 s/sq mm applied sequentially in the X, Y, and Z gradient directions.

Echo train: This is a general term referring to a sequence of echoes and is not itself a unit of measure and should not be expressed as a unit of measure.

EXAMPLE

> D: a length of 5 echo trains
> T: echo train length of 5

k-space: Express this reference to frequency and phase as a hyphenated term when used as either a noun or adjective.

EXAMPLE

> Pulse sequences resulted in data identified in k-space.
> k-space filtering, k-space sampling

Relaxation times: Expressed with a *T* and arabic numbers and lowercase letters, these refer to the relaxation time in MRI.

EXAMPLE

T1	spin-lattice or longitudinal relaxation time
T1p	spin-lattice relaxation time in the rotating frame
T2	spin-spin or transverse relaxation time
T2*	time constant for loss of phase coherence among spins

24.2 Diabetes Terminology and Classification

The terms for classifying diabetes mellitus have evolved over time to include a number of pertinent changes, according to the American Diabetes Association (*www.diabetes.org*).

EXAMPLE

juvenile-onset diabetes	*is now*	type 1 child
		type 1 adult
adult-onset diabetes	*is now*	type 2

The Expert Committee on the Diagnosis and Classification of Diabetes Mellitus adopted the use of arabic numerals for diabetes types in order to improve communication, stating that it is too easy to confuse the roman numeral *II* for the arabic number *11*.

Type 1 diabetes: Formerly *type I, insulin-dependent,* or *juvenile-onset diabetes,* type 1 diabetes is caused by beta-cell destruction. The two forms of type 1 diabetes are immune-mediated and idiopathic.

Type 2 diabetes: Formerly *type II, non-insulin-dependent,* or *adult-onset diabetes,* type 2 diabetes is used for individuals who have insulin resistance and usually relative (rather than absolute) insulin deficiency.

Third-class diseases: The third class of diabetes comprises eight types and encompasses more than 45 specific diseases (examples of disease for each type are shown in parentheses):

EXAMPLE

genetic defects of beta-cell function (mitochondrial DNA)
genetic defects in insulin action (leprechaunism)
diseases of the exocrine pancreas (hemochromatosis)
endocrinopathies (hyperthyroidism)
drug- or chemical-induced (diazoxide)
infections (cytomegalovirus)
uncommon forms of immune-mediated diabetes (stiff man syndrome)
other genetic syndromes sometimes associated with diabetes (Turner syndrome)

Gestational diabetes mellitus: This is defined as any degree of glucose intolerance with its onset or first recognition during pregnancy. The terms *impaired glucose tolerance* and *impaired fasting glucose tolerance* have been retained. Classifications of diabetes mellitus in pregnancy include:

class A	*Gestational diabetes.* Transient.
class B	Initial onset after age 20, less than 10 years' duration, controlled by diet. Patient may become insulin-dependent during pregnancy but not need insulin after delivery.
class C	Onset between ages 10 and 19. Insulin-dependent patient will need increased insulin during pregnancy but will likely return to pre-pregnancy dosage after delivery.
class D	Onset before age 10, with more than 20 years' duration. Patient has hypertension, diabetic retinopathy, and peripheral vascular disease.
class E	Patient has calcification of the pelvic vessels.
class F	Patient has diabetic nephropathy

Infants of diabetic mothers may be described as:

LGA	Large for gestational age. Infants of class A, B, and C mothers are apt to be LGA.
SGA	Small for gestational age. Infants of class D, E, and F mothers are apt to be SGA.

Insulin-dependent, non-insulin-dependent: These terms are no longer used to describe types 1 and 2 because they are classifications based on treatment rather than etiology. However, they should be transcribed *if* dictated.

EXAMPLE

D: The patient has non-insulin-dependent diabetes.
T: The patient has non-insulin-dependent diabetes.
not:
T: The patient has type 2 diabetes.

24.3 Molecular Terms

References to molecular terms can be found in specialty chapters throughout this text, but it is important to be familiar with various molecular terms and the wide degree of variability that exists in expressing these terms. Some molecular terms are better known in their abbreviated forms, as their expansions may be rather obscure. They can often be expressed with a mix of numbers, letters, and cases. They can be full or partial abbreviations, and they differ from standard abbreviations (which are typically uppercase initialisms) in that they can be expressed as contractions of single words, all lowercase letters, a mixture of capital and lowercases letters, and even small caps. Some contain hyphenated suffixes; others do not. Transcriptionists who encounter molecular terminology in the course of dictation should refer to reputable references and resources to confirm appropriate expression, *especially* when documenting any of these complex terms in formal publication.

EXAMPLE

χ_1-antitrypsin
β-catenin
γ-tubulin
glucose-6-phosphate

χ helix
β sheet

Hyphens are used in adjectival usages:

EXAMPLE

β-pleated sheet
glucose-6-posphate dehydrogenase

Hyphens are always used when numbers interrupt the expression:

EXAMPLE

propan-1,2-diol
acyl-5-CoA

The prefixes *levo* (L) and *dextro* (D) are expressed in small capitals.

L-folinic acid
D-glyceraldehyde

Chemical charges (+,-) should be expressed in superscripts. Likewise, numerals indicating quantifies of an element within a molecule should be expressed in superscripts.

HCO_3^-
Fe^{3+}

Section 4: Specialty Standards

Section 5
Resources: Industry Trends and Standards

CHAPTER

25

ASTM Standards for Healthcare Documents

Introduction

Standardization is important in our professional and personal lives. When we make purchasing decisions for standardized items, we can do so with confidence that they will fit and work for our needs. Imagine how complicated it would be if faxes could only be sent and received specific to the same manufacturer, or email could only be sent and received specific to the same Internet provider service. Standards allow for systems, regardless of the manufacturer, to work together. In order to provide procedural consistency and proficiency in performance, processes can also be standardized. This saves time and aggravation, rather than repeatedly taking resources to "reinvent the wheel." ASTM International has long been the leading worldwide organization to establish measurable, accountable standards across multiple industries, including healthcare documentation.

25.1 ASTM History and Objectives

ASTM was founded in 1898, known then as American Society for Testing and Materials. As this title no longer reflects today's diverse worldwide organization, it changed its name to ASTM International. There are 30,000 members from 125 nations in this not-for-profit organization. Over 140 committees from various industries have published more than 12,000 standards in materials, products, systems, and services.

It is important to note that standards-development organizations, such as ASTM, have "rules" to follow so that their standards are fair, relevant, and developed in a way that is objective and nonbiased. The "rules" are established by the American Nationals Standards Institute (ANSI), and organizations that follow the "rules" for developing standards are considered to have ANSI-accredited processes. This distinction is important to understand as many professional associations and trade organizations establish and publish "standards" within the industry they represent. Those "standards" are likely not developed through ANSI-accredited processes but instead they reflect "best practices" or a "standard of practice" for that profession or industry. An example of this would be this *Book of Style* produced by the Association for Healthcare Documentation Integrity (AHDI); it is not an ANSI-accredited standard, but it definitely represents the standard of practice within the medical transcription and healthcare documentation industry.

ASTM is an international, ANSI-accredited, standards-development organization. Standards produced through ASTM are done in a manner to assure a diversity in participation, use consensus agreement, offer opportunities for input, and provide electronic voting with the use of comments (so all members can participate without having to physically attend a meeting). Voting occurs at both the subcommittee level and also the larger committee level (in this case the committee is E31 Healthcare Informatics) to gain acceptance and to tap the extensive expertise from its participating members.

ASTM standards are not mandatory; however, government regulators often give voluntary standards the force of the law by citing them in laws, regulations, legal rulings, and codes.

Healthcare facilities and vendors that incorporate ASTM standards in their processes enjoy the benefits of the work accomplished by the numerous volunteers who participate in the ASTM technical subcommittees. A few of those benefits include:

- Credibility when policies and procedures are consistent with approved ASTM standards.
- Resource efficiency from "reinventing the wheel" when processes are designed to replicate established ASTM standards.
- Demonstrable compliance with the Joint Commission's IM.3.11: Industry and organization standards are used.
- Applied expertise of technical subcommittee participants from many locations to ensure a wider perspective and improved final product.

25.2 E31 Committee on Healthcare Informatics

The ASTM E31 committee on Healthcare Informatics was established in 1970, with its scope to develop standards for health information and its systems. Over the last decade, there has been some reorganization of the subcommittees under E31. Currently there are over 400 E31 members and more than 40 approved ASTM standards within the jurisdiction of this committee. Subcommittees under E31 and their scopes include:

E31.15 Healthcare Information Capture and Documentation: Develops standards to support the systems, processes, and management of data capture and data entry technologies used in quality healthcare documentation.

E31.25 Healthcare Data Management, Security, Confidentiality, and Privacy: Develops standards to support health information interoperability emphasizing EHR (electronic health record) and CCR (continuity of care record) information architecture and content, and to support health information security, confidentiality, and privacy. In addition, the subcommittee will be responsible for collaboration with other Standards Developing Organizations (SDO) and SDO-related entities, including HL7, NCPDP, and X12, to promote harmonization with their related data management and messaging efforts.

E31.35 Healthcare Data Analysis: Develops standards for data analysis and decision logic in the support of direct patient care, patient and provider education, clinical and administrative research, clinical quality, public health, clinical efficiency, management of healthcare costs, and healthcare quality improvement.

The subcommittee E31.15 Healthcare Information Capture and Documentation was originally formed in 1995 (then called Health Information Transcription and Documentation and its number designation was E31.22). The first standard from this subcommittee was successfully balloted in 1997. Through the ASTM standards development process, consensus through balloting is reached by voting within the subcommittee (i.e., E31.15) and the main committee (E31). All negative votes must have an accompanying comment (the reason for the negative vote). These must be resolved either through adoption of changes within the document or a committee vote claiming the negative comment was non-persuasive, therefore not adopting that change within the document. Affirmative votes can also have comments and are also considered when finalizing the document. The final document is often improved from comments submitted through this balloting process. Also, to ensure participation by its members, a minimum of 60% of ballots must be returned to validate the balloting process.

25.3 Standardized Healthcare Document Formats

A standard that was initiated within E31.15 but was completed in another subcommittee was *E2184-02 Standard Specification for Healthcare Document Formats.* This standard addresses the headings, arrangement, and appearance of sections and subsections when used within healthcare documents. This standard was needed as individual healthcare institutions determine their own format requirements and arrangement of the information presented within their documents with a surprising lack of consistency. Even within their own healthcare enterprise, customizations to formats—that is the appearance and arrangement of information displayed within a healthcare report—often occur by campus, departments, and physicians for the same report types. This practice of presenting patient information in a non-standard manner is inefficient and at times risky for healthcare professionals who review those reports for critical information (i.e., allergies, medications, etc.). Providing a uniformity of the information presented within a healthcare report will facilitate the identification and retrieval of health information in a manner that would enhance the quality and efficiency of the health services provided.

Here are some of the other key benefits of standardized healthcare document formats:

- Facilitates information sharing within and among data systems
- Serves as a guide for healthcare providers in the collection of essential data elements
- Promotes greater efficiencies in report generation, no matter how the data is captured
- Expedites the identification and selection of pertinent information needed for communication among members of the healthcare team, and for services such as coding and billing
- Allows for an easier transition to the electronic health record

In both electronic and paper-based health records, the most important step in the standardization of formats is to establish the information needs of the users to fulfill its intended purpose by including all data required in an appropriate, easy-to-use design.

This standard was developed to assist healthcare facilities and providers in achieving this goal of standardizing the formatting of the information presented within a healthcare report. It is important to note, however, that although this standard was published in 2002, the adoption rate has, unfortunately, been low.

Synonymous to standardized healthcare document formats is the creation of healthcare documentation templates. Templates include the required headings, the titles for those headings, and the sequence of them. Templates can be a component of a document, such as the review of systems within a History and Physical Examination report, or they can be the entire report. These templates serve as a guide to required documentation while fostering the creation of a meaningful clinical note.

The CDA4CDT project (*See Chapter 26—Clinical Document Architecture for Common Document Types*) used the same framework established by ASTM but will build templates to allow for the integration of the transcribed notes and the interoperability of its contents within the electronic health record.

With all of the activities surrounding the standardization of healthcare document formats/templates and its important link to document quality and greater operational efficiencies, healthcare institutions should embrace healthcare document standards as a critical step in process improvement. Clearly, with the adoption of the electronic health record and its data conformance requirements, the standardization of healthcare document formats and templates will be embraced by healthcare providers and facilities.

Contributing Author: Brenda J. Hurley, CMT, FAAMT, Chair of ASTM E31.15

CHAPTER

26

Clinical Document Architecture for Common Document Types (CDA4CDT)

Introduction

Undoubtedly, the electronic health record will bring tremendous change to the area of medical transcription. While many MTs are already working in facilities using electronic documents, the electronic health record, as currently envisioned by the healthcare community, is not simply a collection of documents and images in electronic format. The EHR capable of imparting real change to the practice of medicine consists of discrete data that is captured in real-time and accessible from multiple locations by multiple caregivers. Capturing pertinent data about patients and their treatment in the midst of caring for the patient and then storing that data in a readily usable and exchangeable form is one of the biggest challenges in the electronic healthcare arena. Dictation has long been one of the most popular methods of data capture and is still highly preferred by practicing physicians, but this method is the least desirable for an EHR because free-text documents lack structured data.

26.1 CDA4CDT Background and Objectives

The Clinical Document Architecture for Common Document Types (CDA4CDT) project seeks to marry the best of the electronic healthcare record with the advantages of dictation to create documents that are useful to both clinicians and the EHR. AHDI is playing a key role in promoting the use of transcribed documents in the electronic health record by participating in the CDA4CDT project.

In an electronic record-keeping system, data such as blood pressure readings, temperature readings, medications, and allergies are more useful when stored in a database format (i.e., discrete and tabulated) as opposed to being buried within a paragraph of text. Discrete data is "interpretable" by computers and therefore can be quickly graphed to denote trends, evaluated for decision support and real-time alerts, easily collected for epidemiological studies, and reused to build customized reports. Transcribed documents consist of narrative text with no discrete data, which puts the dictation/transcription process at odds with the goals of the future electronic healthcare environment. While discrete data has many advantages over free-style narrative text, dictation still more precisely captures the patient's story, including the nuances that differentiate the care and treatment of two patients with the same diagnosis. In addition, many physicians are reluctant to change their documentation style from dictation to the more time-consuming method of computer data entry. The solution is to create information systems capable of extracting discrete data from free-text documents.

26.2 Health Level Seven (HL7) and Interoperability

Leading the push toward interoperable healthcare information is Health Level Seven (HL7), which is a volunteer organization within the healthcare community that produces standards for the exchange of clinical and administrative data. The mission of HL7 states, "HL7 provides standards for interoperability that improve care delivery, optimize workflow, reduce ambiguity, and enhance knowledge transfer among all of our stakeholders, including healthcare providers, government agencies, the vendor community, fellow SDOs (Standards Developing Organizations) and patients."[1] Contrary to popular belief, HL7 does not create or sell software; rather it publishes the standards (also called specifications or protocols) *used* by software developers to create interfaces between disparate computer systems. For example, using HL7 standards, data from the laboratory information system (typically only accessible by lab personnel) can be transferred to the hospital or clinic's information system, thereby making the data accessible to physicians and nurses. Likewise, data from one hospital can be transferred to an associated facility even though the two facilities use different patient information systems. Information technology professionals use HL7 standards to design computer interfaces that ensure the accurate exchange of information. Each unit of information transferred is called a message. The Reference Information Model (RIM) is the cornerstone of all HL7 messages and describes the relationship of each piece of data to the rest of the data.

The HL7 RIM includes specifications for exchanging clinical and administrative data. Documents such as Word documents (*.doc*), rich text documents (*.rtf*), plain text documents (*.txt*), or portable format documents (*.pdf*) can be transferred across an HL7 interface as a whole, including detailed information *about* the document, but the message does not contain details regarding the information *within* the document. For example, an HL7 message can indicate that a document to be exchanged is an H&P note for a given patient, created on a given date, and authenticated by the attending physician, but the actual contents of the H&P are not computable. Neither the sending nor the receiving computer is able to recognize a blood pressure reading contained within the H&P and extract the reading to be stored in a database of other blood pressure readings for that same patient. The Clinical Document Architecture, Release 2 (CDA R2), standard was developed by HL7 to allow for the exchange of details within a document in a way that both computers can recognize and use those details. A CDA document has a header and a body. The header identifies and classifies the document and provides information on authentication, the encounter, the patient, and the involved providers. The body contains the clinical report, organized into sections whose narrative content can be encoded using standard vocabularies such as LOINC and SNOMED CT.[2] *(See Chapter 27—Standardized Nomenclature for Medicine.)* CDA R2 is a document markup standard that specifies the structure and semantics of a clinical document for the purpose of exchange.[3] CDA uses extensible markup language (XML) to "tag," or identify, specific elements within the text. Both the sending and receiving computers use the XML tags to "parse," or separate, the text into discrete data elements.

26.3 CDA4CDT Workgroup

To facilitate the adoption and promotion of CDA-based electronic documents, a coalition of industry stakeholders formed the CDA4CDT workgroup. Founded by AHDI, MTIA, AHIMA, and M*Modal and managed by Alschuler & Associates, the CDA4CDT workgroup is tasked with creating templates and implementation guides for the most commonly transcribed document types: History and Physical Notes, Progress Notes, Consultation Notes, Radiology Notes, and Operative Notes. These implementation guides will enable EHR vendors and healthcare providers to integrate information contained within a free-text document into an electronic, database-driven, healthcare record system.

26.4 Templates and Implementation Guides

CDA R2 templates and implementation guides are specific to each report type and specify which headings (e.g., *Chief Complaint, History of Present Illness*) must be included in a document of that type and which headings are optional. The type of information to be contained under a specific heading is also defined. CDA documents must be both "human readable" and "machine interpretable," meaning the information should be clearly readable by a human, as any traditional document would be, and it must also contain XML encoding which allows computers to interpret the meaning. An analogy can be made to the encoding of a web page using HTML and XML. The user sees the results of the encoding as a human-readable web page, but the web page actually contains encoded tags which are interpreted by the user's browser. *Figure 1* shows sample text taken from a CDA R2 document with encoding displayed. *Figure 2* is the same text displayed in human-readable form.

```
<title>PHYSICAL EXAMINATION</title>
    <component>
      <section>
        <templateId root="2.16.840.1.113883.10.20.2.4"/>
        <code codeSystem="2.16.840.1.113883.6.1"
codeSystemName="LOINC" code="8716-3" displayName="VITAL
SIGNS"/>
        <title>Vital Signs</title>
        <text>
          <paragraph>Heart Rate: 78, Respiratory Rate: 12,
Temp (degF): 96.7, Oxygen Sat (%): 100.</paragraph>
          <paragraph>Non-invasive Blood Pressure: Systolic:
107, Diastolic: 51, Mean: 64.</paragraph>
        </text>
      </section>
```

Figure 1 Vital signs section taken from a CDA R2 document with encoding displayed.

PHYSICAL EXAMINATION
Vital Signs
Heart Rate: 78, Respiratory Rate: 12, Temp (degF): 96.7, Oxygen Sat (%): 100.
Non-invasive Blood Pressure: Systolic: 107, Diastolic: 51, Mean: 64.

Figure 2 Vital signs section taken from a CDA document with encoding hidden.

The templates and implementation guides specify the encoding for a CDA R2-conformant document. Programmers with knowledge of CDA and XML use the implementation guides to create document templates that can be used by individuals with little or no knowledge of XML. The exact methodology used to incorporate the dictated text with the encoding will be determined by individual EHR and/or transcription vendors, but most likely will involve the transcriptionist's keying data in between simple tags or into document fields. Natural language processing may also be used to add tags to key terms followed by a quality review by an experienced transcriptionist. *Figure 3* shows the same vital signs section of a document template as it might appear to a transcriptionist.

PHYSICAL EXAMINATION
Vital Signs
Heart Rate: < >, Respiratory Rate: < >, Temp (degF): < >, Oxygen Sat (%): < >.
Non-invasive Blood Pressure: Systolic: < >, Diastolic: < >, Mean: < >.

Figure 3 Excerpt taken from a template.

The templates and implementation guides are created based on input from transcriptionists, physicians, information technology professionals, transcription software developers, transcription service owners, and EHR vendors. Because of HL7's inclusive and open approach to standards development, which allows all stakeholders an equal say in the development of the standards, HL7 standards have a solid track record of acceptance and implementation in the marketplace. Other standards developed using the Clinical Document Architecture, Release 2, such as the Continuity of Care Document developed jointly by ASTM and HL7, have been well received in the medical community. Adoption of the CDA4CDT templates and implementation guides will increase the amount of data available to the electronic health record with little to no disruption in physicians' work-flow. The increased data available to electronic record systems will speed the development of interoperable clinical document repositories.

26.5 Implications for the Medical Transcription Sector

The CDA4CDT project has many positive implications for medical transcription-ists. The driving force behind the development of CDA R2 has been the desire to further encode the narrative clinical statements found in clinical reports, and to do so in such a way as to enable comparison of content from documents created on information systems of widely varying characteristics.[4] The interest and effort expended by many stakeholders in the healthcare industry in order to develop CDA R2 and create the implementation guides attests to the ongoing role for MTs in the EHR. Standardization of documents, including headings, subheadings, and content also has positive ramifications for transcriptionists. Documents which are consistent in their format and content can be transcribed more efficiently and with a higher level of accuracy.

Although many providers prefer their own documentation formats, there are many compelling reasons to adopt the CDA R2-conformant templates. Adoption of the template headings and subheadings will benefit all organizations whether or not an EHR implementation is imminent. Creating conforming documents will assure interoperability going forward, aid in the future importation of documents into an EHR, and of course enrich any current EHR implementa-tion. Adoption of template standards also guides the collection of key data that supports reimbursement, clinical research, decision support, and epidemiological surveys. CDA has a low bar of adoption, making it easy to implement the standard stepwise, employing progressively more complex levels of encoding. Because CDA-conforming documents are encoded with XML and supported with style sheets, the human-readable document can easily be adjusted to the provider's stylistic preferences, including font, font size, margins, etc., without affecting the computational value of the document or burdening the transcriptionist with numerous and varying account specification sheets.

AHDI and MTIA are committed to industry efforts to endorse industry standards, promote the propagation of EHRs, and assure a valued place for medical transcriptionists in the documentation arena. Supporting CDA4CDT is an integral part of this ongoing commitment to the medical community and medical transcriptionists.

The following table lists the Required (R) and Optional (O) section headings for a CDA-conforming *History and Physical* as well as a *Consultation Note*. The order of headings is not specified and the following table does not imply any particular order for headings or subheadings. The *Component Name* column indicates the section name using LOINC terminology, which must be included in the encoding, but facilities may choose different heading/subheading descriptions to appear on the printed version of the document.

Note: These implementation guides are currently identified as document standards for *trial use*, which means they have been balloted and approved for 2 years (est. fall 2007) so that they can be tested in the marketplace. Based on user feedback, these guides may undergo revision (after the publication of this text) before they become permanent implementation guides. Users of this text should verify any revisions to the guides beyond that 2-year window after publication of this text.

History and Physical Note[5]

Section Category	R/O	Code	Component Name
Reason for Visit/ Chief Complaint	R	29299-5	REASON FOR VISIT
		10154-3	CHIEF COMPLAINT
		46239-0	REASON FOR VISIT+CHIEF COMPLAINT
History of Present Illness	R	10164-2	HISTORY OF PRESENT ILLNESS
Past Medical History	R	11348-0	HISTORY OF PAST ILLNESS
Medications	R	10160-0	HISTORY OF MEDICATION USE

Section Category	R/O	Code	Component Name
Allergies	R	48765-2	ALLERGIES, ADVERSE REACTIONS, ALERTS
Social History	R	29762-2	SOCIAL HISTORY
Family History	R	10157-6	HISTORY OF FAMILY MEMBER DISEASES
Vital Signs	R	8716-3	VITAL SIGNS (may be a subsection of Physical Examination)
Review of Systems	R	10187-3	REVIEW OF SYSTEMS
Physical Examination	R	29545-1	PHYSICAL FINDINGS
		Optional Subsections	
		10210-3	GENERAL STATUS, PHYSICAL FINDINGS (optional, must be subsection)
		Pending	Additional optional subsections. List includes those in section 3.3.3 (Provider Unspecified History and Physical Note) of the "Additional Information Specification 0004: Clinical Reports Attachment."
Diagnostic Findings	R	30954-2	RELEVANT DIAGNOSTIC TESTS AND/OR LABORATORY DATA
Assessment and Plan	R	AAPLN-X	ASSESSMENT AND PLAN
		ASSMT-X	ASSESSMENT
		18776-5	PLAN
Procedure History	O	10167-5	PROCEDURE HISTORY
Immunizations	O	11369-6	HISTORY OF IMMUNIZATIONS
Problems	O	11450-4	PROBLEM LIST

Consultation Note[6]

Section Category	R/O	Code	Component Name
Reason for Referral/ Reason for Visit	R	42349-1	REASON FOR REFERRAL
		29299-5	REASON FOR VISIT
History of Present Illness	R	10164-2	HISTORY OF PRESENT ILLNESS
Physical Examination	R	29545-1	PHYSICAL FINDINGS
		Optional Subsections	
		10210-3	GENERAL STATUS, PHYSICAL FINDINGS (optional, must be subsection)
		Pending	Additional optional subsections include those in section 3.3.3 (Provider Unspecified History and Physical Note) of the "Additional Information Specification 0004: Clinical Reports Attachment."
Assessment and Plan	R	AAPLN-X	ASSESSMENT AND PLAN
		ASSMT-X	ASSESSMENT
		18776-5	PLAN
Past Medical History	O	11348-0	HISTORY OF PAST ILLNESS
Medications	O	10160-0	HISTORY OF MEDICATION USE
Allergies	O	48765-2	ALLERGIES, ADVERSE REACTIONS, ALERTS
Social History	O	29762-2	SOCIAL HISTORY
Family History	O	10157-6	HISTORY OF FAMILY MEMBER DISEASES
Vital Signs	O	8716-3	VITAL SIGNS (may be a subsection of Physical Examination)
Review of Systems	O	10187-3	REVIEW OF SYSTEMS
Diagnostic Findings	O	30954-2	RELEVANT DIAGNOSTIC TESTS AND/ OR LABORATORY DATA
Procedure History	O	10167-5	PROCEDURE HISTORY
Immunizations	O	11369-6	HISTORY OF IMMUNIZATIONS
Problems	O	11450-4	PROBLEM LIST
Chief Complaint	O	10154-3	CHIEF COMPLAINT

Contributing Author: Laura Bryan, MT (ASCP), CMT, FAAMT

Resources

1. *www.hl7.org*; accessed November 2007.

2. Dolin, Robert H., Alschuler, L.; Boyer, Sandy; Beebe, Calvin; Behlen, Fred M.; Biron, Paul V.; Shabo (Shvo), Amnon, "HL7 Clinical Document Architecture, Release 2," *Journal of the American Medical Informatics Association* 13 (2006): 30-39.

3. ibid.

4. ibid.

5. Alschuler, et al, *CDA Implementation Guide for HL7 Standard for CDA Release 2.0, Levels 1, 2, and 3, History and Physical Notes, (U.S. Realm)* (Ann Arbor, Michigan: HL7, 2008).

6. Alschuler, et al, *CDA Implementation Guide for HL7 Standard for CDA Release 2.0, Levels 1, 2, and 3, Consultation Notes (U.S. Realm)*, (Ann Arbor, Michigan: HL7, 2008).

Systematized Nomenclature for Medicine (SNOMED)

Introduction

Exchanging health information that informs clinical decision-making at the point of care is becoming a critically complex issue for care providers. Increasingly, patients are being treated in many settings across multiple healthcare systems, each with disparate electronic record systems that may or may not be interoperable. Most facilities have some form of a record management system in place, but the limitations of those systems have made it virtually impossible to create an accurate, consistent exchange of data that is both meaningful and available in real time at all access points across the system.

Healthcare IT vendors are equally challenged to keep up with the demand for newer and more diverse platforms that are capable of solving these data exchange issues in a way that is cost-effective and responsive. Tremendous focus has been directed toward developing systems that can communicate with other systems and platforms, and *interoperability* is a turnkey word on the lips of every vendor and every healthcare delivery system representative that is out shopping for one.

Given the presidential mandate to move our nation toward a national health information network, it is only a matter of time before the web of interconnectivity has been laid that will enable nationwide, and eventually global, health data exchange. But what will happen when the channels are created and data streams begin to flow from one system to another? How can the data be captured, encoded, and used for ongoing clinical care as well as research and data mining?

A truly effective electronic health record system, and certainly an effective national health information network, is going to require clinical data to be concrete and defined. A system that is based on open-field free text will be as useless and unmanageable to health care as a paper-based system. The data must be searchable and useable, and to be both, it must be defined. For example, if a provider is allowed to enter a description of the patient's diagnosis on his own, he might manually enter any of the following:

myocardial infarction
acute myocardial infarction
heart attack
cardiac infarction
acute MI
MI

In other words, there are often many ways to describe a single symptom, diagnosis, or event. To address this issue, many EMRs restrict the provider to a single choice (*myocardial infarction*, for example) with further ability to select modifiers (*acute, mild*, etc.) such that the system knows there is a universal and defined way of describing this diagnosis on that system. However, without a single nomenclature system to guide vendors and providers in creating interoperable systems, what good will it do if one system has defined this event as *acute myocardial infarction* and another system has defined it as *heart attack*? When those disparate systems hook up and attempt to communicate, there will be an exchange of data from one system that, while it may mean the same thing, is described in a way that potentially will not be recognized by the other system. A provider whose query to the system for patients presenting with *myocardial infarction* during a specific time period will yield results that are absent any patients whose data could not be mined because of incompatible nomenclature.

27.1 SNOMED Background and Objectives

SNOMED CT® is a universal healthcare nomenclature for clinical terminology. The **S**ystematized **No**menclature for **Med**icine was developed by a division of the College of American Pathologists (CAP), known as SNOMED International, for the purpose of "advancing excellence in patient care delivery" through the promotion and support of SNOMED. The organization touts 40 years of research and effort into development of this standardized nomenclature system for health care.[1]

SNOMED CT (Clinical Terms) is a comprehensive taxonomy of medical language, including diseases, clinical findings, and procedures that allows for a consistent way of identifying, indexing, categorizing, and aggregating health data across multiple systems. Each clinical concept is called a "unit of meaning" and is assigned a numeric code, a unique name (called a **F**ully **S**pecified **N**ame), and a set of descriptions, that includes the "preferred term" and one or more synonyms. The clinical concepts are arranged in hierarchies that are connected by defined relationships and include mapping to ICD-9 (in future, to ICD-10).

In 2003, the Department of Health and Human Services recommended the SNOMED CT as part of a core set of patient medical record information (PMRI) terminology. In the letter regarding PMRI terminology, the National Committee on Vital and Health Statistics said, "The breadth of content, sound terminology model, and widely recognized value of SNOMED CT qualify it as a general-purpose terminology for the exchange, aggregation, and analysis of patient medical information. The broad scope of SNOMED CT itself and the inclusion within it of concepts from other important healthcare terminologies (including the following terminologies developed to support nursing practice: HHCC, NANDA, NOC, NIC, Omaha System, and PNS) allow SNOMED CT to encompass much of the patient medical record information domain." [2]

SNOMED has been adopted as one of the primary source vocabularies of the Unified Medical Language System (UMLS) metathesaurus developed by the United States National Library of Medicine and licensed at no cost to users all over the world. SNOMED International is also working strategically with Health Level Seven (HL7) to coordinate SNOMED CT with the HL7 Reference Information Model.

27.2 Natural Language Processing (NLP)

Natural Language Processing refers to the process by which computer systems convert "natural language," which can refer to speech or free-form text, into codified language that a computer can identify, classify, and understand. Since free-form language can have many implied meanings (as outlined above in reference to *myocardial infarction*), a computer has to be taught to apply a specific set of defined meanings for some or all of the natural language terms it is asked to identify and manipulate.

NLP transforms "natural" or free-form clinical language into structured text. It then abstracts, or identifies and tags, predefined clinical concepts and terms that can be used and reorganized in a variety of ways, including being pulled into standardized formats, mined for research and clinical decision-making, and used in conjunction with computer-assisted coding to facilitate reimbursement. This is where NLP and a standardized nomenclature (like SNOMED) can work hand in hand. NLP can be programmed to map natural language to the codified nomenclature defined by SNOMED so that it can be tagged, mined, and used for statistical data-gathering and clinical decision-making.

27.3 Implications for the Medical Transcription Sector

SNOMED, HL7, and other standardization systems will increasingly become obvious in the transcription domain. When free-license access to SNOMED was made available by the Department of Health and Human Services in 2003, IT vendors jumped at the opportunity to incorporate the nomenclature into electronic health record platforms, and even transcription platform vendors are developing functionality that would enable natural language processing of free-text narrative and MT-assisted tagging of that text for translation into SNOMED. In environments where speech recognition is also deployed, the MT would be positioned at the analysis point of ensuring a seamless transition from dictation to speech-recognized draft to edited finalized draft to SNOMED-coded output. To take it one step further, many are also working on computer-suggested coding as part of this "one-stop shopping" approach to documentation.

A potential SNOMED-enabled NLP process in the transcription model could potentially look like this:

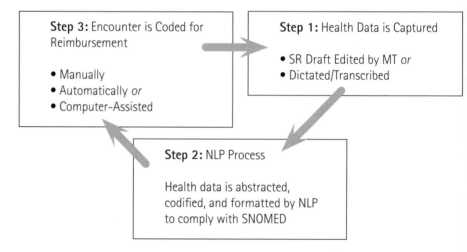

In the above scenario, the MT who evolves to a technology-trained and empowered role in this process would potentially be deployed in the following way:

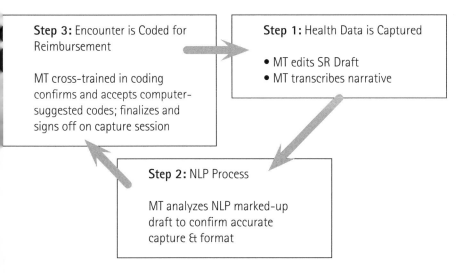

Step 3: Encounter is Coded for Reimbursement

MT cross-trained in coding confirms and accepts computer-suggested codes; finalizes and signs off on capture session

Step 1: Health Data is Captured

- MT edits SR Draft
- MT transcribes narrative

Step 2: NLP Process

MT analyzes NLP marked-up draft to confirm accurate capture & format

SNOMED will not likely be the final manifestation of a comprehensive nomenclature, and it remains to be seen whether it will meet the diverse needs of healthcare delivery, but it is definitely making necessary headway in creating clarity of data exchange, and everyone in healthcare documentation needs to stay abreast of its evolution.

Contributing Author: Lea M. Sims, CMT, FAAMT

Resources

1. *SNOMED International home page.* © 2006. SNOMED International. 20 Dec. 2006. *http://www.snomed.org/index.html*

2. Letter to Secretary of the Department of Health and Human Services from Chair of the National Committee on Vital and Health Statistics. 16 Jul. 2001. SNOMED International website. 20 Dec. 2006. *http://www.snomed.org/snomedct/documents/NCVHS_110503.pdf*

Speech Recognition and SR Editing

Introduction

Speech recognition technology (SRT), also known as automated speech recognition (ASR), continuous speech recognition (CSR) or voice recognition (VR), refers to computer software systems that convert the spoken word to text. This technology is becoming more and more prevalent in the healthcare field, as it is being marketed to institutions and physicians as a way to increase productivity and lower documentation costs. It is also being marketed to (and developed by, in some cases) medical transcription service organizations as a means of increasing documentation productivity and efficiency. Already many MTs in those settings are being redeployed to an editing role, a trend that is expected to increase in the future.

28.1 Speech Recognition Technology (SRT)

28.1.1 Background and Overview

Speech recognition technology has been around now for over two decades. For much of that time, it has been promised to eliminate the need for medical transcriptionists (MTs); meanwhile the need for healthcare documentation and the shortage of qualified MTs has continued to grow. While SRT is used by only a small percentage of healthcare providers in a self-editing (front-end) mode, the use of delayed (back-end) SRT systems is rapidly growing within the healthcare environment. Indeed, for the individuals that SRT was expected to eliminate (MTs), many are now successfully using delayed SRT systems for greater efficiencies by reducing turnaround times for report completion, as they apply their expert medical language skills as editors.[1]

28.1.2 Front-End SRT

Front-end speech recognition is the process of dictating into a PC using software to translate voice to text as the dictation occurs, such that the dictator may make real-time corrections during the dictation process and generate a final document without requiring a third party (i.e., MT or QA editor) to manipulate or modify the document.

In June of 2007, the Gartner Report was released, which purported that traditional dictation and transcription will eventually give way to a "once-and done" (OAD) dictation documentation model performed solely by the physician.[2] The report targeted chief information officers, chief medical information officers, and administrators interested in making dictation and transcription activities more efficient and cost-effective. However, the report further indicated that most significant barrier to widespread adoption of a front-end, OAD model is "the need to change physician behavior," which has inarguably been the barrier to improved documentation outcomes for decades. Most industry experts agree that modification of physician/dictator behavior and documentation habits will present a challenge too great to overcome in ever seeing the industry migrate fully to a front-end solution. It is anticipated, then, that back-end SRT models will be the most likely deployed, adopted, and integrated into the EMR in the future.[3]

In addition, there is still not enough conclusive data to suggest that physicians engaged in a front-end SR scenario are experiencing measurable increases in efficiency and cost-effectiveness. It cannot be confidently determined whether ultimately the physician is better engaged in 15 minutes of front-end dictation and editing or 5 minutes of traditional dictation. Studies have yet to be conducted as to what the ultimate gain or loss of both time and money is being realized where practitioners are using critical time for providing care on the administrative role of documenting that care.

28.1.3 Back-End SRT

Back-end speech recognition is the process of taking a traditionally recorded voice file and passing it through a speech recognition engine to generate a draft document that is then accessed by a third-party editor for correction and modification. Back-end SR is rapidly becoming what many healthcare institutions and transcription service providers believe to be the best-case scenario for integrating an enabling technology in a way that has the greatest chance of impacting documentation volumes. With the advancement of the electronic health record (EHR), today's healthcare professionals are in a challenging and dynamic environment and are under constant pressure to do more with less. The need to explore options to improve service levels and turn-around times while reducing costs is paramount.[4]

It is the back-end scenario where transcriptionists will find themselves engaged in an emerging and evolving role for documentation. It is the most highly skilled MT with the greatest degree of interpretive knowledge and informed judgment who is going to most successfully migrate to a meaningful role in SR editing. Transcriptionists whose skills are sub par – those who still require significant QA oversight and monitoring – will find that if the SR engine is capable of producing a draft document of the same or greater quality and accuracy, then the MT has become expendable in the process. It is the high-quality MT capable of recognizing, identifying, and correcting the nuances and potential errors of the speech-recognized draft who will partner with SRT to produce a client-ready deliverable.

28.1.4 Factors Impacting Adoption/Implementation

While SRT, particularly the back-end model, can and has been integrated with great success in many cases, there are a great many factors that can impact whether SRT is integrated in a way that yields a measurable return on investment (ROI) and the anticipated productivity gain for all parties involved (provider, service owner, and SR editor).

Dictation Habits: The inconsistency of speech patterns can and does pose a great problem for smooth, efficient integration of SRT. Speech converts to text when the speech patterns are consistent.[3] If a dictator, regardless of speed or accent, is able to deliver a consistent speech pattern that the SR engine can recognize and accurately correlate to clinical language, the outcome is a draft deliverable that requires only minimal editing by the SR editor, and thus, a productivity gain for both the engine and the editor. However, the reality is that a great majority of dictators are not SR-ready or SR-compatible. Their speech patterns are irregular and unpredictable, making it impossible for the SR engine to learn and acclimate to the dictator. This results in a draft document that has a high probability of inconstancy and error – one that will require significant time at the editing stage, resulting in a productivity loss for both the engine and the editor. If the ultimate goal of SRT is to generate a greater volume of client-ready, accurate outcomes than can be delivered from traditional transcription models, this can only be accomplished when there is a high degree of accuracy from the first draft.

Return on Investment Statistics: When providers or service organizations compare the cost of traditional transcription versus SR editing, they need to also factor in the costs of hardware/software amortization, residual usage fees, editing costs, training and implementation costs, etc., that are specific and unique to SR integration and would not be incurred in a traditional transcription model. A 40% savings in transcription production costs may look like a huge win, but that might only equate to a 10% overall savings once all other costs are added back in.[3] The only way there will be a significant savings is if the integration of the technology has resulted in real, measurable productivity gains – gains that are seen consistently across the board and not merely in isolated cases.

Efficiency and Skill Set of the Editor: The goal of engaging an MT in an editing role is that the MT will be able to edit a document at least twice as fast as he/she can transcribe it. When this does not occur, the reason generally correlates to (1) a translation challenge on the part of the engine to produce a good first draft, (2) a lack of efficient editing skill on the part of the SR editor, or (3) the SR editor is so fast and efficient as a traditional MT that there is little measurable productivity gain in migrating to the role of editor.

Variability of Technology: Productivity gains can also be impacted by the platform and interface of the technology itself. The best scenarios involve SR technologies that accurately and consistently format the document in a way that facilities quick and efficient editing. How well the SR tools support the navigation of the document on the part of the editor can also impact the turn-around of that document. Time spent reformatting and struggling with the navigation capabilities of the platform can result in frustrating productivity loss on the part of the editor.

28.2 SR Editing

28.2.1 Transition from MT to Editor

Performing SRT editing successfully requires a somewhat more specialized skillset than that involved in traditional, manual transcription. There is a different eye/ear/brain coordination dynamic at work in SRT editing compared to transcribing, which often makes it more challenging to identify errors in an SRT-draft document. It is more common in SRT editing for the brain to be "tricked" into thinking that the eye has seen what the ear has heard.[5] With an SRT-draft document, the power of suggestion can sometimes make it more difficult for an editor to hear and recognize an inconsistency or error.

MTs transitioning out of traditional transcription and into the role of SR editor should be aware that it typically takes 30 to 90 days to acclimate to the new process of document navigation and editing before realizing any measurable productivity gains. It is also important to be aware of all of the following skills and proficiencies deemed necessary for transition to SR editing (*See Appendix D: Model Job Descriptions*).

PROFESSIONAL/BUSINESS SKILLS

- Understanding of the medicolegal implications and responsibilities of the healthcare record, ensuring compliance with local, state, and federal rules and regulations, along with security standards and privacy practices
- Ability to multi-task and work under pressure with time constraints
- Ability to work independently with minimal or no supervision
- Organizational skills for file management
- Actively participates in continuing education
- Maintains and assesses equipment and work area with minimal supervision
- Demonstrates an understanding Editing of area systems, priorities, timelines and goals that contribute to the mission of the department
- Basic understanding of departmental technology

TECHNICAL/SYSTEM SKILLS

- Strong technical proficiency in computer applications so those measurable gains through system efficiencies are continually maximized in conjunction with speech recognition and other technologies available
- Ability to operate computer, multiple software applications, transcription equipment, and other office equipment necessary, including the ability to accept voice/text files in multiple formats and word processing software
- Desire to keep up to date and learn latest technology advancements and trends
- Continually develops understanding of multiple computer applications and document management programs in order to effectively contribute and adapt to the changing healthcare environment

QUALITATIVE/TRANSCRIPTION SKILLS

- Developing ability to work in all work types and specialties
- Knowledge of medical terminology, anatomy and physiology, disease processes, signs and symptoms, medications, and laboratory values
- Developing quality transcription work with a goal of maintaining accuracy score of 98% or higher
- Knowledge of medical transcription guidelines (*The Book of Style for Medical Transcription*) and practices
- Developing ability to understand diverse accents, dialects, and varying dictation styles, commonly confused terms, and knowledge of homonyms
- Proficient in referencing and researching with full library of references (books/electronic) and Internet access
- Acute auditory sensitivity and keen hand/eye coordination, as would be expected in medical transcription
- Edit a speech recognized draft document against actual dictation

- Edit documents consistently in order to maximize the efficiencies gained through recognition
- Utilize all available reference tools to ensure the accuracy of the transcribed document
- Recognize, interpret, and evaluate inconsistencies, discrepancies, and inaccuracies in medical text drafts and/or dictation appropriately to clarify, flag, or report them, as needed
- Adhere to policies and procedures to contribute to the efficiency of the transcription department
- Transcribe reports as required

INTERPERSONAL SKILLS
- Excellent written and oral communication skills, including grammar, punctuation, and style, in order to provide quality feedback to the transcriptionist
- Communicate and interact productively with management personnel with objective feedback as needed

28.2.2 Resolution of Standards/Style Conflicts

One of the inevitable challenges of migrating to an automating technology is in ensuring a smooth transition that does not compromise accuracy and quality. Already organizations who are migrating to SR capture and back-end editing are encountering conflicts between SR capture and documentation standards, particularly those standards recommended throughout this text. There are many instances where traditional transcriptionists edit the report to reflect these standards in ways that an SR engine cannot be trained to recognize and duplicate. The result is a draft document that is generated without application of these standards, requiring considerable time and editing on the part of the SR editor. This can include everything from what to do when a physician includes a patient name in the body of the report, when numbers are dictated at the beginning of the sentence, when laboratory values are dictated without indication of a break or pause between tests, etc. In each of these instances (and in so many others indicated throughout this book) the traditional MT would know to edit or recast these sentences to ensure appropriate application of the standard. The SR engine, however, cannot be trained to make the same informed, interpretive judgment, and the engine will capture these scenarios exactly as they are dictated.

The dilemma for the organization trying to deploy SRT in a way that results in productivity gains and improved TAT outcomes is in trying to balance the need for quality with a need to reduce those instances where significant editing is required of the SR draft. Obviously, the more detailed editing, recasting, and standards formatting is required by the editor, the lower the productivity gain for all parties. Yet, SR integration and implementation cannot come at the expense of quality documentation outcomes.

AHDI strongly recommends that organizations utilizing and implementing SRT approach standards conflicts with informed wisdom. Regardless of the need to ensure capture efficiency and productivity, accurate capture of the patient care encounter and clarity of communication is paramount. These considerations must precede and override any decision to sacrifice quality for automation. However, AHDI also recognizes that there may be standards recommended for traditional documentation that may not make sense in an SR environment, and any attempt to force them into an SR model may do nothing but hinder the capabilities of the technology to bring measurable documentation solutions to healthcare delivery. With that in mind, AHDI recommends that organizations faced with a specific style or standards conflict approach the conflict with the following contemplative consideration:

1. Can the SR engine be trained to recognize and apply that standard consistently? In other words, can the SR engine be trained to make the informed edit that the MT would know to make?

   if not:

2. Can the dictator be engaged to resolve the conflict by changing a dictation habit?

   if not:

3. Does the conflict represent an area where clinical accuracy or clarity of communication will be compromised if not corrected?

If after careful consideration and investigation of each of these questions, it is determined that the style issue is critical enough to accuracy and communication that it *must* be ensured in the record, then the organization has no choice but to engage the SR editor in making those corrections of the SR draft. If the style issue is not deemed to be of critical concern, AHDI would recommend that the organization forego the standard to facilitate capture efficiency. In no way, however, do we recommend a blanket policy to forego standards to facilitate an unhindered editing process. Each style or standards issue must be approached and investigated safely, again with the primary concern of ensuring that quality is not compromised.

Bibliography

The following texts served as the primary sources of clinical information and evolving language standards for this edition:

Iverson et al. *The AMA Manual of Style: A Guide for Authors and Editors*, 10th edition. American Medical Association. Oxford University Press. © 2007.

Sabin, William A. *The Gregg Reference Manual*, 10th edition. McGraw-Hill Irwin. © 2004.

Tortora, G. and Derrickson, B. *Principles of Anatomy and Physiology*, 11th edition. Wiley Higher Education. © 2006.

Dirckx, J. *Laboratory Tests & Diagnostic Procedures in Medicine*. Health Professions Institute. © 2004

Golish, J. and Michota, F. *Diagnostic Procedure Handbook*. Lexicomp, Inc. and Lippincott, Williams, and Wilkins. © 2001.

Dircks, J. *H&P: A Nonphysician's Guide to the History and Physical Examination*, 3rd Edition. Health Professions Institute. © 2001.

Other sources cited throughout this text:

Tessier, C. "What's Wrong with This Picture?" *Journal of the American Association for Medical Transcription*, Vol.12, No. 4, July-August 1993, pp. 3, 32-33,36-38.

Rhodes, H. "Modifying the Patient Record: Corrections, Revisions, Additions and Addenda" *The AAMT Book of Style, 2nd Edition*, Appendix G, pp. 481-488.

Taylor, B.N. *Guide for the Use of the International System of Units*. May 2007. 11 Nov. 2007. < *http://physics.nist.gov/Pubs/SP811/contents.html*>

Sneath et al. *International Code of Nomenclature of Bacteria*. American Society for Microbiology. Revised 1990. 18 December 2007. *http://www.ncbi.nlm.nih.gov/books/bv.fcgi?indexed=google&rid=icnb.TOC*

Moses, Scott MD. "*The Family Practice Notebook: Psychiatry*" 8 September 2007. 21 December 2007. *http://www.fpnotebook.com/PSY84.htm*

Health Level Seven. Accessed November 2007. *http://www.hl7.org*

Dolin, Robert H., Alschuler, L.; Boyer, Sandy; Beebe, Calvin; Behlen, Fred M.; Biron, Paul V.; Shabo (Shvo), Amnon, "HL7 Clinical Document Architecture, Release 2," *Journal of the American Medical Informatics Association* 13 (2006): 30-39

Alschuler, et al. *CDA Implementation Guide for HL7 Standard for CDA Release 2.0, Levels 1, 2, and 3, History and Physical Notes*, (U.S. Realm). Ann Arbor, Michigan: HL7, 2008.

Alschuler, et al. *CDA Implementation Guide for HL7 Standard for CDA Release 2.0, Levels 1, 2, and 3, Consultation Notes* (U.S. Realm). Ann Arbor, Michigan: HL7, 2008.

SNOMED International home page. © 2006. SNOMED International. 20 Dec. 2006. *http://www.snomed.org/index.html*

Letter to Secretary of the Department of Health and Human Services from Chair of the National Committee on Vital and Health Statistics. 16 Jul. 2001. SNOMED International website. 20 Dec. 2006. *http://www.snomed.org/snomedct/documents/NCVHS_110503.pdf*

Hurley, Brenda J. CMT FAAMT. *Speech Recognition Technology: The New Efficiency Tool for MTs?* Association for Healthcare Documentation website. 12 January 2008. *http://www.ahdionline.org/scriptcontent/Downloads/SRT.pdf*

Hieb, Barry R. MD. *The Evolving Model of Clinical Dictation and Transcription.* 13 June 2007/ID Number G00148961. Gartner, Inc.© 2007

Catuogno, George. *SRT 2007: Where are We Now?* Health Data Matrix. Vol. 26 Issue 5. October 2007. Association for Healthcare Documentation Integrity and the Medical Transcription Industry Alliance. © 2007

Gerzel, Bob. *A 360° Look at SRT.* Health Data Matrix. Vol 26 Issue 5. October 2007. Association for Healthcare Documentation Integrity and the Medical Transcription Industry Alliance. © 2007

Speech Recognition Technology page. Association for Healthcare Documentation website. 12 January 2008. *http://www.ahdionline.org/scriptcontent/srt.cfm*

National Patient Safety Goals, as published by The Joint Commission: *http://www.jointcommission.org/PatientSafety/NationalPatientSafetyGoals/*

Final Privacy Rule, as published in the Federal Register, August 14, 2002:
http://www.hhs.gov/ocr/hipaa/privrulepd.pdf

Office of Civil Rights—Privacy Questions & Answers:
http://answers.hhs.gov/cgi-bin/hhs.cfg/php/enduser/std_alp.php

Office of Civil Rights—HIPAA Assistance:
http://www.hhs.gov/ocr/hipaa/assist.html

AHIMA Practice Brief: Facsimile Transmission of Health Information:
http://library.ahima.org/xpedio/groups/public/documents/ahima/pub_bok2_000116.html

History and Physical

CHIEF COMPLAINT
Status post motor vehicle accident.

HISTORY OF PRESENT ILLNESS
The patient is a 17-year-old white male who is status post a high-speed motor vehicle accident in which he was ejected from the vehicle. He denies loss of consciousness, although the EMT people report that he did have loss of consciousness. The patient was stable en route. Upon arrival, he complained of headache.

PAST MEDICAL HISTORY
Medical: None. Surgical: None.

REVIEW OF SYSTEMS
Cardiac: No history.
Pulmonary: Some morning cough (patient is a smoker).

MEDICATIONS
None.

ALLERGIES
No known drug allergies.

PHYSICAL EXAMINATION
VITAL SIGNS: Blood pressure 120/80, pulse 82, respirations 20, and temperature 36.8°.
HEENT: Contusion over right occiput. Tympanic membranes benign.
NECK: Nontender.
CHEST: Atraumatic, nontender.
LUNGS: Clear to auscultation and percussion.
ABDOMEN: Flat, soft, and nontender.
BACK: Atraumatic, nontender.
PELVIS: Stable.
EXTREMITIES: Contusion over right forearm. No underlying bone deformity or crepitus.
RECTAL: Normal sphincter tone; guaiac negative.
NEUROLOGIC: Glasgow coma scale 15. Pupils equal, round, reactive to light. Patient moves all 4 extremities without focal deficit.

DIAGNOSTIC STUDIES
Serial hematocrits 44.5, 42.4, and 40.4. White blood count 6.3. Ethanol: None. Amylase 66. Urinalysis normal. PT 12.6, PTT 29. Chem-7 panel within normal limits. X-rays of cervical spine and lumbosacral spine within normal limits.

X-rays of pelvis and chest within normal limits.

ASSESSMENT
1. Closed head injury.
2. Rule out intra-abdominal injury.

PLAN
The patient will be admitted to the trauma surgery service for continued evaluation and treatment for closed head injury as well as possible intraabdominal injury.

Consultation

REASON FOR CONSULTATION
This 92-year-old female states that last night she had a transient episode of slurred speech and numbness of her left cheek for a few hours. However, the chart indicates that she had recurrent TIAs 3 times yesterday, each lasting about 5 minutes, with facial drooping and some mental confusion. She had also complained of blurred vision for several days. She was brought to the emergency room last night, where she was noted to have a left carotid bruit and was felt to have recurrent TIAs. The patient is on Lanoxin, amoxicillin, Hydergine, Cardizem, Lasix, Micro-K, and a salt-free diet. She does not smoke or drink alcohol.

Admission CT scan of the head showed a densely calcified mass lesion of the sphenoid bone, probably representing the benign osteochondroma seen on previous studies. CBC was normal, aside from a hemoglobin of 11.2. ECG showed atrial fibrillation. BUN was 22, creatinine normal, CPK normal, glucose normal, and electrolytes normal.

PHYSICAL EXAMINATION
On examination, the patient is noted to be alert and fully oriented. She has some impairment of recent memory. She is not dysphasic, nor is she apraxic. Speech is normal and clear. The head is noted to be normocephalic. Neck is supple. Carotid pulses are full bilaterally, with left carotid bruit. Neurologic exam shows cranial nerve function II through XII to be intact, save for some slight flattening of the left nasolabial fold. Motor examination shows no drift of the outstretched arms. There is no tremor or past-pointing. Finger-to-nose and heel-to-shin performed well bilaterally. Motor showed intact neuromuscular tone, strength, and coordination in all limbs. Reflexes 1+ and symmetrical, with bilateral plantar flexion, absent jaw jerk, no snout. Sensory exam is intact to pinprick, touch, vibration, position, temperature, and graphesthesia.

IMPRESSION
Neurological examination is normal, aside from mild impairment of recent memory, slight flattening of the left nasolabial fold, and left carotid bruit. She also has atrial fibrillation, apparently chronic. In view of her age and the fact that she is in chronic atrial fibrillation, I would suspect that she most likely has had embolic phenomena as the cause of her TIAs.

RECOMMENDATIONS
I would recommend conservative management with antiplatelet agents unless a near-occlusion of the carotid arteries is demonstrated, in which case you might consider it best to do an angiography and consider endarterectomy. In view of her age, I would be reluctant to recommend Coumadin anticoagulation. I will be happy to follow the patient with you.

Operative Report

PREOPERATIVE DIAGNOSES
1. Right spontaneous pneumothorax secondary to barometric trauma.
2. Respiratory failure.
3. Pneumonia with sepsis.

POSTOPERATIVE DIAGNOSES
1. Right spontaneous pneumothorax secondary to barometric trauma.
2. Respiratory failure.
3. Pneumonia with sepsis.

NAME OF OPERATION
Right chest tube insertion.

INDICATIONS
Spontaneous right pneumothorax secondary to barometric trauma from increased
PEEP. An early morning chest x-ray showed approximately 30% pneumothorax
on the right.

INFORMED CONSENT
Not obtained. This patient is obtunded, intubated, and septic. This is an emergent procedure with two-physician emergency consent signed and on the chart.

PROCEDURE
The patient's right chest was prepped and draped in sterile fashion. The site of
insertion was anesthetized with 1% Xylocaine, and an incision was made. Blunt
dissection was carried out 2 intercostal spaces above the initial incision site. The
chest wall was opened, and a 32-French chest tube was placed into the thoracic
cavity after examination with the finger, making sure that the thoracic cavity had
been entered correctly. The chest tube was placed on wall suction and subsequently sutured in place with 0 silk. A postoperative chest x-ray is pending at
this time. The patient tolerated the procedure well and was taken to the recovery
room in stable condition.

ESTIMATED BLOOD LOSS
10 mL.

COMPLICATIONS
None.

Discharge Summary

ADMITTING DIAGNOSES
1. Second-degree heart block with 2:1 conduction.
2. Right bundle branch block.
3. Left anterior fascicular block.
4. Adult-onset diabetes.

HISTORY OF PRESENT ILLNESS
The patient is a 69-year-old white female who has been followed in my clinic for adult-onset diabetes. She is known to have a right bundle branch block and left anterior fascicular block on previous EKG. She presented to my office complaining of increased lethargy over the preceding week.

PHYSICAL EXAMINATION
Physical exam demonstrated bradycardia with pulse in the 40s. EKG revealed second-degree heart block with 2:1 conduction and a ventricular rate in the 40s. The patient denied any lightheadedness, syncope, chest pain, shortness of breath, palpitations, history of myocardial infarction, or rhythm disturbance.

HOSPITAL COURSE
The patient was admitted directly to the hospital and admitted to a monitored floor. MI was ruled out, and cardiology consult was obtained. At that time, it was felt that the patient was in need of a permanent pacemaker. She underwent dual-chamber pacemaker insertion on the following day without complications. She has done well postoperatively, without any symptoms, and has remained in normal sinus rhythm with pacer capturing throughout observation. She is presently without complaints except for some nasal congestion and tenderness over the pacer insertion site. However, there is no erythema or discharge at the operative site. The patient is clinically stable for discharge.

DISCHARGE MEDICATIONS
1. Ecotrin 1 p.o. b.i.d. with meals.
2. Keflex 500 mg p.o. q.i.d. for 4 days.
3. Iron sulfate 325 mg p.o. b.i.d.

PLAN
The patient is to see me again in 2 weeks. She will call if symptoms recur.

Progress Note

The patient is being seen today in followup for a bad cough, sinus congestion, and nasal discharge, worse since his last visit. He also complains of a sore on the bottom of his right foot, and he has a bulge in the left groin.

PHYSICAL EXAM
HEENT shows posterior pharyngeal drainage. The neck is supple, with tender adenopathy. TMs are clear. Lungs have some forced expiratory rhonchi. Examination of the bottom of the right foot shows a corn. I pared away some of the overlying callus. Valsalva maneuver shows a prominent left inguinal hernia; testicular exam is normal.

IMPRESSION
1. Sinusitis.
2. Corn, right foot.
3. Left inguinal hernia.

PLAN
We put him on amoxicillin 250 mg t.i.d. for 10 days. Advised him to pare the corn and use a Dr. Scholl's foot pad. We will refer him to a general surgeon regarding the left inguinal hernia. Return in 2 weeks if sinusitis is not improved.

NOTE: In order to conserve space in the chart, some physician offices, clinics, and other healthcare facilities format their progress notes by using section headings followed by colons, with findings beginning on the same line. Defer to facility preference for formatting.

SOAP Note

SUBJECTIVE
The patient is brought in for a 6-month checkup. She is doing very well. She is seeing Dr. Green for evaluation of her feet. He gave her a clean bill of health. She is on breast milk as well as cereal.

OBJECTIVE
HEENT exam is normal. Lungs are clear. Cardiac examination is within normal limits. Musculoskeletal exam is normal. Abdomen is benign. Genitalia are normal.

ASSESSMENT
Normal exam.

PLAN
Continue breast-feeding; no dietary modifications are necessary. DPT and Hib will be given.

NOTE: In order to conserve space in the chart, some physician offices, clinics, and other healthcare facilities format their SOAP notes by using section headings followed by colons, with findings beginning on the same line. Defer to facility preference for formatting.

EEG

DESCRIPTION
This is the record in a 12-month-old infant on no regular medications, who received chloral hydrate before the test. The EEG is well organized and shows symmetrical activity of normal amplitude, which is persistent throughout. There is no focal or paroxysmal abnormality. Provocative procedures were not carried out. The child remained asleep throughout most of the recording.

IMPRESSION
Normal electroencephalogram.

Radiology

THYROID UPTAKE AND SCAN
Uptake is markedly elevated at 82% at 24 hours. Images show that the left lobe is considerably enlarged, about 5 times normal size, whereas the right lobe is about normal in size. There is uniform uptake throughout both lobes.

IMPRESSION
The findings are consistent with Graves disease, with asymmetric involvement of the lobes, the left being quite enlarged, whereas the right is not enlarged.

Flow Cytometry

Examination of Wright-stained cytoprep slides of the submitted bone marrow specimen shows a predominant population of maturing myeloid cells with smaller numbers of maturing erythroid cells. Only rare small lymphocytes are observed. No prominent abnormal lymphocytic population is identified. By flow cytometric immunophenotyping, within the lymphocytic region, there is a preponderance of T lymphocytes with only a small number of B lymphocytes. No monoclonal IgM-lambda-expressing B-lymphocytic population is identified by this flow cytometric study. Nevertheless, these findings should be correlated with the bone marrow biopsy for definitive diagnosis (since some aggregates of lymphoma, especially paratrabecular lymphoma, may not be very well aspirated).

Cytology

SPECIMEN
Vaginal smear.

CLINICAL DATA
Postmenopausal vaginal bleeding.

GROSS DESCRIPTION
Received is 1 alcohol-fixed smear.

MICROSCOPIC DESCRIPTION
One Papanicolaou-stained smear is examined. The smear is highly cellular, consisting predominantly of superficial vaginal/exocervical epithelial cells intermixed with large numbers of neutrophils. Occasional trichomonas organisms are seen. No dysplastic cells are seen.

DIAGNOSIS
Pap smear showing marked acute inflammation with Trichomonas vaginalis being present (Pap smear, vagina).

Pathology

SPECIMEN
Fine-needle aspiration, right kidney.

CLINICAL DATA
Hypertension workup, asymptomatic right renal mass.

GROSS DESCRIPTION
In the department of radiology, under CT guidance, I performed a single pass into a right kidney mass. This resulted in production of less than 1 mL of bloody fluid. From this fluid were created 3 air-dried smears and 4 alcohol-fixed smears. In addition, the syringe and needle were rinsed in B-5 solution for producing a bloody slur totaling approximately 0.75 mL. This material will be filtered through a tea bag and submitted in its entirety in a single cassette.

MICROSCOPIC DESCRIPTION
Four Papanicolaou-stained smears, 3 Wright-stained smears, and 3 H&E-stained sections from a B-5 fixed cell button are reviewed. Seen are rather large clusters of cohesive, moderate-sized cells which are oval to spindle shaped. These cells contain nongranular, nonvacuolated cytoplasm, and cytoplasmic borders are indistinct. Gland-like lumina and evidence of squamous differentiation are lacking, and no significant areas of necrosis are found. The nuclei are rounded to oval and show a finely granular pattern of chromatin staining. Other nuclei show prominent euchromatin. Nuclei containing prominent nucleoli are not found. There is minimal nuclear pleomorphism noted, and virtually no mitotic figures are encountered. No papillary structures are seen. No calcifications are encountered. Metaplastic bone and cartilage formation are not found. No pigmentation is noted.

DIAGNOSIS
Renal cell carcinoma (hypernephroma), right kidney.

Autopsy

The patient was a 70-year-old white male with a history of adenocarcinoma of the right upper lobe, treated with lobectomy in 1985, and coronary artery disease, treated with coronary artery bypass graft in 1986. The patient presented to University Medical Center in October of 1988 with mental status changes and was found to have a right frontal lobe metastasis. The patient received steroids and x-ray therapy at that time and was discharged to home. He returned to our medical center on the 19th of October with decreasing mental status and shortness of breath. The patient was found to have a left upper lobe pneumonia and possible right lower lobe pneumonia, urinary tract infection, sinus tachycardia, ventricular ectopy, and mental status changes. He was admitted for antibiotic therapy and supportive care. The patient was made DNR (do not resuscitate) and developed agonal rhythm early on the morning of 21 October and quietly expired.

GROSS AUTOPSY FINDINGS
The body is that of a cachectic white male appearing the stated age of 70 years, measuring approximately 5 feet 8 inches in height and weighing approximately 130 pounds. Hair is white with bitemporal baldness. The eyes are of a brownish-gray color, with 3 mm pupils. The nose is unremarkable. The mouth is opened and edentulous. The neck shows the trachea to be in the midline. There is no palpable cervical adenopathy. The thorax is symmetrical. There is a well-healed midline chest incision measuring 29 cm in length and a well-healed incision at the right fourth intercostal space measuring 21 cm. The abdomen is flat. There are right and left well-healed inguinal incisions measuring 12 cm each. There is no evidence of ascites, organomegaly, or palpable masses. The extremities reveal petechiae and scabs over both arms, abrasions over both knees, and petechiae over both ankles. There are puncture wounds noted at the right and left wrists and antecubital fossae and over the right ankle. The genitalia are those of a normal adult circumcised male. The back discloses a moderate amount of livor mortis, and a mid-thoracic spine and sacral decubitus. Rigor mortis is present in the upper and lower extremities.

INTERNAL EXAMINATION
The usual Y-shaped incision is made, disclosing musculature of normal hydration, as well as a panniculus measuring 0.5 cm. There is a wire suture in the central portion of the sternum. The organs of the thoracic and abdominal cavities are in their normal anatomic positions.

Thyroid: The thyroid shows a red-brown color and smooth contour. There is no evidence of tumor.

Respiratory system: There are diffuse obliterative adhesions of the pleura on the right and focal adhesions of the pleura on the left. A hydrothorax is present bilaterally, measuring less than 50 mL. The lungs weigh 1200 g on the left and 600 g on the right. The right lung shows a ragged, spongy consistency, with an area of consolidation in the lower lobe. The left lung shows firm, rubbery consolidation, with parenchymal cavitation in the upper lobe and a red, spongy, congested appearance in the lower lobe. Bronchi and bronchioles are lined by a thin, red-gray mucosa covered by pink, frothy material. No tumor is noted in the lungs. There is no evidence of pulmonary emboli.

Cardiovascular system: The heart weighs 600 g and shows evidence of biventricular dilatation. The pericardial sac is densely adherent to the epicardium and shows a 2 cm abscess cavity at the AV (atrioventricular) junction, along the left lateral/posterior wall. The myocardium is red-brown and mottled and shows multifocal fibrosis in the left ventricle and septum. In the left ventricle, the myocardium measures 1.5 cm in thickness and in the right ventricle 0.5 cm, exclusive of papillary muscles. The endocardium is smooth and moist and discloses no fibrosis or petechiae. The valve leaflets are thin and pliable and demonstrate no vegetations. The circumferences of the valves are tricuspid 11, pulmonary 8, mitral 11, aortic 6. The chordae tendineae are thin, discrete, and of normal length. The left coronary ostium is patent; the right coronary ostium appears to be attenuated. The aorta and main systemic vessels show slight arteriosclerotic change with plaques.

Spleen: The spleen weighs 200 g. The capsule is smooth. The cut surface is deep red in color and markedly hyperemic.

Liver: The liver weighs 1750 g and is of a red-brown color. The capsule is smooth, and the organ is firm. The parenchyma is homogeneous and of a red-brown color. The architecture is intact.

Gallbladder: The gallbladder is present, thin walled, and nondilated. It contains no stones.

Pancreas: The pancreas weighs 75 g. It is a light pinkish-tan organ that is lobular and cuts with normal resistance.

Gastrointestinal tract: There are no adhesions noted in the abdominal cavity. There is minimal free fluid in the peritoneal cavity; this measures less than 30 mL. The esophagus is patent and normal throughout; it enters the stomach in a normal fashion. The stomach is contracted and contains 20 mL of blood. There is a mesenteric tumor nodule noted adjacent to the jejunum. The appendix is present and unremarkable. The adrenals are normal in size, shape, and anatomic position.

Genitourinary system: The right kidney weighs 225 g, and the left kidney weighs 225 g. The capsules strip with ease. The subcapsular surfaces are finely granular and bear a few pitted scars. The right kidney shows multiple areas of yellow-tan, minute nodules measuring approximately 1 mm apiece. The renal arteries are unremarkable. The ureters are thin walled and nondilated. The urinary bladder is contracted and thick walled, containing less than 5 mL of cloudy urine. The prostate is unremarkable.

Central nervous system: The scalp is reflected in the usual manner, and the bony calvarium appears intact. The pachymeninges are thin, fibrous, and glistening. There is no evidence of previous laceration, contusion, or healed fracture. The cerebral hemispheres are rounded and reveal slightly atrophic convolutions and sulci. The venous tributaries are markedly congested. The brain weighs 1250 g. The vessels at the base of the brain are unremarkable. The pituitary is present in its usual anatomic position. Further examination of the brain parenchyma must follow thorough fixation.

Position

AHDI opposes the growing trend among healthcare facilities toward adopting a "verbatim" transcription policy, one that limits medical transcriptionists (MTs) to transcribing exactly what is dictated, regardless of error, and flagging all discrepancies for review by the dictator. AHDI believes this restricted role for documentation specialists ignores the contribution to risk management that MTs are trained and equipped to provide. A skilled, engaged MT partners with the dictating provider to ensure an accurate, timely, and secure record. Healthcare providers and facilities would be well served to recognize this contribution and empower MTs to be actively engaged in the story-telling of the patient encounter, noting discrepancies in grammar, style, and clinical information, and correcting those discrepancies that fall within the scope of the MT's knowledge and informed judgment.

Rationale

Routing discrepancies back to the dictator that could have been reasonably corrected by the transcriptionist has a direct impact on turn-around time and reimbursement. A significant delay in document work flow from patient encounter to reimbursement results when any record is flagged for provider review and correction. In an environment where even minor discrepancies must be flagged for review, the impact on turn-around time leads to backlog and delayed billing. Such a restrictive policy for editing and correction can be costly to the facility and burdensome to the medical records department who has to facilitate those corrections. MTs are risk management professionals equipped with an interpretive medical language skill set that should be *deployed*, not restricted, in the medical records setting to (a) ensure the accurate capture of clinical data, and (b) facilitate the forward progress of the record through the system.

Guidelines for MT Editing

AHDI recognizes that MTs are *not* engaged in provision of patient care and cannot be expected to have insight into the patient encounter beyond what is provided by the dictator. However, many discrepancies encountered in dictation represent areas of obvious error where correction falls within the scope of the interpretive skill set and clinical knowledge of the MT.

AHDI provides the following editing guidelines to MTs when addressing discrepancies in dictation:

Editing

Verbatim transcription of dictation is seldom possible. MTs should prepare reports that are as correct, clear, consistent, and complete as can be reasonably expected, without imposing their personal style on those reports. Editing is inappropriate in medical transcription when it alters information without the editor's being certain of the appropriateness or accuracy of the change, when it second-guesses the originator, when it deletes appropriate and/or essential information, and when it tampers with the originator's style. Edit grammar, punctuation, spelling, and similar dictation errors as necessary to achieve clear communication. Likewise, edit slang words and phrases, incorrect terms, incomplete phrases, English or medical inconsistencies, and inaccurate phrasing of laboratory data.

Dictation Problems

A variety of dictation problems may occur, and medical transcriptionists' being alert to them is a form of risk management. Watch for and correct obvious errors in dictation, including grammar, spelling, terminology, and style. When uncertain, draw suspected errors to the attention of the originator and/or supervisor. When the change would be significant, particularly if it would influence medical meaning, the MT should leave a blank and flag it. Never "close up" the space where the unintelligible word, phrase, or sentence belongs, making it appear that a transcript is complete. Likewise, do not transcribe the questionable dictation, adding [sic] to indicate it is transcribed verbatim. When the transcriptionist cannot determine how to edit the incorrect dictation properly, sometimes the best choice is to leave a blank and flag it. Appropriate use of blanks should prompt careful followup and contribute to patient care and risk management. A medical transcriptionist who identifies an inconsistency in dictation should resolve it if this can be done with competence and confidence. If the discrepancy cannot be resolved with certainty, the report should be flagged and brought to the attention of the supervisor or the report's originator for resolution.

Honoring a physician's dictation style, recognizing error or inconsistency in the record, correcting errors appropriately, refraining from correcting or altering what cannot be confirmed, protecting the integrity of the patient encounter, and ensuring the confidentiality of the record define what a skilled, qualified medical transcriptionist is engaged in every day. AHDI encourages facilities who currently embrace verbatim transcription to replace this policy with one that provides clear guidelines for appropriate editing that empowers their MTs to be a contributory part of the risk management process.

© 2007- *Association for Healthcare Documentation Integrity*

Appendix C: Usage Glossary

abdominal	pertaining to the abdomen
abominable	detestable; unpleasant or disagreeable
abduction	moving away from (often dictated as "a-b-duction")
adduction	drawing toward (often dictated as "a-d-duction")
aberrant	wandering; abnormal
apparent	clear or obvious; visible
abject	existing in a low condition, as in *abject poverty*
object	to oppose (v); something on which one is focused (n)
ablation	surgical removal
oblation	religious offering
accent	characteristic pronunciation
ascent	rising or moving upward; upward slope or incline
assent	to agree with (v); agreement (n)
accept	to receive willingly; to regard as proper
except	other than; to leave out or exclude
access	means of approach; the ability or right to approach
axis	center
excess	more than usual
acetic	sour
acidic	acid-forming
aesthetic	characterized by increased awareness of beauty
ascitic	pertaining to an accumulation of serous fluid in the abdominal cavity
asthenic	pertaining to or characterized by a lack or loss of energy
esthesic	mental perception of sensation
esthetic	improvement in appearance
adapt	to modify to fit a circumstance or requirement
adopt	to take or make one's own
adverse	contrary to one's interests; undesirable, unwanted, as in *adverse reaction*
averse	having a feeling of dislike or revulsion, as in *averse to taking risks*
advice	opinion about what should be done (n)
advise	to counsel, recommend, or inform (v)

aerogenous	gas-producing
erogenous	arousing erotic feelings, as in *erogenous zone*
affect	to influence (v), as in *he affected her deeply*; external expression of emotion (n), as in *a flat affect* (psych)
effect	to bring about (v), as in *effect a change*; result (n), as in *cause and effect*
afferent	toward a center
efferent	outward from a center
affusion	act of pouring a liquid on
effusion	liquid which escapes into tissue
infusion	introduction of a liquid solution through a vein or tissue
alfa	international spelling for alpha, as in interferon alfa
alpha	first letter of the Greek alphabet; the first one; the beginning
allude	make reference to
elude	evade
elute	extract or remove
allusion	indirect but pointed meaning or reference
elusion	the act of avoiding capture
elution	separation by washing of one solid from another
illusion	erroneous perception of reality
alkalosis	increased alkalinity of blood and tissues
ankylosis	immobilization of a joint
all	the whole amount
awl	a pointed instrument
a lot	to a considerable quality or extent
allot	to distribute or assign a share of something
alternate	a person acting in the place of another, as in *an alternate delegate* (n); to do by turns (v) alternating happening by turns, as in *alternating movements*
alternative	a choice between two possibilities, as in *the only alternative*
among	relationship in a group of more than 2
between	relationship of 1 entity to another

anecdote	an amusing or interesting short story
antidote	a remedy for counteracting a poison
anergia	inactivity
inertia	inability to move spontaneously
anuresis	retention of urine in the bladder
enuresis	involuntary bed-wetting
aphagia	refusal or inability to swallow
aphakia	absence of the lens of the eye
aphasia	speech disorder that involves a defect or loss of the power of expression by speaking, writing, or signing; also inability to comprehend spoken or written language
aplasia	lack of development of an organ or tissue
apposition	placing side by side or next to
opposition	contrary action or condition
appraise	set a value upon
apprise	inform or make known
assure	to cause to feel sure; to make safe or secure
ensure	to make sure or certain
insure	to protect against loss
astasia	inability to stand due to lack of muscle coordination
ectasia	dilation or expansion attacks spells; assaults
aura	a sensation or motor phenomenon preceding a paroxysmal attack (seizure)
aural	pertaining to the ear
ora	plural of os
oral	pertaining to the mouth
orale	point in the midline maxillary suture that is lingual to the central incisors
avert	to turn aside or turn away
evert	to turn inside out
invert	to turn inside out or upside down; to reverse the order
overt	open to view
ball valve	a heart valve
bivalve	consisting of two similar but separable parts

Usage Glossary

Beaver Deaver	brand name of a series of blades, knives, and keratomes retractor
bolus bullous	a single, rather large mass or quantity of a drug or medication that is administered either orally or intravenously relating to bullae
caliber calipers	the diameter of a projectile (bullet) or of a canal or tube a compass-like instrument used for measuring thicknesses
callous callus	hard like a callus; hardened in mind or feelings, as in *a callous attitude* a hardened or thickened area of skin; the meshwork of woven bone that forms at the site of a healing fracture, as in callus formation
carotid parotid	artery gland
caudal coddle	a position more toward the tail; often used as a synonym for inferior to pamper
cease seize	to stop doing; to come to an end to grab; to take by force; to convulse
cecal fecal thecal	pertaining to the cecum pertaining to feces pertaining to an enclosing case or sheath, as in *thecal sac*
cede seat seed	yield or grant, as in the tennis player was forced to cede the point to her opponent to cause or assist to sit down; to fix firmly in place, as with components of a joint replacement semen; a small shell used in application of radiation therapy
celiotomy ciliotomy	surgical incision into the abdominal cavity surgical division of the ciliary nerves
cell cella sella	smallest unit of life capable of existence an enclosure or compartment a saddle-shaped depression, as in *sella turcica*

cellular	consisting of cells; porous
sellar	pertaining to the sella turcica
cerise	deep to vivid purplish red
cereus	a genus of cactus
scirrhous	pertaining to or of the nature of a hard cancer
serous	pertaining to or resembling serum
cholic	an acid; relating to bile
colic	acute abdominal pain
chordae	plural of chorda; any cord or sinew
chordee	downward bowing of the penis
cilium	a hairlike projection from a cell
psyllium	the seed of a plant that is used as a mild laxative
circumcise	to remove the foreskin of the penis
circumscribe	to mark off carefully
cirrhosis	liver disease
xerosis	abnormal dryness, as seen in the eyes, skin, or mouth
cite	to quote as an authority or example; to mention as an illustration
-cyte	cell
sight	the function of seeing
site	a place or location
clonus	alternating muscular contraction and relaxation in rapid succession
conus	resembling a cone in shape
cornice	a decorative band
CNS	central nervous system
C&S	culture and sensitivity
collum	the neck
column	a pillar-like structure
complement	that which completes or makes perfect
compliment	an expression of praise or admiration
compose	to be a constituent of
comprise	to be composed of or include

continence	self-restraint; the ability to retain urine or feces
continents	land masses of the world
continual	recurring frequently
continuous	going on without interruption
council	an executive or advisory body
counsel	advice given as a result of a consultation
corollary	something that naturally follows
coronary	pertaining to the heart
creatine	high-energy phosphate
creatinine	product excreted in urine
keratin	scleroprotein formed in epidermis, hair, nails, and horny tissues
cremation	consumption by fire
crenation	abnormal notch found on microscopic exam of an erythrocyte
crus	a term used to designate a leg-like part
crux	a decisive point, as in *crux of the matter*
cytotoxin	a toxin or antibody that has a toxic action on cells of a specific organ
Cytoxan	an antineoplastic drug
sitotoxin	food poisoning
decision	a choice made among options
discission	an incision or cutting into
denervation	loss of nerve supply
enervation	loss of nervous energy
innervation	supply of nerves to a part
dental	relating to teeth or dentistry
dentil	one of a series of small rectangular blocks forming a molding
denticle	a conical pointed projection
identical	the same
desperate	frantic
disparate	markedly distinct in quality
device	equipment or mechanism designed for a purpose
devise	to plan, design, or contrive

diaphysis	the body or shaft of a long bone that ossified from a primary center
diathesis	inborn tendency to develop certain diseases or other abnormal conditions
diarrhea	abnormally loose and frequent bowel movements
diuria	a crystalline substance derivable from two molecules or urea
diuresis	excretion of abnormally high amounts of urine
discreet	a judicious reserve in one's speech or behavior
discrete	separate or individually distinct, as in *discrete mass*
dissension	strong disagreement; discord
distention	state of being distended or enlarged
dose	a quantity to be administered at a single time
dosage	a regimen or the regulated administration of doses over time
dysphagia	difficulty in swallowing
dysphasia	difficulty in speaking
dystaxia	difficulty in controlling voluntary movement
dystectia	defective closure of the neural tube, resulting in malformation
eczema	type of dermatitis
exemia	loss of fluid from blood vessels
ejection	expelling, throwing out
ingestion	taking of food or liquid into the body through the mouth
injection	a shot; congestion
elicit	to bring out or evoke, as in *elicit a response*
illicit	illegal, as in *illicit drugs*
emanate	to flow out or proceed from; to originate from
eminence	a prominence or projection, particularly of bone
eminent	important, well known, prominent
imminent	impending or about to occur
enema	injection of fluid into the rectum
intima	innermost structure
intimal	pertaining to the inner layer of a blood vessel

erasable	removable with an eraser
irascible	easily provoked to anger
facial	pertaining to the face
fascial	pertaining to or of the nature of fascia
faucial	pertaining to the passage from the mouth to the pharynx
false	not true
falx	a sickle-shaped organ or structure, as in *falx cerebri*
farther	physical distance, as in *driving farther than planned*
further	metaphoric distance, as in of time or degree – *further her career*
fascicle	a band or bundle of fibers, as in muscle or nerve
vesical	pertaining to the bladder
vesicle	a small sac containing fluid, as in *the lesions seen in chickenpox*
faze	to cause to be disconcerted, as in *the problem didn't faze him*
phase	a stage of development
phrase	a group of words
fibers	slender structures or filaments
fibrose	to form fibrous tissue
fibrous	composed of or containing fibers
filamentous	composed of long threadlike structures
velamentous	in the form of a sheet or veil
filiform	thread-shaped; a slender bougie
phalliform	shaped like a penis
piliform	shaped like or resembling hair
flanges	projecting borders or edges
phalanges	plural of phalanx; bones of the fingers or toes
fornix	arch-shaped roof of an anatomical space
pharynx	the throat (often mispronounced as "fair-nix")
fovea	a cup-shaped pit or depression
folia	plural of folium, a leaf-like structure
phobia	a fear or morbid dread

gaited	walking or running in a certain manner, as in *a gaited horse*
gated	an entrance or opening, as in *gated magnetic resonance cardiac imaging*
glands	cells that function as secretory or excretory organs
glans	a conical-shaped structure, as in *glans penis*
graft	tissue implanted from one point to another
graph	a diagram with connecting points
hear	to listen
here	where you are right now
hemolysis	disruption of the integrity of the erythrocyte
homolysis	lysis of a cell by extracts of the same type of tissue
heterotopia	displacement of parts or organs; presence of tissue in an abnormal location
heterotrophia	nutritional disorder
heterotropia	strabismus
HNP	herniated nucleus pulposus
H&P	history and physical
humerus	long bone in upper arm
humorous	funny
ileac	pertaining to the distal portion of the colon
iliac	pertaining to the superior portion of the hip bone
ileum	distal portion of the colon
ilium	superior portion of the hip bone
inanimate	without life or spirit, as in *an inanimate object*
innominate	nameless, as in *an innominate artery*
inanition	loss of vitality
inattention	failure to pay attention
inhibition	self-restriction of freedom of activity
incidence	rate or frequency of occurrence
incidents	single occurrences, events, or happenings
instance	case or example

infarction	necrosis caused by obstruction, as in *myocardial infarction*
infection	invasion of the body by organisms that can cause disease
inflection	change in vocal pitch or loudness; bending forward
infraction	incomplete fracture; breaking of a rule
installation	placing in a position or office
instillation	injecting slowly
irradiate	to treat with radioactivity
radiate	to spread out from a center, as in *the pain radiates into the lower leg*
jewel	a precious stone
joule	a unit of energy
jowl	a fold of flesh hanging from the jaw
karyon	nucleus
kerion	a secondarily infected granulomatous lesion
keloid	a hyperplastic scar
keroid	resembling horn or corneal tissue
kempt	referring to a neat appearance
kept	past tense of keep
labial	pertaining to a lip or lip-like structure
labile	unstable, as in labile blood pressure
lassitude	listlessness
latitude	freedom of choice; plane of reference
leap	to jump, as in over an object
LEEP	loop electrosurgical procedure (gyn)
lesser	smaller when comparing two things, as in *lesser evil*
lessor	one who conveys property by a lease
liable	responsible for
libel	defamation by written or printed words
libido	sexual desire
livedo	bluish discoloration of skin
lice	parasites
lyse	to break up or disintegrate, as in *lysis of adhesions*

lie	to recline, rest, or stay; to take a position of rest
lay	to put or place (requires an object)
lightening	decreasing in weight or color
lighting	illumination
lightning	a flash of light produced by electricity in the atmosphere
liver	large gland in the abdomen
livor	discoloration appearing on the body after death
loop	an oval or circular ring formed by bending a vessel or cylindrical organ
loupe	a magnifying glass
loose	not securely attached
lose	to misplace
meiosis	method of cell division
miosis	contraction of the pupil of the eye
mitosis	method of indirect cell division
mycosis	presence of parasitic fungi in the body
myiasis	infection due to invasion by larvae of dipterous insects
meiotic	pertaining to special cell division
miotic	causing contraction of the pupil of the eye
mitotic	pertaining to indirect division of a cell
myopic	nearsighted
menorrhagia	excessive uterine bleeding
menorrhalgia	painful menstruation; dysmenorrhea
metrorrhagia	uterine bleeding of abnormal amount, occurring at abnormal times
mnemonic	something intended to assist memory
pneumonic	related to or affecting the lungs
modeling	learning by observation and imitation
mottling	a condition of spotting with patches of color
mucous	adjective form of mucus; pertaining to or resembling mucus
mucus	free slime of the mucous membranes

myoclonic	demonstrating one of a series of shock-like muscular contractions, as in *a seizure*
myotonic	exhibiting delayed relaxation of a muscle after a strong contraction, or prolonged contraction after mechanical stimulation
nucleide	a compound of nucleic acid with a metallic element
nuclide	a species of atom
osteal	bony
ostial	pertaining to an ostium
pain	discomfort, distress, or agony
pane	a segment of window glass
pair	two of something
pare	to trim or remove skin
palate	roof of the mouth
palette	an oval board with a thumb-hole used by artists to mix their paints
pallet	a portable platform; a temporary bed made of folded blankets
palpable	may be felt with the hand
palpebral	pertaining to the eyelid
palpation	feeling with the fingers
palpitation	an abnormal, rapid heartbeat
papillation	a covering of small round protuberances
parotic	near the ear
perotic	characterized by perosis
porotic	favoring growth of connective tissue
peal	to ring, as a bell
peel	to strip away a layer
perfusion	the act of pouring over or through
profusion	abundance
protrusion	a jutting-out from the surrounding surface
perineal	pertaining to the perineum
peritoneal	pertaining to the peritoneum
peroneal	pertaining to the outer or fibular side of the leg

perspective	one's ideas; a way of looking at something
prospective	in the future, potential
phenol	carbolic acid
phenyl	derived from benzene
pheresis	removal from a donor; separation and retransfusion
-phoresis	word ending indicating transmission
plain	not fancy; radiograph, as in *plain abdomen*
plane	anatomic level, as in *the sagittal plane*
pleuritis	inflammation of the pleura
pruritus	itching
pleural	pertaining to the pleura of the lung
plural	more than one
precede	to go before
proceed	to continue on
precedent	coming before; an example
president	a governmental leader
prescribe	to order; to advise
proscribe	to banish or denounce; to forbid
principal	a leader, as in *high school principal*; a main participant, as in *principal diagnosis*; the main body of an estate or financial holding
principle	a basic truth; a rule or standard
prostate	a gland of the male urinary tract
prostrate	stretched out with the face upon the ground
prostatic	relating to the prostate gland
prosthetic	pertaining to an artificial device that replaces a body part
psoriasis	a dermatosis
siriasis	sunstroke
psychosis	mental disorder
sycosis	pustular inflammation of hair follicles

quiet	without noise
quite	completely
radical	extreme, drastic, or innovative; elements/atoms in uncombined state
radicle	smallest branch of a vessel
rectus	straight structure
rhexis	rupture of an organ
rictus	fissure or cleft; a gaping expression
ructus	a belching of wind
refection	recovery
reflection	bending back
refraction	deviation of light
regard	to look at or observe; to relate or refer to
regards	good wishes
regime	a form of government
regimen	a system of treatment designed to achieve certain ends
role	the part one plays
roll	to turn over (v); a list for attendance purposes (n)
saccadic	simultaneous movements of both eyes that are involuntary
psychotic	pertaining to a severe mental disorder
scatoma	a tumor-like mass in the rectum
scotoma	an area of depressed vision in the visual field
scleredema	unusual swelling of the facial area
scleroderma	chronic thickening and hardening of the skin
xeroderma	a mild form of ichthyosis
cereal	breakfast dish made from grains or wheat
serial	arranged in a series
sural	pertaining to the calf of the leg
shoddy	of poor workmanship or quality
shotty	resembling buckshot, as in *shotty nodes*
statue	a three-dimensional work of art
statute	a law enacted by a legislative body

subtle	so slight as to be difficult to detect or analyze
supple	moving or bending with agility; limber

Medical Transcriptionist Job Descriptions

Professional Levels

In an independent benchmarking study of the medical transcription profession by the Hay Management Consultants (HayGroup), three distinct professional levels for medical transcriptionists were identified and described as presented below. The HayGroup is a worldwide human resources consulting firm with extensive expertise in work analysis and job measurement.

Compensation

Subsequent to this benchmark study of the job content levels of MTs, the HayGroup conducted a compensation survey, analyzing pay as it relates to these levels. (Hay's survey methodology complied with federal antitrust regulations regarding healthcare compensation surveys.) The results include information on transcription pay at the corporate level (healthcare organizations and MT businesses) and compensation for independent contractors. The data are further presented by geographic region, size of business, types of pay programs (pay for time worked and pay for production), and reward programs (benefits, etc.). The Hay report, "Compensation for Medical Transcriptionists," is contained in a 30-page booklet, available to members upon request.

Position Summary

Professional Level 1
Medical language specialist who transcribes dictation by physicians and other healthcare providers in order to document patient care. The incumbent will likely need assistance to interpret dictation that is unclear or inconsistent, or make use of professional reference materials.

Professional Level 2
Medical language specialist who transcribes and interprets dictation by physicians and other healthcare providers in order to document patient care. The position is also routinely involved in research of questions and in the education of others involved with patient care documentation.

Professional Level 3
Medical language specialist whose expert depth and breadth of professional experience enables him or her to serve as a medical language resource to originators, coworkers, other healthcare providers, and/or students on a regular basis.

Nature of Work

Professional Level 1
An incumbent in this position is given assignments that are matched to his or her developing skill level, with the intention of increasing the depth and/or breadth of exposure. OR The nature of the work performed (type of report or correspondence, medical specialty, originator) is repetitive or patterned, not requiring extensive depth and/or breadth of experience.

Professional Level 2
An incumbent in this position is given assignments that require a seasoned depth of knowledge in a medical specialty (or specialties). OR The incumbent is regularly given assignments that vary in report or correspondence type, originator, and specialty. Incumbents at this level are able to resolve non-routine problems independently, or to assist in resolving complex or highly unusual problems.

Professional Level 3
An incumbent in this position routinely researches and resolves complex questions related to health information or related documentation. AND/OR Is involved in the formal teaching of those entering the profession or continuing their education in the profession. AND/OR Regularly uses extensive experience to interpret dictation that others are unable to clarify. Actual transcription of dictation is performed only occasionally, as efforts are usually focused in other categories of work.

Knowledge, Skills & Abilities

Professional Level 1

1. Basic knowledge of medical terminology, anatomy and physiology, disease processes, signs and symptoms, medications, and laboratory values. Knowledge of specialty (or specialties) as appropriate.
2. Knowledge of medical transcription guidelines and practices.
3. Proven skills in English usage, grammar, punctuation, style, and editing.
4. Ability to use designated professional reference materials.
5. Ability to operate word processing equipment, dictation and transcription equipment, and other equipment as specified.
6. Ability to work under pressure with time constraints.
7. Ability to concentrate.
8. Excellent listening skills.
9. Excellent eye, hand, and auditory coordination.
10. Ability to understand and apply relevant legal concepts (e.g., confidentiality).

Professional Level 2

1. Seasoned knowledge of medical terminology, anatomy and physiology, disease processes, signs and symptoms, medications, and laboratory values. In-depth or broad knowledge of a specialty (or specialties) as appropriate.
2. Knowledge of medical transcription guidelines and practices.
3. Excellent skills in English usage, grammar, punctuation, and style.
4. Ability to use an extensive array of professional reference materials.
5. Ability to operate word processing equipment, dictation and transcription equipment, and other equipment as specified, and to troubleshoot as necessary.
6. Ability to work independently with minimal or no supervision..
7. Ability to work under pressure with time constraints.
8. Ability to concentrate.
9. Excellent listening skills.
10. Excellent eye, hand, and auditory coordination.
11. Proven business skills (scheduling work, purchasing, client relations, billing).
12. Ability to understand and apply relevant legal concepts (e.g., confidentiality).
13. Certified medical transcriptionist (CMT) status preferred.

Professional Level 3

1. Recognized as possessing expert knowledge of medical terminology, anatomy and physiology, disease processes, signs and symptoms, medications, and laboratory values related to a specialty or specialties.
2. In-depth knowledge of medical transcription guidelines and practices.
3. Excellent skills in English usage, grammar, punctuation, and style.
4. Ability to use a vast array of professional reference materials, often in innovative ways.
5. Ability to educate others (one-on-one or group).
6. Excellent written and oral communication skills.
7. Ability to operate word processing equipment, dictation and transcription equipment, and other equipment as specified, and to troubleshoot as necessary.
8. Proven business skills (scheduling work, purchasing, client relations, billing).
9. Ability to understand and apply relevant legal concepts (e.g., confidentiality).
10. Certified medical transcriptionist (CMT) status preferred.

MT Editor Job Description

The medical transcription editor must be a highly skilled Level-2 medical transcriptionist with proven skills in all work types, specialties, accents, and dialects. The MT must possess acute auditory and acoustical sensitivity in coordination with keen hand/eye coordination, as would be expected in an experienced medical proofreader. The editor must also be proficient in referencing and researching, along with excellent communication skills to give consistent constructive feedback to the transcriptionists.

Supervisor Defined

Different facilities use different titles, e.g., editors, proofers, and proofreaders. The editor would report to a lead editor or transcription supervisor, as directed by the facility.

Minimum knowledge, skills, and abilities required:
- Must be a qualified professional Level-2 transcriptionist.
- Demonstrate ability to work in all work types and specialties.
- Demonstrate quality transcription work, consistently maintaining an accuracy score of 98% or higher.
- Certified transcriptionist preferred.
- Advanced knowledge of medical terminology, anatomy, physiology, disease processes, signs and symptoms, medications, and laboratory values.
- In-depth knowledge of medical transcription guidelines (The AAMT Book of Style) and practices.
- Excellent written and oral communication skills, including grammar, punctuation, and style, in order to provide quality feedback to the transcriptionist.
- Excellent acoustical skills.
- Demonstrate an understanding of the medicolegal implications and responsibilities of the healthcare record, ensuring compliance with local, state, and federal rules and regulations, along with security standards and privacy practices.
- Ability to understand diverse accents, dialects, and varying dictation styles.
- Proficient in referencing and researching.
- Full library of references (books/electronic) and Internet access.
- Ability to multi-task and work under pressure with time constraints.
- Ability to work independently with minimal or no supervision.
- Ability to operate computer, multiple software applications, transcription equipment, and other office equipment necessary, including the ability to accept voice/text files in multiple formats and word processing software.

- Organizational skills for file management.

Principal duties and responsibilities:

- Edit the transcribed document against actual dictation.
- Edit documents consistently and fairly according to transcription guidelines, standards of style, and formats of practice.
- Using preferred standard quality scoring guidelines, calculate and score reports consistently and fairly, weighing the varying degrees of errors against the documentation length.
- Utilize all available reference tools to ensure the accuracy of the transcribed document.
- Provide timely and consistent quality feedback to inform and update the transcriptionists regarding quality issues and areas of concern to help eliminate repetition of errors.
- Recognize, interpret, and evaluate inconsistencies, discrepancies, and inaccuracies in medical dictation and appropriately clarify and flag or report them, as needed.
- Identify potential risk management situations.
- Adhere to policies and procedures to contribute to the efficiency of the transcription department.
- Access patient's health information as needed for further clarification.
- Transcribe reports as needed.

Speech Recognition Medical Transcription Editor (SRMTE)
Job Description

Issue
This position statement outlines key areas of proficiency necessary for a speech recognition medical transcription editor. It is important to note that speech recognition is an evolving technology and may include other auto-generated medical texts and technologies. The level of accuracy achieved through the recognition process will impact the competency requirement of the medical transcriptionist.

AHDI Position
The speech recognition medical transcription editor (SRMTE) edits speech-recognized drafts and may also transcribe reports by physicians and other healthcare providers in order to document patient care. The responsibilities for a person with basic MT qualifications may vary depending on their demonstration of skill in various work types, specialties, accents, and dialects.

Assignments are given to match his/her skill level with the intention of increasing the depth and/or breadth of exposure, continually improving quality and productivity. As the SRMTE gains expertise in speech-recognition editing, they may serve as a resource to coworkers and dictators within the editing/transcription team researching questions, educating, and coaching coworkers toward an improved level of efficiency and skill.

Minimum knowledge, skills, and abilities required

PROFESSIONAL/BUSINESS SKILLS
- Understanding of the medicolegal implications and responsibilities of the healthcare record, ensuring compliance with local, state, and federal rules and regulations, along with security standards and privacy practices.
- Ability to multi-task and work under pressure with time constraints.
- Ability to work independently with minimal or no supervision.
- Organizational skills for file management.
- Actively participates in continuing education
- Maintains and assesses equipment and work area with minimal supervision.
- Demonstrates an understanding of area systems, priorities, timelines and goals that contribute to the mission of the department.
- Basic understanding of departmental technology.

TECHNICAL/SYSTEM SKILLS:

- Strong technical proficiency in computer applications so those measurable gains through system efficiencies are continually maximized in conjunction with speech recognition and other technologies available.
- Ability to operate computer, multiple software applications, transcription equipment, and other office equipment necessary, including the ability to accept voice/text files in multiple formats and word processing software.
- Desire to keep up to date and learn latest technology advancements and trends.
- Continually develops understanding of multiple computer applications and document management programs in order to effectively contribute and adapt to the changing healthcare environment.

QUALITATIVE/TRANSCRIPTION SKILLS:

- Developing ability to work in all work types and specialties.
- Knowledge of medical terminology, anatomy and physiology, disease processes, signs and symptoms, medications, and laboratory values.
- Developing quality transcription work with a goal of maintaining accuracy score of 98% or higher.
- Knowledge of medical transcription guidelines (*The Book of Style for Medical Transcription*) and practices.
- Developing ability to understand diverse accents, dialects, and varying dictation styles, commonly confused terms, and knowledge of homonyms.
- Proficient in referencing and researching with full library of references (books/electronic) and Internet access.
- Acute auditory sensitivity and keen hand/eye coordination, as would be expected in medical transcription.
- Edit a speech recognized draft document against actual dictation.
- Edit documents consistently in order to maximize the efficiencies gained through recognition.
- Utilize all available reference tools to ensure the accuracy of the transcribed document.
- Recognize, interpret, and evaluate inconsistencies, discrepancies, and inaccuracies in medical text drafts and/or dictation appropriately to clarify, flag, or report them, as needed.
- Adhere to policies and procedures to contribute to the efficiency of the transcription department.
- Transcribe reports as required.

INTERPERSONAL SKILLS:

- Excellent written and oral communication skills, including grammar, punctuation, and style, in order to provide quality feedback to the transcriptionist.
- Communicate and interact productively with management personnel with objective feedback as needed.

MT QA Manager Job Description

The quality assurance manager must be a highly skilled editor with proven experience in the medical transcription profession. He or she must have demonstrated fair and unbiased judgment with the ability to review and coordinate a random review process of documents. This includes the process of monitoring, measuring, and reporting transcribed documents by transcriptionists and documents reviewed by editors.

Supervisor Defined

Different facilities use different titles, e.g., quality assurance coordinator, team leader, lead editor, or quality assurance specialist. The quality assurance manager would report to the transcription supervisor or as directed by the facility.

Minimum knowledge, skills, and abilities required:

- Must be a highly qualified editor.
- Demonstrated leadership/management skills.
- Demonstrate ability to work in all work types and specialties.
- Demonstrate quality transcription work, consistently maintaining an accuracy score of 98% or higher.
- Certified transcriptionist preferred.
- Advanced knowledge of medical terminology, anatomy, physiology, disease processes, signs and symptoms, medications, and laboratory values.
- In-depth knowledge of medical transcription guidelines (The Book of Style for Medical Transcription) and practices.
- Excellent written and oral communication skills, including grammar, punctuation, and style, in order to provide consistent quality feedback to the transcriptionists, editors, and supervisors.
- Excellent acoustical skills.
- Demonstrate an understanding of the medicolegal implications and risk management responsibilities of the healthcare record, ensuring compliance with local, state, and federal rules and regulations.
- Ability to understand diverse accents, dialects, and varying dictation styles.
- Proficient in referencing, researching, reporting, tracking, and monitoring.
- Ability to multi-task with multiple priorities and time frames.
- Ability to work independently with minimal or no supervision.
- Ability to operate computer, multiple software applications, transcription equipment, and other equipment necessary, including the ability to accept voice/text files in multiple formats and word processing software.

- Organizational skills for file management.
- Mathematical skills, including calculations and statistics.
- Ability to communicate QA concerns/questions effectively with client/user.

Principal duties and responsibilities:

- Direct efforts toward quality documentation, including providing procedures, training, and resources for transcription team members.
- Establish guidelines for identifying qualified applicants for transcription and quality assurance staff positions.
- Develop standards for employee performance review related to quality documentation.
- Establish criteria for quality reviews.
- Establish policies and procedures that contribute to the efficiency of the transcription department.
- Through a standard random selection process, select randomly transcribed or edited reports for review.
- Review the transcribed report against actual dictation, applying industry-specific standards provided by current resources and references.
- Using preferred standard quality scoring criteria, calculate and score reports consistently and fairly, weighing the varying degrees of errors against the documentation length.
- Provide timely and consistent feedback to the medical transcriptionist or editor in order to eliminate repetition of errors, build skills, and mentor the medical transcriptionist/editor.
- Recognize, interpret, and evaluate inconsistencies, discrepancies, and inaccuracies in the medical dictation, and appropriately clarify and/or report them as required.

Appendix E: Industry Abbreviations

The following is a list of abbreviations and credentials used within the healthcare documentation domain and/or medical records industry:

AHDI   Association for Healthcare Documentation Integrity (*www.ahdionline.org*) *formerly* the American Association for Medical Transcription

AHIMA   American Health Information Management Association (*www.ahima.org*)

ASTM   American Society for Testing and Materials

CCA   Certified Coding Associate

CCS   Certified Coding Specialist

CCS-P   Certified Coding Specialist – Physician Based

CHP   Certified in Healthcare Privacy

CHS   Certified in Healthcare Security

CHPS   Certified in Healthcare Privacy & Security

CMT   Certified Medical Transcriptionist

EHR   electronic health record

EMR   electronic medical record

FTE   full-time employees

FTP   file transfer protocol

HIM   health information management

HIMSS   Healthcare Information and Management Systems Society (*www.himss.org*)

HIPAA   Health Insurance Portability and Accountability Act

HL7   Health Level 7

IP   internet protocol (as in *IP address*)

ISP	internet service provider
ISMP	Institute for Safe Medication Practices (*www.ismp.org*)
JC	The Joint Commission (*www.jointcommission.org*)
MGMA	Medical Group Management Association (*www.mgma.org*)
MRI	Medical Records Institute (*www.medrecinst.com*)
MT	medical transcriptionist
MTIA	Medical Transcription Industry Association (*www.mtia.com*)
MTS	medical transcription service
MTSO	medical transcription service owner
QA	quality assurance
RHIA	Registered Health Information Administrator
RHIT	Registered Health Information Technologist
RMT	Registered Medical Transcriptionist
SR	speech recognition
SRT	speech recognition technology
ROI	return on investment
TAT	turn-around time
TEPR	Toward the Electronic Patient Record
VPN	virtual private network
VR	voice recognition
VRT	voice recognition technology

AHDI Abbreviations: The following is a list of abbreviations used specifically through and by the association and its members:

ACE   Annual Convention and Exposition

BOD   Board of Directors

CEC   continuing education credit

HOD   House of Delegates

NMTW   National Medical Transcriptionist Week

Index

A

classification systems, 329–331
  angina, 329
  atrial fibrillation, 331
  coronary artery angiography, 331
  dermatology/allergy/immunology, 369–371
  diabetes, 453–454
  heart failure, 330
  myocardial infarction, 330
  obstetrics/gynecology/pediatrics, 406–408,
    413–415
  oncology and, 356–361
  ophthalmology, 422
  orthopedics/neurology, 388–390, 398–399
  psychiatry, 439
  pulmonary/respiratory, 448–449
classification terms, numbers and, 239
clauses, 73–76
  adjective, 75
  adverb, 76
  dependent/subordinate, 74
  elliptical clauses, 76
  essential, 119
  independent, 73–74, 112
  intervening, 92
  nonessential, 119
  noun, 75
Clinical Document Architecture, Release 2 (CDA
    R2), 467–470
Clinical Document Architecture for Common
    Document Types (CDA4CDT), 3, 462,
    465–473
  background and objectives, 465–466
  HL7 and interoperability and, 466–467
  implications for the medical transcription sec-
    tor, 469–473
  templates and implementation guides,
    467–469
  workgroup, 467
clock referents, numbers and, 239
clotting factor variants, 348
clusters of differentiation (CDs), 371
cm, 199, 277
code names, pharmacology and, 298
codes, pacemaker, 328

collective nouns, 59, 96
College of American Pathologists (CAP), 476
colons, 121–123
  first word capitalization following, 147–148
  numbers and, 231
  ratios expressed with, 266
colony-stimulating factors
  dermatology/allergy/immunology, 376–377
  drug nomenclatures, 310–312
combining numerals with words, 234–235
commas
  numbers and, 231, 235
  separating, 110–118
    adjectives, 110–111
    dates, 115
    dialogue, 117
    genetics, 116
    geographic names and addresses, 116
    independent clauses, 112
    introductory elements, 113
    items in a simple series, 111–112
    laboratory values, 118
    numbers, 113–118
    omitted word(s), 117
    titles, 115
    units of measure, 117
  setting off, 118–121
    afterthoughts, 120
    appositives, 119
    interrupting elements, 119
    nonessential expressions, basic rules for,
      118–119
    transitional words and phrases, 120–121
common names, 423–424
common nouns, 58
common prefixes, units of measure, 287
common-gender antecedents, 100
compass points, capitalization and, 164
competency, tests for, 439
complements, subject, 70
complete predicate, 68
complete subject, 68
complex sentence, 77
Component Name column, 470

delivery, 405–406
dementia, tests for, 440
demographics, 29–30
demonstrative pronouns, 61
deoxyribonucleic acid, 333
Department of Health and Human Services
    (HHS), 37, 50–51, 411, 477, 478
departments, divisions and specialties, capitaliza-
    tion and, 155–157
dependent/subordinate clauses, 74
depression, tests for, 439
derived quantities, 274
derived units, 274
dermatology/allergy/immunology, 365–379
    CD cell markers, 371
    classification systems for, 369–371
    colony-stimulating factors, 376–377
    cytokines/chemokines, 371–372
    HLA/histocompatibility, 373
    immunoglobulins, 374
    interferons, 374–375
    interleukins, 375–376
    lymphocytes, 377–379
    terminology for, 365–368
    testing and procedures for, 368
designations
    capitalization and, 149–153, 154, 161–162
    chromosomes, 339–340
    copy, 17–18
diabetes terminology and classification, 453–454
diagnoses, 18–19
    plurals and, 174–175
    psychiatric and DSM, 437
Diagnostic and Statistical Manual of Mental
    Disorders (DSM), 436–437
diagnostic terms, for ophthalmology, 417–419
diagnostic testing and procedures
    cardiology and, 321–329
    cardioversion/defibrillation, 328–329
    echocardiography, 327
    EKG and tracing, 323–326
    laboratory tests, 322–323
    orthopedics/neurology, 393–398
    pacemaker codes, 328

diagonal, 138
dialogue, 117
dictation
    habits, 483
    missing/inaudible, 31–32
    problem, 49–50
Dictation Best Practices Tool Kit, 49–50
dictator style, 31
dictator/transcription initials, 15–16
diction, 101
Dietary Supplement Health and Education Act of
    1994, 314
differential blood count, 346
digits, multiple, 232–233
diopter, 420
direct objects, 68, 69
direct quotation, 435
direct quotes, 32
directional and positional terms, 382
disc areas, 418
disc diameters, 418
disc/disk, 393
discharge summaries, 5–6, 21
disclosures, 37–38
diseases
    named after people, capitalization of, 155
    third class, 453
disk spaces, intervertebral, 270
disk/disc, 393
disorder terms, psychiatric, 437
disorganized, 437
distance acuity, 419
-distim suffixes, 311, 377
ditto marks, 220
division symbol, 220
divisions
    capitalization and, 155–157
    word, 125
dL, 277
DNA, 333–334
DNR, 215
do not resuscitate, 215
Do Not Use abbreviations, 207–211
.doc documents, 466

Epworth Sleepiness Scale, 448–449
equal/equal to symbols, 220
equipment
    eponymous, capitalization of, 155
    for ophthalmology, 419–421
equivalence/duality, 139
ERG (electroretinogram), 421
erythrocytes, 344–345
erythropoietin blood factors, 312
esophageal leads, 324
essential clauses, 119
EU Data Privacy Directive, 43
euro, 248
evaluation and diagnostic terms, for ophthalmol-
    ogy, 417–419
evaluations, gynecologic, 402
events, awards and legislation, capitalization and,
    162–163
every one, 92
everybody, 92
everyone, 92
everything, 92
evolved potential testing, 395–397
-ex suffixes, 132
exam/examination, 218
examination, mental status, 438
except, 92
exceptions, numbers and, 230–236
exclamation point, 110
exclamatory sentence, 79
exertional angina, 329
Expert Committee on the Diagnosis and
    Classification of Diabetes Mellitus, 453
exponential expressions, 279
expressions
    nonessential, 118–119
    numeric, proportions and, 264
    parenthetical, capitalization and, 148–149
extensible markup language (XML), 43

F

FAB classification, 358–359

facility policy, abbreviations and, 195
Fahrenheit, 284
false singulars, 177
The Family Practice Notebook: Psychiatry (Moses),
    440
family titles, capitalization and, 150–151
faxes, sending and receiving, 45–46
Federal Register, 54
Federal Rule of Evidence 803, 52
Federation Internationale de Gynécologie et
    Obstérique, 407
FIGO staging, 360, 407
file transfer, electronic, 47
Final Privacy Rule, 54
finding, negative, 32
fingerbreadth, 384
first, 230, 257
first words, capitalizing, 146–149
first-time reference, abbreviations and, 196
flagging the report, 33–34
flow cytometry, 352–353
fluctuation/fluctuance, 384
fluids, intravenous, numbers and, 258–259
followthrough, 132
followup, 132
font, 11
for, 112
for example, 121, 124
foreign nouns, 95
foreign terms, plurals and, 177–182
formal and vernacular names, viruses and, 432
formats, 8–19, 461–463
    character spacing, 12–13
    continuation pages, 17
    copy designation, 17–18
    diagnosis, 18–19
    dictator/transcription initials, 15–16
    headings/subheadings, 13–15
    margins, 9–10
    paragraphs, 11
    salutation, 10
    signature blocks, 15
    time/date stamping, 16–17
    type style, 11–12

former, 132
formerly, 427
-form/-forme suffixes, 367
forms
    irregular, plurals and, 171–172
    short, abbreviations and, 214–219
forms and routes, pharmacology and, 301–303
forms/symbols, acceptable, abbreviations and,
        213–223
formulas, chemical nomenclature and, 296
Forrester classification system, 330
forward slash (/), 138–142. *see also* virgule or
        forward slash (/)
fractions, 134, 142, 243–245
French Catheter Scale, 251
frequency, 394
from... through, 134
from... to, 132
front-end SRT, 481
FSN (fully specified name), 476
fully specified name (FSN), 476
fundal height, 405
future perfect tense, 83
future tense, 83
F-wave study, 398

G

g, 276, 277
GAF (global assessment of functioning), 439
gamma, 312
Garden classification, 388
GARF (global assessment of relational function-
        ing), 439
Gartner Report, 482
gas abbreviations, 443
G-CSFs (granulocyte colony-stimulating factors),
        311, 376
gene nomenclature
    human, 333–338
    nonhuman, 341–342
generic names
    capitalization and, 158

pharmacology and, 299
genes
    and gene symbols, 334–336
    tumor suppressor, 338
genetic testing, 409–411
genetics, 116, 333–342
    chromosomes, 338–341
    human gene nomenclature, 333–338
    nonhuman gene nomenclature, 341–342
    obstetrics/gynecology/pediatrics, 408–411
genotype and phenotype, 336–337
genus names, 425–427
geographic names, 97
    abbreviations and, 200
    and addresses, 116
    capitalization and, 160–161
gerund, 72
gerund phrase, 73
gestational age, 404
gestational diabetes mellitus, 454
Glasgow coma scale, 398
Gleason tumor grade, 360
global assessment of functioning (GAF), 439
global assessment of relational functioning
        (GARF), 439
GM-CSFs (granulocyte-macrophage colony-
        stimulating factors), 311, 376
Goldmann perimetry, 421
GPA (gravida, para, abortus), 402–404
grade, 422
gram (unit of measure), 276, 277
gram staining, 429
grammar, 24, 57–79
    abbreviations, 200–205
    clauses, 73–76
    parts of a sentence, 68–70
    parts of speech, 57–67
    phrases, 70–73
    sentence classification, 77–79
gram-negative, 155
-gramostim suffixes, 311
granulocyte colony-stimulating factors (G-CSFs),
        311, 376

granulocyte-macrophage colony-stimulating factors (GM-CSFs), 311, 376
-*grastim* suffixes, 311
gravida, para, abortus (GPA), 402–404
greater linear dimension, 418
greater/greater than/less than symbols, 220
Greek letters, 221
group designation for chromosomes, 339–340
growth hormone, 307
guessing, 30
Guide for the Use of the International System of Units, 288
gynecologic evaluations, 402
gynecology, 401–415. *see also* obstetrics/gynecology/pediatrics

H

habits, dictation, 483
half normal saline solution, 258–259
Harvard criteria for brain death, 398
head diameter, 252, 386
headings
    in referenced report, capitalization and, 165–166
    and subheadings, 13–15
health information, protected. *see* protected health information (PHI)
Health Information Transcription and Documentation, 461
Health Level Seven (HL7), 3, 11, 52, 53–54, 461, 469, 477, 478
    HL7 Clinical Document Architecture, Release 2 (Dolin, et al), 473
    HL7 Reference Information Model, 477
    HL7 RIM, 466–467
    interoperability and, 466–467
Healthcare Data Analysis, 461
healthcare document formats, standardized, 461–463
Healthcare Informatics, 8
heart failure, classification systems and, 330
heart sounds, 318

height, fundal, 405
helping verbs, 64
hematocrit, 345
hematology, 343–353
    blood groups/types, 343–344
    erythrocytes, 344–345
    flow cytometry, 352–353
    histocompatibility, 350–351
    leukocytes, 345–346
    lymphocytes, 346–347
    platelets and hemostasis, 347–350
    smears and stains, 351–352
hemoglobin, 345
hemophilias, 349
hemostasis, 347–350
hepatitis, 432–433
hepatitis nomenclature, 432–433
herbals and supplements, nomenclatures for, 314–315
here are, 98
here is, 98
hertz, 277
HGNA (Human Gene Nomenclature Committee), 333
HHCC, 477
HHS. *see* Department of Health and Human Services (HHS)
HIPAA, 37, 38–39, 42, 43, 44, 45–46, 52
    accountable parties under, 36–37
HIPAA Health Insurance Portability and Accountability Act of 1996, 35
HIPAA Privacy Final Rule – Amendment of Protected Health Information, 52
histocompatibility, 350–351, 373
historic present tense, 82
History
    of present illness, 467
history
    obstetrical, 402–404
    and physical examinations, 19
    and physical note, 470–471
History and Physical Examination, 3, 462
history and physical examination, 6
History and Physical Notes, 467

indexing, audio, 33
indicative mood, 84
indirect objects, 68, 69
infinitive, 73
infinitive phrase, 73
information
    contradictory, 32
    protected, 36
information integrity, 49–54
    authentication issues, 50–51
    corrections, revisions and addenda, 51–54
    problem dictation, 49–50
initialisms, 194
    capitalization and, 166
initials, dictator/transcription, 15–16
injection, 418
INN (international proprietary name), 314
instruments, surgical, 386–387
    eponymous, capitalization of, 155
insulin, drug nomenclatures, 308–309
insulin-dependent diabetes, 453, 454
integrity of information, 49–54
intensive pronouns, 60
interferons
    dermatology/allergy/immunology, 374–375
    drug nomenclatures, 309
interleukin 3 (IL-3) factors, 311, 377
interleukins, 375–376
    drug nomenclatures, 310
International Code of Nomenclature of Bacteria
    (Sneath), 433
International Organization for Standards, 272
international proprietary name (INN), 314
International Society of Blood Transfusion (ISBT),
    343
International System of Units (SI), 262, 272
interoperability, 466–467
interpersonal skills, 486
interrogative pronouns, 60
interrogative sentence, 79
interrupting elements, 119
intervening clauses, 92
intervening phrases, 92
intervertebral disk spaces, 270

intransitive verbs, 63
intravenous fluids, numbers and, 258–259
introductory elements, 113
inverted sentences, 98
irreconcilable words and phrases, 32
irregular forms, plurals and, 171–172
ISBT (International Society of Blood Transfusion),
    343
ISMP, 207, 217
    abbreviations, 211–213
isotopes, drug nomenclatures, 312–313
italics, 11–12
    viruses, 431
items in a simple series, 111–112
IV fluids, numbers and, 258–259

J

Jaeger system, 419
jargon, 25–27
Jewett classification of bladder carcinoma, 360
Joint Commission, 19, 20, 21, 22, 50, 460
    abbreviations and, 206–211
joint possession, 189
*Journal of the American Association for Medical
    Transcription*, 54
*Journal of the American Medical Informatics
    Association*, 473
Jr./Sr., 115, 218
jugular venous pulse, 320–321
juvenile-onset diabetes, 453

K

Karnofsky rating status, 360
karyotypes, 341
Kelvin, 285
-kin suffixes, 310
Kirschner wires, 243, 253, 387
k-space, 452
Kurtzke disability score, 399
K-wires, 243, 253, 387

quotes, direct, 32

R

radiation therapy, 362–363
radiology, 451–452
Radiology Notes, 467
radiotherapy, 362
Rancho Los Amigos cognitive function scale, 399
ranges, 134, 261–262, 267–270
    blood pressure with, 268–269
    EKG leads, 269
    hyphen *vs.* to, 267
    intervertebral disk spaces, 270
    with large numbers, 268
    money, 269
    with over or out of, 268
    percents in, 263
rather than, 92
ratios, 261–262, 266
    colons and, 266
    to or hyphen and, 266
re- prefix, 451
reading vision, 419
receiving faxes, 45–46
record privacy, 35–41
    accountable parties under HIPAA, 36–37
    audit trails, 39
    confidentiality, 36
    inclusion of PHI, 40–41
    penalties, 38–39
    permitted disclosure, 37–38
    precedence of state laws, 39
    protected health information, 36
    reporting of disclosures, 38
    retention of PHI, 39–40
record security, 44–48
    electronic file transfer, 47
    electronic system security, 46–47
    physical transport of PHI, 45
    sending and receiving faxes, 45–46
    storage of PHI, 48
records, ancillary, 31

referenced report headings, capitalization and, 165–166
references, legal and academic, capitalization of, 152–153
referents
    clock, 239
    numeric, 237–259
    time, 254–258
reflective pronouns, 59, 60
reflexes, 385–386
refraction, 420
regimens, multi-drug, 313
region-based terms, 382
regular type, 11
relative pronouns, 60
relaxation times, 452
-relin suffixes, 307
-relix suffixes, 307
report, notification and flagging, 33–34
report headings, referenced, capitalization and, 165–166
report section titles, abbreviations and, 197–198
report types, 3–8
    autopsy, 4
    consultation, 4–5
    correspondence, 5
    death summary, 5
    discharge summary, 5–6
    history and physical examination, 6
    operative, 7
    pathological, 7–8
    progress note, 8
    SOAP note, 8
reporting of disclosures, 38
resolution of standards/style conflicts, 486–487
resources, 22
respirations per minute, 444
respiratory, 441–449. *see also* pulmonary/respiratory
retention of PHI, 39–40
return on investment (ROI), 483–484
revisions, integrity and, 51–54
Rhodes, Harry, 54
ribonucleic acid, 334

psychiatric/psychological, 439–440

testing, genetic, 409–411

tests, laboratory, 322–323

than/as, 89–90

that, 119

that is, 121, 124

the, 248

The AAMT Book of Style, 2nd Edition, 54

therapy, radiation, 362–363

there are, 98

there is, 98

therefore, 120

these, 122

thinking, critical, 30

third class diseases, 453

third interspace leads, 324

thousand, 235

thread diameter, 252, 386

thrombolysis in myocardial infarction (TIMI), 331

through, 392

thus, 122

thyroid hormones, 308

time, 98

    turn-around, 19–21

    units of, 282–283

time, military, 254–255

time referents, 254–258

time span, 255

time zones, 255–256

time/date stamping, 16–17

times, seasons and holidays, capitalization and, 165

TIMI (thrombolysis in myocardial infarction), 331

titles, 115

    abbreviations and, 197–198

    capitalization and, 149–153

    family, 150–151

    personal, 149–150, 174

    plurals, 174

    publications and articles, 151–152

TNM staging system for malignant tumors, 354–355

to, 392

    hyphen *vs.*, 267

    ratios expressed with, 266

together with, 92

tonight/yesterday, 214, 256

TPAL system, 403–404

tracing, 323–326

trade names, 298

transcription initials, 15–16

transcription skills, 485–486

transitional words and phrases, 120–121

transitive verbs, 63

transport of PHI, 45

treatment, pulmonary/respiratory, 444–447

tumor suppressor genes, 338

tumors, malignant, 354–355

turn-around times, 19–21

.txt documents, 466

type 1 diabetes, 453

type 2 diabetes, 453

type style, 11–12

U

ulcers, decubitus, 370

UMLS (Unified Medical Language System), 477

uncertain meanings, abbreviations and, 198

underlined type, 11

Unified Medical Language System (UMLS), 477

Uniform Rules of Evidence, 51

Union Internationale Contre le Cancer, 354

United States Library of Medicine, 477

United States Pharmacopeia (USP), 272, 305

    equipment sizes, 251

units and properties, basic, 273, 281

units of measure, 97, 117, 271–288

    abbreviations and, 199

    convention (nonmetric) units, 280–285

    derived, 274

    metric units, 272–280

    quick reference guides, 286–288

    by type, 286

units of time, 282–283

irreconcilable words and phrases, 32
missing/inaudible dictation, 31–32
negative findings, 32
when to edit, 24–30
  back formations, 27–28
  contextual inconsistencies, 29
  demographics, 29–30
  grammar/punctuation, 24
  incorrect terms, 28
  slang, jargon and brief forms, 25–27
  spelling, 25
  syntax, 24–25
  transposition of terms and values, 29
which, 119
who *vs.* whom, 88–89
wires, 251–253, 386–387
with, 97
word(s), omitted, 117
word choice, 101
word division, 125
Word documents (.doc), 466
words
  capitalizing first, 146–149
  combining with numerals, 234–235
words and phrases
  irreconcilable, 32
  transitional, 120–121
World Health Assembly, 272
World Health Organization, 299
www.hl7.org, 473

X

X12, 461
XML (extensible markup language), 43, 467–468
x-rays, 451
X/x symbols, 223

Y

year(s), 257
  in date, 115
yesterday, 256

Z

z, 393
zero, 236
zero, less than, 263–264
zip code, 116

Medical Transcription Education Program Approval

What is Medical Transcription Program Approval?

The medical transcription program approval process was instituted by the Association for Healthcare Documentation Integrity (AHDI, formerly AAMT) to encourage compliance with AHDI's *Model Curriculum for Medical Transcription*, maintain sound educational programming, produce competent entry-level medical transcriptionists, and provide assurance to the public of consistency and quality outcomes for medical transcription education. Programs must comply with specific educational and institutional criteria as established by AHDI. There is no formal accreditation process for medical transcription programs.

What are the steps that lead to Program Approval?

1. Interested programs should obtain a copy of the *AHDI Model Curriculum* and download the *Medical Transcription Program Approval Manual* from the AHDI website – *http://www.ahdionline.org/scriptcontent/eduprogramapproval.cfm*

2. Programs must submit a $200 nonrefundable deposit with a Letter of Intent and a copy of the Gap Analysis for review. Copies of both are available at the web address listed above under #1. The Gap Analysis will be reviewed and returned to the program director with any recommendations before formally moving forward with remainder of full application fees due.

3. Programs complete the application process and submit binders containing complete compliance data to be reviewed and the remainder of the approval fee to the AHDI office in Modesto. Compliance data may not be submitted piecemeal, and must be sent at least 8 weeks prior to the anticipated next quarterly meeting of ACCP. Binders are then sent to volunteer peer reviewers and a recommendation is made to the ACCP (Approval Committee for Certificate Programs).

4. The ACCP meets quarterly to review applications. They issue a decision – approved, approved with condition, approval withheld, or approval denied – and the decision is shared with the programs following completion of the meeting.

How long is approval good for?

Program approval is valid for 3 years from the date of approval. Before the end of the 3-year period, the program needs to re-apply.

Is there a cost involved in Program Approval?

The total cost for approval is $1500 for AHDI members and $1800 for nonmembers.

Is there a list of currently approved programs available?

To see a list of currently approved programs visit *www.ahdionline.org/scriptcontent/ mtapproved.cfm*

Got Credentials?

Why Not?

A growing number of companies in the US are recognizing the link between certified professionals and quality documentation outcomes. Many are now seeking, reimbursing, and compensating the credential in the marketplace. Advance Magazine's 2007 Salary Survey showed that "The number of certified medical transcriptionists (CMTs) rose about 1 percent from last year, and the pay for CMTs grew from $31,949 last year to a $37,864 in 2007."[1]

Registered Medical Transcriptionist (RMT)

The Registered Medical Transcriptionist credential was developed to assure consumers and employers that successful candidates are qualified to practice medical transcription. It is based on the skills and knowledge described in the AHDI Model Job Description Level 1 MT and the competencies outlined in the AHDI Model Curriculum. This credential is ideal for recent graduates of transcription training programs and practitioners with limited work experience.

Certified Medical Transcriptionist (CMT)

Certified Medical Transcriptionists have demonstrated the knowledge and skill set of a Level 2 MT as described in the AHDI Model Job Description. Possession of the CMT credential confirms the commitment to lifelong learning and professional development. Successful CMT candidates have a minimum of 2 years of acute care transcription experience.

What Your Colleagues Are Saying

The process of preparing for and taking the RMT test greatly increased my confidence and reinforced all that I had learned during my medical transcription course, making me feel ready to enter the work force. I had no trouble passing the pre-employment test with the company I am now working for as a full-time MT.
– Mary McLaughlin, RMT since 2007

Obtaining the CMT certification proved to be a valuable stepping stone in my career. I received a promotion shortly afterwards. As we centralized our pool of transcriptionist I felt the CMT credential aided in my credibility as a supervisor. I went on to obtain a Bachelors in Nursing and currently teach transcription at a community college as well.
– Cheryl Klopcic, CMT since 1999

Striving for something that seems unreachable is a great challenge – accomplishing it is a great reward!
– Debbie Bright-Chunn, BS, RHIT, CMT since 2003

I took the CMT exam for personal gratification and a sense of accomplishment. My employer does give a 2% bonus for being certified but that was not a huge motivation in itself, just an added bonus.
– Sandi Ash, CMT since 2003

How to Get Started

Visit *www.ahdionline.org* and click on Professional Development

1. Jusinski, Lynn. "2007 Salary Survey Results: How Does Your Salary Measure Up?" *Advance for HIM.*
   <http://health-information.advanceweb.com/Editorial/Content/editorial.aspx?CC=105027&CP=1>.

Membership in AHDI

This book was created by the Association for Healthcare Documentation Integrity (AHDI), formerly AAMT. The Association has been the professional organization representing medical transcriptionists since 1978. AHDI sets standards of practice and education for medical transcriptionists, administers a credentialing program, has established a code of ethics, and advocates on behalf of the profession.

Membership in AHDI provides you with invaluable benefits such as:

- *Health Data Matrix (Bimonthly Publication)*
- *Plexus (Bimonthly Publication)*
- Professional Practices Network
- Product Discounts
- Vendor Affiliate Discounts
- Vitals *(Weekly Electronic Newsletter)*
- 20% Discount on Stedman's Products
- 5% Discount and Free Shipping on all Elsevier Products
- ACE Discounted Registration
- Credentialing Discounts
- *ADVANCE* Magazine
- Bank of America Credit Card
- Modesto's First Credit Union open membership
- Reduced Cost Insurance Program
- HealtheCareers Job Bank
- E-Mentoring
- Online CECs
- Online Membership Directory

Extra Benefits:
- Mentoring Privileges
- Voting Privileges
- Leadership Opportunities
- Networking Opportunities
- Legislative Representation
- Professional Recognition
- AHDI Website
- Position Papers

For more information regarding membership, credentialing, or products and services, visit *www.ahdionline.org* or call our toll free number 800-982-2182.